Global Health
and the Future Role of the United States

Committee on Global Health and the Future of the United States

Board on Global Health

Health and Medicine Division

A Consensus Study Report of
The National Academies of
SCIENCES · ENGINEERING · MEDICINE

THE NATIONAL ACADEMIES PRESS
Washington, DC
www.nap.edu

THE NATIONAL ACADEMIES PRESS 500 Fifth Street, NW Washington, DC 20001

This activity was supported by BD (Becton, Dickinson and Company), Medtronic, Grant No. CCO-160111-015127 from the Merck Foundation, the National Institutes of Health, Grant No. 2016 AVH 305 from The Rockefeller Foundation, Grant No. APC-6M-0002 from the U.S. Agency for International Development, Grant No. HHSP233201400020B/HHSP23337049 from the U.S. Centers for Disease Control and Prevention, Grant No. HHSP233201400020B/ HHSP23337048 from the U.S. Food and Drug Administration, and The U.S. President's Emergency Plan for AIDS Relief. Any opinions, findings, conclusions, or recommendations expressed in this publication do not necessarily reflect the views of any organization or agency that provided support for the project.

International Standard Book Number-13: 978-0-309-45763-7
International Standard Book Number-10: 0-309-45763-7
Digital Object Identifier: https://doi.org/10.17226/24737
Library of Congress Control Number: 2017950553

Additional copies of this publication are available for sale from the National Academies Press, 500 Fifth Street, NW, Keck 360, Washington, DC 20001; (800) 624-6242 or (202) 334-3313; http://www.nap.edu.

Printed in the United States of America

Suggested citation: National Academies of Sciences, Engineering, and Medicine. 2017. *Global health and the future role of the United States*. Washington, DC: The National Academies Press. doi: https://doi.org/10.17226/24737.

The National Academies of
SCIENCES · ENGINEERING · MEDICINE

The **National Academy of Sciences** was established in 1863 by an Act of Congress, signed by President Lincoln, as a private, nongovernmental institution to advise the nation on issues related to science and technology. Members are elected by their peers for outstanding contributions to research. Dr. Marcia McNutt is president.

The **National Academy of Engineering** was established in 1964 under the charter of the National Academy of Sciences to bring the practices of engineering to advising the nation. Members are elected by their peers for extraordinary contributions to engineering. Dr. C. D. Mote, Jr., is president.

The **National Academy of Medicine** (formerly the Institute of Medicine) was established in 1970 under the charter of the National Academy of Sciences to advise the nation on medical and health issues. Members are elected by their peers for distinguished contributions to medicine and health. Dr. Victor J. Dzau is president.

The three Academies work together as the **National Academies of Sciences, Engineering, and Medicine** to provide independent, objective analysis and advice to the nation and conduct other activities to solve complex problems and inform public policy decisions. The National Academies also encourage education and research, recognize outstanding contributions to knowledge, and increase public understanding in matters of science, engineering, and medicine.

Learn more about the National Academies of Sciences, Engineering, and Medicine at **www.nationalacademies.org.**

The National Academies of

SCIENCES • ENGINEERING • MEDICINE

Consensus Study Reports published by the National Academies of Sciences, Engineering, and Medicine document the evidence-based consensus on the study's statement of task by an authoring committee of experts. Reports typically include findings, conclusions, and recommendations based on information gathered by the committee and the committee's deliberations. Each report has been subjected to a rigorous and independent peer-review process and it represents the position of the National Academies on the statement of task.

Proceedings published by the National Academies of Sciences, Engineering, and Medicine chronicle the presentations and discussions at a workshop, symposium, or other event convened by the National Academies. The statements and opinions contained in proceedings are those of the participants and are not endorsed by other participants, the planning committee, or the National Academies.

For information about other products and activities of the National Academies, please visit www.nationalacademies.org/about/whatwedo.

COMMITTEE ON GLOBAL HEALTH AND THE FUTURE OF THE UNITED STATES

JENDAYI E. FRAZER (*Co-Chair*), Council on Foreign Relations, Washington, DC
VALENTIN FUSTER (*Co-Chair*), Mount Sinai Medical Center, New York, NY
GISELA ABBAM, General Electric Healthcare, London, United Kingdom
AMIE BATSON, PATH, Seattle, WA
FREDERICK M. BURKLE, JR., Harvard University, Kailua, HI
LYNDA CHIN, Institute for Health Transformation, University of Texas System
STEPHANIE L. FERGUSON, Lynchburg College and Stanford University, Amherst, VA
LIA HASKIN FERNALD, School of Public Health, University of California, Berkeley
PETER LAMPTEY, FHI 360, Accra, Ghana
RAMANAN LAXMINARAYAN, Centers for Disease, Dynamics, and Policy, New Delhi, India
MICHAEL H. MERSON, Duke Global Health Institute, Duke University, Durham, NC
VASANT NARASIMHAN, Novartis, Basel, Switzerland
MICHAEL T. OSTERHOLM, Center for Infectious Disease Research and Policy, University of Minnesota, Minneapolis
JUAN CARLOS PUYANA, University of Pittsburgh, PA

Study Staff

MEGAN SNAIR, Study Director
CECILIA MUNDACA-SHAH, Senior Program Officer
EESHAN KHANDEKAR, Research Associate
ELAINE HYNDS, Senior Program Assistant
PATRICK KELLEY, Director, Board on Global Health (*until August 2016*)
JULIE PAVLIN, Director, Board on Global Health (*from November 2016*)

Consultants

RONA BRIERE, Arlington, VA
ANNA NICHOLSON, Chapel Hill, NC

Reviewers

This Consensus Study Report was reviewed in draft form by individuals chosen for their diverse perspectives and technical expertise. The purpose of this independent review is to provide candid and critical comments that will assist the National Academies of Sciences, Engineering, and Medicine in making each published report as sound as possible and to ensure that it meets the institutional standards for quality, objectivity, evidence, and responsiveness to the study charge. The review comments and draft manuscript remain confidential to protect the integrity of the deliberative process.

We thank the following individuals for their review of this report:

Cynthia Beall, Case Western Reserve University
Paul Biondich, Regenstrief Institute
Charles Carpenter, Brown University
Barbara J. Culliton, The Culliton Group
Sue Curry, University of Iowa
Christopher Elias, Bill & Melinda Gates Foundation
Amanda Glassman, Center for Global Development
Clarion Johnson, Private Consultant
Jennifer Kates, Kaiser Family Foundation
Rebecca Katz, Georgetown University
Ilona Kickbusch, Graduate Institute Geneva
J. Stephen Morrison, Center for Strategic and International Studies
Loyce Pace, Global Health Council
Gerald W. Parker, Texas A&M AgriLife Research
Jeffrey Sturchio, Rabin Martin

Charles D. Wells, Sanofi
Gavin Yamey, Duke Global Health Institute

Although the reviewers listed above provided many constructive comments and suggestions, they were not asked to endorse the conclusions or recommendations of this report nor did they see the final draft before its release. The review of this report was overseen by **David Challoner,** University of Florida, and **Martin Philbert,** University of Michigan. They were responsible for making certain that an independent examination of this report was carried out in accordance with the standards of the National Academies and that all review comments were carefully considered. Responsibility for the final content rests entirely with the authoring committee and the National Academies.

Preface

The U.S. government has long been at the forefront of shaping the international policy agenda and establishing institutions like The U.S. President's Emergency Plan for AIDS Relief (PEPFAR) and the Global Fund to Fight AIDS, Tuberculosis and Malaria, which make the world safer for America's citizens by improving health and producing more stable societies in other countries, and more humane for millions of people facing heavy disease burdens. The United States has worked with other nations to create Gavi, the Vaccine Alliance, which played an important role in reducing mortality from vaccine-preventable disease (a major contributor to the Millennial Development Goals). Working with philanthropies, the United States has also supported the creation of the Global Polio Eradication Initiative, which has brought the world to the brink of declaring permanent victory over the polio virus. Furthermore, U.S. industry, foundations, and nongovernmental organizations have been on the frontlines in responding to global health emergencies and advancing the research and innovation that has helped curtail the world's most dangerous pathogens.

Collaborative international efforts, especially strengthening the capacity of national health systems, are essential to prevent and prepare for an array of threats, from infectious disease pandemics to the silent killers of chronic noncommunicable diseases. The committee grappled with striking the right balance in fulfilling its mandate to examine the United States' role on the future of global health while reflecting that the United States—as a member of the global community of states—has common challenges and lessons to learn from others to influence our future.

The committee prioritized global health challenges with the potential for catastrophic loss of life and impact on society and the economy—such as pandemics, persistent communicable diseases (HIV/AIDS, tuberculosis, and malaria), and noncommunicable diseases (cardiovascular health and select cancers)—as well as areas where significant U.S. investment has created gains that should be consolidated and sustained—such as promoting women's and children's health, building capacity, and global health innovation and implementation. The Committee on Global Health and the Future of the United States concluded that the U.S. government should maintain its leadership position in global health as matter of urgent national interest and as a global public benefit that enhances America's international standing.

While additional investment is required, more money alone is not the answer. The report offers 14 significant recommendations to strengthen U.S global health programs, recognizing that many other areas are worthy of attention. In order to maximize work toward the prioritized global health challenges (see Chapters 3 to 6) the committee focused on how to better leverage U.S. resources by doing business differently, especially through the use of improved research and development processes and digital health (see Chapter 7), smart financing mechanisms to maximize returns on U.S. investments (see Chapter 8) and demonstrating leadership within the global health architecture and governance (see Chapter 9).

We would like to thank the members of the committee for their devotion of time and energy to this project. It was a privilege and a pleasure to work with our fellow committee members, to learn from them in their respective areas of expertise, and to engage with them in hearty discourse about the issues at hand. Many other experts also gave generously of their time and expertise to contribute to our information gathering, and their contributions are deeply appreciated. Specific participants in this process are listed in the acknowledgments on the following page. We would like to add a special note of gratitude to the National Academies of Sciences, Engineering, and Medicine and especially to Megan Snair, Cecilia Mundaca-Shah, Eeshan Khandekar, Elaine Hynds, and other members of the project staff for their laudable efforts shepherding and supporting the committee through every aspect of the process.

Jendayi Frazer and Valentin Fuster, *Co-Chairs*
Committee on Global Health and the Future of the United States

Acknowledgments

This Consensus Study Report would not have been possible without the invaluable contributions from many experts and stakeholders dedicated to global health. The committee would like to thank all of the speakers (whose full names and affiliations are found in Appendix C) and participants who played a role in the public workshops, as well as the many others who provided valued insight and responded to rapid requests for information to accommodate our short and demanding timeline, many of whom are listed below:

Soji Adeyi, World Bank
Daniel Bausch, Tulane University School of Public Health and Tropical Medicine
Deborah Birx, The U.S. President's Emergency Plan for AIDS Relief
Robert E. Black, Johns Hopkins Bloomberg School of Public Health
Matthew Brown, National Institutes of Health
Robert Einterz, AMPATH Consortium
Amanda Glassman, Center for Global Development
David Hohman, Office of Global Affairs
Jennifer Kates, Kaiser Family Foundation
Kamiar Khajavi, U.S. Agency for International Development
Ron Klain, Revolution LLC
Joseph Larsen, Biomedical Advanced Research and Development Authority
Ruth Levine, Hewlett Foundation

Timothy K. Mackey, University of California, San Diego, School of Medicine
Thomas Mampilly, U.S. Centers for Disease Control and Prevention
Michael Miller, Kyle House Group
Troy Moon, Vanderbilt University School of Medicine
Thomas Novotny, U.S. Department of Health and Human Services
Dykki Settle, PATH
Maria "Bea" Spadacini, U.S. Agency for International Development

The committee would also like to thank the sponsors for their generous financial support: the Merck Foundation, the National Institutes of Health, The Rockefeller Foundation, the U.S. Agency for International Development, the U.S. Centers for Disease Control and Prevention, the U.S. Food and Drug Administration, and The U.S. President's Emergency Plan for AIDS Relief, with additional support from BD (Becton, Dickinson and Company) and Medtronic. Finally, deep appreciation goes to the Lauren Shern and Porter Coggeshell on the Report Review Committee; Daniel Bearss and Ellen Kimmel at the Research Center of the National Academies of Sciences, Engineering, and Medicine for their assistance in fact checking the report; Patrick Kelley, for envisioning this consensus study; and Victor Dzau, for his assistance and support of this project.

Contents

PART 1: SECURING AGAINST GLOBAL THREATS

PART 2: ENHANCING PRODUCTIVITY AND ECONOMIC GROWTH

APPENDIXES

Boxes, Figures, and Tables

BOXES

FIGURES

TABLES

Acronyms and Abbreviations

AMC	Advanced Market Commitment
AMPATH	Academic Model Providing Access to Healthcare
AMR	antimicrobial resistance
ASPR	Assistant Secretary for Preparedness and Response
BARDA	Biomedical Advanced Research and Development Authority
CARB-X	Combating Antibiotic-Resistant Bacteria Pharmaceutical Accelerator
CDC	U.S. Centers for Disease Control and Prevention
CDER	Center for Drug Evaluation and Research
CEPI	Coalition for Epidemic Preparedness Innovation
CGD	Center for Global Development
CIADM	Centers for Innovation in Advanced Development and Manufacturing
COPD	chronic obstructive pulmonary disease
CVD	cardiovascular disease
DAH	development assistance for health
DALY	disability-adjusted life year
DART	disaster assistance response team
DCA	Development Credit Authority
DHS	U.S. Department of Homeland Security
DIB	development impact bond

DoD	U.S. Department of Defense
DOTS	directly observed treatment, short-course
DREAMS	Determined, Resilient, Empowered, AIDS-free, Mentored, and Safe
DRM	domestic resource mobilization
DRR	disaster risk reduction
EOC	emergency operating center
EPMCD	Ending Preventable Maternal and Child Deaths
ESTH	environment, science, technology, and health officer
FAO	Food and Agriculture Organization
FDA	U.S. Food and Drug Administration
FEMA	U.S. Federal Emergency Management Agency
FETP	Field Epidemiology and Training Program
FSO	foreign service officer
FY	fiscal year
G7	Group of Seven
GAIN Act	Generating Antibiotic Incentives Now Act
Gavi	Gavi, the Vaccine Alliance
GBAS	global bidding and assignment system
GBV	gender-based violence
GDL	Global Development Lab
GDP	gross domestic product
GFF	Global Financing Facility
GHE-S	government health expenditure as a source
GHI	Global Health Initiative
GHP	global health programs
GHSA	Global Health Security Agenda
Global Fund	Global Fund to Fight AIDS, Tuberculosis and Malaria
GMEP	Global Malaria Eradication Program
GNI	gross national income
HESN	Higher Education Solutions Network
HHS	U.S. Department of Health and Human Services
Hib	*Haemophilus influenza* serotype b
HIV/AIDS	human immunodeficiency virus/acquired immunodeficiency syndrome
HPP	Hospital Preparedness Program
HPV	human papillomavirus
IFFIm	International Finance Facility for Immunization

IHR	International Health Regulations
IMCI	Integrated Management of Childhood Illness
IOM	Institute of Medicine
JEE	joint external evaluation
LMIC	low- and middle-income country
LSDI	Lubombo Spatial Development Initiative
MDB	multilateral development bank
MDG	Millennium Development Goal
MDR-TB	multidrug-resistant tuberculosis
MEPI	Medical Education Partnership Initiative
MERS-CoV	Middle East respiratory syndrome coronavirus
NASEM	National Academies of Sciences, Engineering, and Medicine
NCD	noncommunicable disease
NEPI	Nursing Education Partnership Initiative
NGO	nongovernmental organization
NIAID	National Institute of Allergy and Infectious Diseases
NIH	National Institutes of Health
NTD	neglected tropical disease
ODA	overseas development aid
OECD	Organisation for Economic Co-operation and Development
OFDA	Office of U.S. Foreign Disaster Aid (USAID)
OGA	Office of Global Affairs (HHS)
OGHD	Office of Global Health Diplomacy (U.S. Department of State)
OIE	World Organisation for Animal Health
OTA	Other Transaction Authority
PACCARB	Presidential Advisory Council on Combating Antibiotic-Resistant Bacteria
PCAST	President's Council of Advisors on Science and Technology
PEER	Partnerships for Enhanced Engagement in Research
PEF	Pandemic Emergency Financing Facility
PEPFAR	The U.S. President's Emergency Plan for AIDS Relief
PHEIC	public health emergency of international concern
PHEMCE	Public Health Emergency Medical Countermeasure Enterprise

PHEP	Public Health Emergency Preparedness
PMI	President's Malaria Initiative
PPE	personal protective equipment
PPP	public–private partnership
PrEP	pre-exposure prophylaxis
PRRR	Pink Ribbon Red Ribbon
PRV	Priority Review Voucher
R&D	research and development
RBF	results-based financing
RBM	Roll Back Malaria
RCT	randomized controlled trial
SARS	severe acute respiratory syndrome
SDG	Sustainable Development Goal
SFI	Sustainable Finance Initiative
SIB	social impact bond
TB	tuberculosis
TFAH	Trust for America's Health
TOSSD	total official support for sustainable development
UKAID	United Kingdom Department for International Development
UN	United Nations
UNAIDS	Joint United Nations Programme on HIV/AIDS
UNICEF	United Nations International Children's Emergency Fund
USAID	U.S. Agency for International Development
USDA	U.S. Department of Agriculture
VIA	visual inspection with acetic acid
WEF	World Economic Forum
WHA	World Health Assembly
WHO	World Health Organization
XDR-TB	extensively drug-resistant tuberculosis

Summary

By investing in global health over the next 20 years, there is a chance to save the lives of millions of children and adults. Beyond these health benefits to individuals, global health is directly linked to economic productivity and growth worldwide. According to the *Lancet* Commission on Investing in Health, the return on investments in global health can be substantial—as the benefits can exceed the costs by a factor between 9 and 20, for low-income and lower middle-income countries, respectively. Worldwide, investing in core capacities to prevent, detect, and respond to infectious disease outbreaks through the development of multidisciplinary "One Health" systems focused on the interface of human and animal health can result in an estimated savings of $15 billion annually from the prevention of outbreaks alone. In light of these benefits, as well as the continual emergence and reemergence of infectious diseases and the growing threat of antimicrobial resistance, a sustainable commitment to global health security is an imperative for all nations.

The United States has long been a leader in global health, including through such high-profile programs as The U.S. President's Emergency Plan for AIDS Relief (PEPFAR); the President's Malaria Initiative; the Global Fund to Fight AIDS, Tuberculosis and Malaria; Gavi, the Vaccine Alliance; and more recently the Global Health Security Agenda. However, resources are not unlimited, and the case for continued commitment must be made. Against the backdrop of the influential legacy of the United States on the global health stage, the new administration is now faced with the choice of whether or not to ensure that gains in global health—won with billions of

U.S. dollars, years of dedication, and strong programs—are sustained and poised for further growth.

THE CASE FOR CONTINUED COMMITMENT TO GLOBAL HEALTH

The tremendous growth in international travel and trade that has occurred over the last several decades heightens the urgency of continued investments in global health. The resulting increased interconnectedness of the world and interdependency of countries, economies, and cultures have brought improved access to goods and services, but also a variety of health threats.

Foreign assistance is often considered a type of charity, or support for the less fortunate. Although this can be true for the poorest and most vulnerable populations, the majority of such aid, especially when directed toward health, is an *investment* in the health of the recipient country, as well as that of the United States and the world at large. This investment motivation for the United States is two-pronged—to secure protection against global health threats and to promote productivity and economic growth in other countries. While the burden of infectious diseases rests predominantly with low-income countries, these diseases represent global threats that could have dire consequences for any country, including the United States, in terms of both human and economic costs. Approximately 284,000 deaths were attributed to the 2009 H1N1 influenza outbreak, for example, and 2 million excess deaths are projected for a future moderate influenza pandemic. In only a few short months in 2003, the outbreak of severe acute respiratory syndrome (SARS) cost the world $40–$54 billion, while in 2014, the United States alone committed $5.4 billion in response to the Ebola outbreak, $119 million of which was spent on domestic screening and follow-up of airline passengers.

The increasing prevalence of noncommunicable diseases (NCDs) also has negatively affected global economies, threatening societal gains in life expectancy, productivity, and overall quality of life. The productivity losses associated with disability, unplanned absences from work, and increased accidents incur costs as much as 400 percent higher than the costs of treatment. Research also has shown that investors are less likely to enter markets where the labor force suffers a heavy disease burden. Thus, healthy populations are important on multiple levels. Investing in human capital contributes significantly to economic growth, prosperity, and stability in countries and creates more reliable and durable partners in the world. This strategy has proven successful, as evidenced by the fact that 11 of the top 15 trading partners of the United States are former recipients of foreign assistance.

In this context, the National Academies of Sciences, Engineering, and

TABLE S-1 Committee Recommendations and Corresponding Actions

Recommendation	Actions
1	Improve international emergency response coordination.
2	Combat antimicrobial resistance.
3	Build public health capacity in low- and middle-income countries.
4	Envision the next generation of The U.S. President's Emergency Plan for AIDS Relief.
5	Confront the threat of tuberculosis.
6	Sustain progress toward malaria elimination.
7	Improve survival in women and children.
8	Ensure healthy and productive lives for women and children.
9	Promote cardiovascular health and prevent cancer.
10	Accelerate the development of medical products.
11	Improve digital health infrastructure.
12	Transition investments toward global public goods.
13	Optimize resources through smart financing.
14	Commit to continued global health leadership.

Medicine were charged with conducting a consensus study to identify global health priorities in light of current and emerging global health threats and challenges and providing recommendations to the U.S. government and other stakeholders for increasing responsiveness, coordination, and efficiency in addressing these threats and challenges by establishing priorities and mobilizing resources. With support from a broad array of federal agencies, foundations, and private partners, an ad hoc 14-member committee was appointed to carry out this task over the course of 6 months.

RECOMMENDATIONS

Based on a rigorous and evidence-based consensus process, committee members formulated a set of 14 recommendations that, if implemented, will deliver a strong global health strategy and allow the United States to maintain its role as a global health leader (see Table S-1).[1] The arguments supporting these recommendations are summarized in the section below on four priority areas for action.

[1] The full text of these recommendations can be found in Chapter 10 of this report.

Priority Areas for Action

The landscape of global health is vast, and with new and sometimes disparate priorities across the health sector, considering each issue or disease in its own silo can be counterproductive. Such a narrow perspective hinders the ability to leverage investments in other programs and adapt resources from existing programs when a new threat arises. Thus, while prioritization of resources is necessary, it is also essential to embrace more holistic, system-focused concepts of integration, capacity building, and partnership to achieve results more comprehensively. With this understanding, the committee identified four priority areas for global health action that it believes, if addressed, will result in the greatest positive effect on global health.

1. *Achieve global health security*
   In the last 10 years, outbreaks of potentially pandemic influenza, Middle East respiratory syndrome coronavirus (MERS-CoV), Ebola, and most recently Zika have threatened populations around the world. In each case, global and national responses, including those of the United States, have been reactionary, uncoordinated, ineffective, and highly costly. Absent the establishment of fundamental public health protections and preparedness capabilities at home and abroad, the world will never be ready to prevent, detect, and respond to such outbreaks. A solid commitment in the form of a sustainable mechanism for addressing these global threats is a critical need. The committee urges the administration to create a coordinating body within the U.S. government with the authority and budget to develop a proactive, cost-effective, and comprehensive approach to preparedness for and response to international public health emergencies. In addition, the committee calls for continued investments at the national level—and increased investments at the international level—to improve capabilities to confront the growing and alarming threat of antimicrobial resistance. Finally, the U.S. government should strengthen preparedness and response capacity in low- and middle-income countries through training and information exchange efforts (see Recommendations 1, 2, and 3).

2. *Maintain a sustained response to the continuous threats of communicable diseases*
   Dedicated efforts of national governments, foundations, and the global community have resulted in millions of lives saved from AIDS, tuberculosis (TB), and malaria, yet all three diseases continue to pose immediate and longer-term threats to the health of populations around the world. More than 36 million people are living with HIV, with 2 million new infections occurring each year. TB disproportionately affects the

poorest populations of the world, killing 1.4 million each year, while dangerous resistant strains are becoming more prevalent and easily spread. The mortality rate due to malaria has decreased by more than 60 percent in the last 10 years, but those infected can lose 25 percent of their family's income as a result of their lost productivity, affecting the prosperity of the society at large as well. The committee believes that a sustained focus on HIV/AIDS and malaria and a reevaluation of the commitment to fighting TB are imperative to prevent reversal of the gains achieved in the last few decades and avoid the further spread of resistant strains for all three diseases (see Recommendations 4, 5, and 6).

3. *Save and improve the lives of women and children*
Efforts to save the lives of women and children across the globe have historically been an important focus for the U.S. government. Although child and maternal mortality rates have decreased since 2000, each year nearly 6 million children die before their fifth birthday, and more than 300,000 women die from pregnancy- and childbirth-related causes. The vast majority of these deaths are preventable. The committee urges the U.S. government to continue its commitment to this survival agenda but also expand it to incorporate early childhood development as a key element. If current survival-focused programs can be complemented by a strong multisector focus on childhood development, the committee sees an opportunity to foster healthy families, resulting in turn in resilient societies and growing economies (see Recommendations 7 and 8).

4. *Promote cardiovascular health and prevent cancer*
Infectious diseases often captivate the media, but an equally important concern is rising rates of NCDs, such as cardiovascular disease (CVD) and cancer, in countries around the world, regardless of income level. The costs of managing these diseases are rising as well. CVD alone is projected to cost the world $1 trillion annually in treatment costs and productivity losses by 2030. However, because of their historical focus on infectious diseases, many health systems in low- and middle-income countries are not adequately equipped to care for patients with NCDs. The need to fill these gaps often goes unmet because of other priorities, but their prevention and treatment can be built into existing platforms for other areas, such as HIV/AIDS or maternal and child health. The committee calls for improved mobilization and coordination of private partners at the country level and across the U.S. interagency community to implement strategies proven to ensure the highest impact. These strategies include targeting CVD risk factors, early detection and treat-

ment of hypertension and cervical cancer, and immunization against vaccine-preventable cancers (see Recommendation 9).

Maximizing Returns on Investments in Global Health

To have the greatest effect in the above priority areas, the committee identified three cross-cutting areas for action to maximize the returns on investments, achieve better health outcomes, and use funding more effectively: (1) catalyze innovation through both the accelerated development of medical products and integrated digital health infrastructure; (2) employ more nimble and flexible financing mechanisms to leverage new partners and funders in global health; and (3) maintain U.S. status and influence as a world leader in global health while adhering to evidence-based science and economics, measurement, and accountability (see Recommendations 10 through 14). Achieving true improvements in global health will require changing the way global health business is conducted to better enable innovation. Adequately protecting U.S. citizens at home and abroad necessitates not only investment in U.S. infrastructure, but also continued awareness of global issues and active engagement in the international global health arena. Many of the events and elements of the changing global health landscape described throughout this report have created an environment for a centralized and comprehensive strategy for U.S. global health diplomacy. To these ends, a change in approach and long-term visioning across the various U.S. agencies involved in global health will be necessary, with an emphasis on integration and partnership.

The committee wishes to emphasize that strong collaboration and cooperation among donors, national governments, nongovernmental organizations, and private companies will be essential to achieving the proposed global health goals. Health effects extend far beyond the health sector, and addressing them will therefore require cross-sectoral interaction and synergy. While existing multilateral institutions continue to be crucial, engaging in new and more productive partnerships with other donor governments and the private sector can augment multilateral networks and lead to more successful outcomes moving forward. These joint investments should be geared toward harmonized approaches to global public goods and general global health goals shared by all countries. Finally, to have the greatest effect, all global health work should incorporate essential principles of community inclusion and cultural competency.

CONCLUSION

The United States cannot ignore the reality that the health and well-being of other countries affect both directly and indirectly the health, safety, and economic security of Americans. For many years, strong bipartisanship has backed U.S. engagement in global health, with active support from the faith community, private industry, foundations, and civil society. To sustain the proud U.S. legacy in global health, the committee encourages the administration to focus on the above key areas and cross-cutting opportunities and to implement the recommendations set forth in this report. The committee believes that implementing evidence-based interventions, modifying country engagement strategies, exploring new investment mechanisms, and taking a more proactive and systematic approach to global health priorities will make the U.S. government's current efforts in global health more efficient and cost-effective. The United States must preserve and extend its legacy as a global leader, partner, and innovator in global health through forward-looking policies, a long-term vision, country and international partnerships, and, most importantly, continued investment. Doing so will not only lead to improved health and security for all U.S. citizens but also ensure the sustainable thriving of the global population.

1

Introduction

While much progress has been made over the last decade toward achieving the Millennium Development Goals (MDGs),[1] the number and complexity of global health challenges has persisted. Growing forces for globalization have increased the interconnectedness of the world and the interdependency among countries, economies, and cultures. Monumental growth in international travel and trade has brought improved access to goods and services for many, but such growth carries with it an ongoing and ever-present global threat of zoonotic spillover and infectious disease outbreaks, including in recent years avian influenza, Ebola, Zika, and chikungunya. This threat intensifies each year in the face of diminished budgets, especially when considering the corresponding increase in urbanization and population density worldwide. Simultaneously, noncommunicable diseases (NCDs) have continued to grow in prevalence and impact on economies, threatening societal gains in life expectancy and quality (WEF, 2017). Many countries now face a rising burden of NCDs such as cardiovascular disease and cancer, while still trying to eliminate such diseases as tuberculosis (TB), malaria, and human immunodeficiency virus/acquired immunodeficiency syndrome (HIV/AIDS). Unfortunately, many health care systems in these countries are not designed to care for noncommunicable

[1] The Millennium Development Goals are "The world's time-bound and quantified targets for addressing extreme poverty in its many dimensions-income poverty, hunger, disease, lack of adequate shelter, and exclusion-while promoting gender equality, education, and environmental sustainability. They are also basic human rights-the rights of each person on the planet to health, education, shelter, and security" (Millennium Project, 2006).

TABLE 1-1 U.S. Program Successes for Global Health

Program	Successes in the 21st Century
The U.S. President's Emergency Plan for AIDS Relief (PEPFAR)	• In 2016, 11,490,518 people received life-saving antiretroviral therapy (PEPFAR, 2016a). • In 2016, 6,184,237 orphans and vulnerable children were supported (PEPFAR, 2016a). • In 2016, nearly 2 million babies were born HIV-free (PEPFAR, 2016b). • In 2016, 220,000 health workers were trained to deliver HIV and other services (PEPFAR, 2016b).
President's Malaria Initiative (PMI)	• Between 2005 and 2013, nearly 140 million antimalarial treatments were provided (Summers, 2013). • In 2015, 16 million people were protected through the spraying of more than 4 million homes with insecticides (USAID, 2016a). • Since 2005, under-5 mortality has decreased between 8 and 67 percent; 4 countries have decreased under-5 mortality by more than 50 percent (USAID, 2016a).
Biomedical Advanced Research and Development Authority (BARDA)	• Since 2006, 21 products have been stockpiled for emergency use (Larsen and Disbrow, 2017). • Since 2006, 6 products have achieved FDA approval or licensure against chemical, biological, radiological, or nuclear threats (Larsen and Disbrow, 2017).
U.S. Agency for International Development's (USAID's) Acting on the Call: Ending Preventable Child and Maternal Deaths	• Since 2008, the lives of 4.6 million children have been saved (USAID, 2017). • Since 2008, the lives of 200,000 women have been saved (USAID, 2017). • As compared to 1990, 18,000 fewer children and 630 fewer women die every day as a result of USAID and WHO interventions (USAID, 2016b).

NOTE: FDA = U.S. Food and Drug Administration; WHO = World Health Organization.

diseases and current infrastructure lacks a focus on integrated care, a properly trained workforce, and effective population-level policies—elements that can significantly improve these serious health burdens.

Over the last few decades, the United States has significantly contributed to global health successes in key priority areas, such as HIV/AIDS, malaria, research and development for health security threats, and saving the lives of mothers and children, as illustrated in Table 1-1. Even more recent commitment is evident through the creation and dedication of the Global Health Security Agenda (GHSA) and efforts to combat antimicrobial resistance (AMR) at the national and international levels. While the world's attention is easily captured by infectious disease events like Ebola or Zika, it is also important to address the burdens of chronic diseases plaguing populations and adversely affecting their economic growth. Identifying cross-cutting solutions to address all facets of health is necessary for sustainable progress. The gains bought with billions of U.S. dollars are poised to be sustained and grown, or phased down and lost. A loss of focus in key priority areas—responding to disease outbreaks; sustaining gains in HIV/AIDS, TB, and malaria; ignoring the health of women and children; or disregarding the growing imperative of the NCD burden—would be a tremendous opportunity loss for the United States and humanity.

HISTORICAL CONTEXT FOR THIS STUDY

For decades, the United States has been involved in foreign aid and global health in some capacity. Various efforts and programs were expanded following the creation of The U.S. President's Emergency Plan for AIDS Relief (PEPFAR) in 2003 and the President's Malaria Initiative (PMI) in 2005. Since the establishment of these two initiatives, along with the Global Fund to Fight AIDS, Tuberculosis and Malaria in the early part of the 21st century, the field of global health has seen tremendous growth and has evolved through a proliferation of nonprofit and private foundations, with a keen interest in and commitment to improving the health of vulnerable populations around the world. While these changes were occurring over the past two decades, the National Academies of Sciences, Engineering, and Medicine conducted two consensus studies on this topic, charged with advising future government leadership on areas of prioritization within the growing field of global health.

Past Institute of Medicine Reports on Global Health

Twenty years ago, the Institute of Medicine's (IOM's) Board on International Health was commissioned to produce the first report directly addressing the United States' interest in and commitment to improving human health on a global scale. The report *America's Vital Interest in Global Health: Protecting Our People, Enhancing Our Economy, and Advancing Our International Interests* (1997) construed global health as "health problems, issues, and concerns that transcend national boundaries, and may best be addressed by cooperative actions" (IOM, 1997, p. 2). Twelve years later, an independent committee was formed by the IOM Board on Global Health to prepare a new report, *The U.S. Commitment to Global Health: Recommendations for the New Administration* (2009), to advise the incoming Obama administration. The 2009 committee was tasked with assessing

U.S. efforts in global health and making recommendations about future priorities and opportunities to improve health worldwide, while also protecting and promoting U.S. interests. Due to the breadth of the statement of task and the time constraints of the study, the committee's approach was to focus on the directions needed for the future. The committee was not able to conduct an in-depth review of these two previous reports and the progress made since their release. However, several themes from those reports emerged in initial discussions to inform the committee's deliberations, with some outlined in this chapter (see Appendix A for more detail on the previous IOM reports' recommendations and the advancements in global health since their release).

The IOM's 1997 report *America's Vital Interest in Global Health* showed that, even 20 years ago, there was an appreciation for the interconnectedness of the world and the interdependency of the United States with other countries. As the report underscored, "the direct interests of the American people are best served when the United States acts decisively to promote health around the world" (IOM, 1997, p. 2). Also included in that report were calls for better structuring of market incentives for the needed development of critical medical products, an area that the global health community still struggles with today. Since then, however, the Office of the Assistant Secretary for Preparedness and Response established the Biomedical Advanced Research and Development Authority (BARDA) through the 2006 Pandemic and All-Hazards Preparedness Act,[2] which incentivizes the private sector to collaborate, develop, and ensure surge capacity for drug and vaccine manufacturing through cost-sharing mechanisms and partnerships with the U.S. government. The U.S. Food and Drug Administration's (FDA's) priority review voucher program, established in 2007 (Ridley, n.d.), also spurs development by allowing for expedited FDA review of certain types of new drugs (e.g., products to treat Ebola became eligible in 2014). Additionally, with the recent launch of the Coalition for Epidemic Preparedness Innovation in January 2017, it is clear this need for drug and vaccine development in an uncertain market is still a priority and will require international public- and private-sector collaboration.

The 2009 IOM report *The U.S. Commitment to Global Health* followed an explosion of global health programs and an increase in total global health funding between 2000 and 2008. To generate and share knowledge, as well as build capacity, the report called on the U.S. research sector to collaborate with global partners, establish information sharing networks, and support academia and health systems in low- and middle-income countries (LMICs) through country-led workforce development and the creation of national health plans (IOM, 2009). Progress in health research collabora-

[2] Pandemic and All-Hazards Preparedness Act, Public Law 109-417, Sec. 401.

tion since 2009 includes the Partnerships for Enhanced Engagement in Research (PEER) (2011), a competitive program that awards scientists from LMICs (and partners them with U.S. government–funded researchers) to support research and capacity building. Additionally, the formation of the medical education partnership initiative and nursing education partnership initiative, developed through the PEPFAR program to address the severe workforce shortage of health workers in high-burden HIV/AIDS countries, has enhanced workforce capacity (see Chapter 4).

Perhaps the most notable recommendation of the 2009 report was to improve coordination across the U.S. government by creating a White House Interagency Committee on Global Health, chaired by a senior official designated by the president, to be tasked with leading, planning, prioritizing, and coordinating the budget for major U.S. government global health programs and activities. This concept was implemented through the launch of the Global Health Initiative (GHI) in 2009 by President Obama. However, with an initiative spanning so many agencies and health areas, its success depended on strong authority and budget given to the GHI organizers. Unfortunately, it received neither, and by 2012, the committee found that GHI had little more than a Web presence coordinating priority area global health programs. Though full U.S. government interagency coordination and cooperation in global health was not realized in the past 10 years, many smaller-scale coordination efforts have been successful, such as Feed the Future, PEPFAR, PMI, and most recently the GHSA. The committee feels that coordinating efforts within a manageable scope with dedicated funding, leadership, and accountability is feasible and should be a key consideration as the new administration looks to the future to shape U.S. global health programs.

STUDY CHARGE, APPROACH, AND SCOPE

In follow-up to the 1997 and 2009 IOM reports on global health priorities, a broad array of stakeholders sponsored the National Academies of Sciences, Engineering, and Medicine to conduct a similar consensus study to review changes in the global health landscape over the last 10 years and assess future priorities. In addition, this expert committee was tasked with making recommendations on how to improve responsiveness, coordination, and efficiency within the U.S. government and across the global health field. Finally, the committee was charged with guiding the new administration, as well as other funders and global health actors, in setting future priorities and mobilizing resources (see Box 1-1 for the full statement of task). The sponsors of this study included the Merck Foundation, the National Institutes of Health (NIH), PEPFAR, The Rockefeller Foundation, the United States Agency for International Development (USAID),

BOX 1-1
Statement of Task

In the 8 years since an Institute of Medicine (IOM) ad hoc committee deliberated to produce the report *The U.S. Commitment to Global Health: Recommendations for the Public and Private Sectors*, the factors that shape the U.S. global health agenda have continued to evolve. Reflective of this and of the opportunity presented by a new administration, the National Academies of Sciences, Engineering, and Medicine will convene an ad hoc consensus committee to reassess and update the public- and private-sector roles in contributing to and deriving benefit from improved global health in its broadest sense—meaning, health beyond health care.

The U.S. Commitment to Global Health and its predecessor, the 1997 IOM study titled *America's Vital Interest in Global Health: Protecting Our People, Enhancing Our Economy, and Advancing Our International Interests*, both influenced public and private funding and the shaping of priorities for global health. While these reports resulted in many improvements, some of their recommendations are yet to be fulfilled.

The committee will begin its task by reviewing where the two prior reports resulted in more effective investments in global health initiatives and where recommendations were not taken up. The committee will then assess the current global health landscape and how it has evolved over the last 8 years. After reviewing these issues, the committee will offer conclusions and recommendations to guide the new administration, as well as other funders and global health actors, in setting future priorities and mobilizing resources. The committee will also review U.S. governmental external leadership and internal coordination of the global health enterprise and offer recommendations on how to improve responsiveness and efficiency. The audience for this report will include the private sector (in the United States, other industrialized countries, and developing countries), the U.S. and for-

the U.S. Food and Drug Administration, with additional support provided by BD (Becton, Dickinson and Company) and Medtronic, demonstrating the diversity of entities that understand the importance of global health issues and trends. The recommendations that the committee has developed are far reaching and applicable to multiple agencies and stakeholders, including nongovernmental organizations (NGOs), private-sector companies, and national ministries of health in other countries. However, as the U.S. government maintains its role as a leader in global health, the committee directs many of these recommendations to the new administration and federal agency leaders and hopes the U.S. government will continue to lead through action, and in partnership and collaboration with the numerous public and private stakeholders on the global health stage.

eign governments, and international organizations. Beyond demographic trends, the committee will consider relevant global changes over this period, including

- increased forces for globalization that foster the movement of people (including health care workers), microbes, food, and pharmaceuticals, increasing America's interdependency with other countries;
- aspects of globalization that increase the opportunities and challenges associated with greater global engagement in medical research and development;
- the 2015 culmination of the timeframe for the Millennium Development Goals and the initiation of the era of the Sustainable Development Goals;
- the commitment to an AIDS-free generation;
- the commitment to quality universal health care;
- the increasing privatization of health care delivery in many parts of the world;
- achieved and likely advances in technology and health systems design that could improve the potential for disease prevention, recognition, response, and eradication; technological advances that could raise the potential for naturally occurring and man-made biological agents to accidently or intentionally spread beyond national borders;
- the growing frequency of global infectious disease epidemics affecting health and family welfare, trade, migration, and security;
- the growing global epidemic of antimicrobial drug resistance and the lack of a commensurate response;
- the increasing relative importance of injury and chronic noncommunicable diseases (e.g., heart disease, diabetes, mental illness) in the developing world; and
- the unfinished and neglected tropical disease agenda.

Approach

The 14-member committee, appointed in August 2016, deliberated over the course of 5 months and four in-person meetings, in addition to working electronically and via phone, to compile this report and its 14 recommendations. Two of the meetings included information-gathering sessions from sponsor representatives and additional subject area content experts. The agendas from these two meetings can be found in Appendix C. To better understand the challenges and successes of programs implemented in other countries, the committee also distributed an information-gathering request via SurveyGizmo to 12 USAID health directors and 40 U.S. Centers for Disease Control and Prevention (CDC) country directors, asking respondents to give qualitative responses to questions regarding their work with U.S. global health programs (see Box 1-2). Forty-eight responses were received, and responses can be accessed via this project's Public Access

BOX 1-2
Language Used to Solicit Input on U.S. Global Health Policies and Programs

The National Academies of Sciences, Engineering, and Medicine's Committee on Global Health and the Future of the United States would like to invite your input on U.S. global health policies and programs in the last 8 years and opportunities for the future. Input will be accepted through Friday, November 4, 2016.

The input is intended to help ensure that the committee hears from project implementers and those at the country level about their experiences working with other U.S. agencies on global health as well as national governments and community organizations in country. Submissions will be made available to inform members of the committee. By submitting input, you agree that it will be included in the study's Public Access File and may be quoted in whole or in part in the committee's report.

SurveyGizmo and Widgix, LLC, is not affiliated in any way with, or endorsed by, the National Academies of Sciences, Engineering, and Medicine, and your submission to this website is subject to SurveyGizmo's terms of use.

1. What region is the focus of the majority of your work?
   a. Afghanistan and Pakistan
   b. Africa
   c. Asia
   d. Europe and Eurasia
   e. Latin America
   f. Middle East

2. Have you worked on any main presidential initiatives for global health in the last 4-8 years (e.g., PEPFAR, President's Malaria Initiative, Ending Preventable Child and Maternal Deaths, Global Health Security Agenda, Feed the Future, or others)?
   a. Yes
   b. No

3. (If answered yes) Because you answered yes to the above question, what has been your experience with implementing these programs at the country level?

4. If you could make recommendations for the next U.S. administration on global health, what would they be?

5. Do you have any other comments you would like the National Academies committee to consider?

File.[3] Furthermore, the committee conducted an extensive literature review on relevant topics.

Scope and Limitations

Global health challenges span a broad range of health conditions, risk factors, and policy issues. The wide range of health conditions that afflict the global population was investigated in the 2015 Global Burden of Disease Study, which found that 315 conditions contributed to the majority of global disability-adjusted life years (DALYs)[4] in 2015 (Kassebaum et al., 2016). The same study identified 79 behavioral, environmental, occupational, and metabolic risk factors to health that can be addressed (Forouzanfar et al., 2016). Beyond specific disease and risk factors there is increasing recognition of the influence of climate change and the environment on global health. While these challenges are all important, the committee has decided to focus this report on areas it believes the United States can have the most immediate and substantial impact, given the limited resources available. The committee focused on areas that met three specific criteria: (1) areas in which the United States has existing investments and deep expertise, (2) areas that are identified as high priority by current efforts such as the Sustainable Development Goals and the Global Burden of Disease Study, (3) and areas where specific interventions with strong evidence have been identified. By focusing the analyses and recommendations the committee hopes that it enables U.S. government agencies to optimally deploy scarce resources to interventions with the greatest potential impact to improve health outcomes in a cost-effective manner.

Though this report was not able to highlight every major global health issue, the committee emphasizes that the omission of certain topics is not meant to understate their critical nature. Sectors such as mental health and substance abuse, environmental health (including food safety, air pollution, and water and sanitation issues), refugee health, and health workforce challenges will be crucial factors affecting global health in coming years. In fact, the global burden of mental illness accounted for up to 13 percent of global DALYs (Vigo et al., 2016), and injuries resulted in approximately 8.5 percent of global deaths in 2015 (Wang et al., 2016). Sustaining a health workforce will be important as well. Populations are growing, and health systems are struggling to keep up. The World Health Organization

[3] To obtain the Public Access File, send an email to paro@nas.edu to request information from the Public Access Records Office.

[4] The burden of disability associated with a disease or disorder can be measured in units called disability-adjusted life years (DALYs). DALYs represent the total number of years lost to illness, disability, or premature death within a given population. See more at https://www.nimh.nih.gov/health/statistics/global/index.shtml (accessed April 1, 2017).

estimates the world will be short 12.9 million health care workers by 2035 (WHO, 2013). This shortage could have serious repercussions, which the committee acknowledges as a pressing issue in all countries. As the United States continues to reform health care and medical and public health professional education, it will need to work multilaterally to better understand the causes and effects of workforce reduction in health care.

Despite the focused approach proposed in this report, the committee also strongly believes the United States has an important leadership role to play in shaping policy across global health challenges—even when specifically resourced operational programs are not possible. For example, helping to shape the policy debate on the role of climate change on global health is absolutely critical in light of recent experiences such as the Zika virus. The effects of climate change on health will be felt in the form of malnutrition, drought, extreme temperatures, worsened air quality, and infectious disease spillover—and mitigation of these effects will require work well beyond the health sector, necessitating multidisciplinary collaboration and action (USGCRP, 2016). As such, the committee recognized that an effort on climate change and health would require work and expertise outside the scope of this study, but agrees a multidisciplinary investigation is needed. Across the global health landscape, experts in the U.S. government should continue to participate and shape the discourse on these important topics.

ORGANIZATION OF THE REPORT

Throughout this report are references to changes that are required for the United States to better participate as a leader in global health in the 21st century. While acknowledging that much progress has been made in the field in the past 10 years, the committee believes there is still much to be done. This report presents the committee's findings, conclusions, and recommendations for future global health priorities of the U.S. administration and its global health partners. The structure of the report reflects the two key themes motivating the investment in global health by the United States: securing against global threats and enhancing productivity and economic growth. The final section on Maximizing Returns is cross-cutting as its contents encompass methods that should be applied to all of the focus areas within this report (see Figure 1-1).

Chapter 1 provides an overview of the report, as well as important highlights from the previous IOM reports on this topic. Chapter 2 explains prior global health investment and the current spending while also discussing important changes in the global landscape to provide context for later chapters. The first main section of the report, "Securing Against Global Threats," includes Chapters 3 and 4, and focuses on the broad issues of global health security to the United States and the global community. While

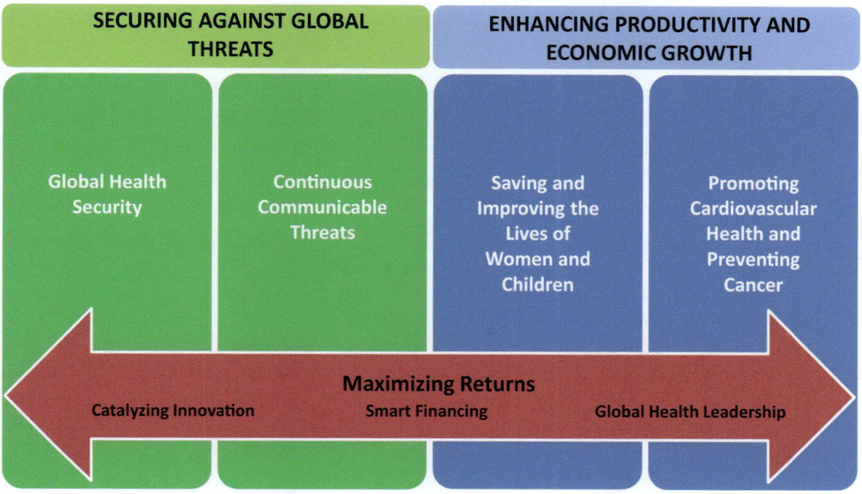

FIGURE 1-1 Overview of the report structure.

Chapter 3 discusses threats that are immediate, such as pandemic influenza and infectious disease outbreaks, including Ebola, Chapter 4 discusses more persistent and continuing infectious disease threats such as HIV/AIDS, tuberculosis, and malaria. The second section, "Enhancing Productivity and Economic Growth," includes Chapters 5 and 6, and explores the justification and methods for building capacity in countries of all income levels to create strong and stable countries. While many arguments can be made that addressing infectious diseases would also have an impact on productivity and economic growth of countries, they often receive disproportionate attention. As a result, the committee has designed the second main section to highlight areas of health that typically do not fall in the spotlight. Chapter 5 addresses the need and justification for saving and improving the lives of women and children, and Chapter 6 discusses the necessity of curbing the burden of NCDs—with a focus on cardiovascular disease and cancer. Finally, the last section of the report, "Maximizing Returns," encompasses important longer-term approaches and changes to the ways the United States engages in global health to improve effectiveness and cost-efficiency of spending efforts. Within this section, Chapter 7 addresses methods for catalyzing innovation through medical product development and integrated digital health infrastructure. Chapter 8 examines various methods of innovative financing used by many global health players to be more nimble and catalytic in foreign investments. Chapter 9 discusses the critical need for the United States to stay engaged in and committed to international partnerships and organizations focused on, or influencing global health, and also explores how the United States can more strategically incorporate health into foreign policy. Finally, Chapter 10 provides a concluding summary of the whole report, highlighting all 14 recommendations.

REFERENCES

Forouzanfar, M. H., A. Afshin, L. T. Alexander, H. R. Anderson, Z. A. Bhutta, S. Biryukov, M. Brauer, et al. 2016. Global, regional, and national comparative risk assessment of 79 behavioural, environmental and occupational, and metabolic risks or clusters of risks, 1990-2015: A systematic analysis for the Global Burden of Disease Study 2015. *The Lancet* 388(10053):1659-1724.

IOM (Institute of Medicine). 1997. *America's vital interest in global health: Protecting our people, enhancing our economy, and advancing our international interests.* Washington, DC: National Academy Press.

IOM. 2009. *The U.S. commitment to global health: Recommendations for the new administration.* Washington, DC: The National Academies Press.

Kassebaum, N. J., M. Arora, R. M. Barber, Z. A. Bhutta, J. Brown, A. Carter, D. C. Casey, et al. 2016. Global, regional, and national disability-adjusted life years (DALYs) for 315 diseases and injuries and healthy life expectancy (HALE), 1990-2015: A systematic analysis for the Global Burden of Disease Study 2015. *The Lancet* 388(10053):1603-1658.

Larsen, J., and G. Disbrow. 2017. Project Bioshield and the Biomedical Advanced Research Development Authority: A ten year progress report on meeting U.S. preparedness objectives for threat agents. *Clinical Infectious Diseases* 64(10):1430-1434.

Millennium Project. 2006. *What they are.* Washington, DC: The United Nations Millennium Project. http://www.unmillenniumproject.org/goals (accessed March 10, 2017).

PEPFAR (The U.S. President's Emergency Plan for AIDS Relief). 2016a. *Impact.* https://data.pepfar.net (accessed March 9, 2017).

PEPFAR. 2016b. *PEPFAR latest global results.* Washington, DC: The U.S. President's Emergency Fund for AIDS Relief.

Ridley, D. n.d. *Priority review vouchers.* http://priorityreviewvoucher.org (accessed April 2, 2017).

Summers, T. 2013. *President's malaria initiative: Big success from a quiet team.* Washington, DC: Center for Strategic and International Studies.

USAID (U.S. Agency for International Development). 2016a. *10: A decade of progress.* Washington, DC: U.S. Agency for International Development.

USAID. 2016b. *Acting on the call: Ending preventable child and maternal deaths: A focus on equity.* Washington, D.C.: U.S. Agency for International Development.

USAID. 2017. *Maternal and child health.* https://www.usaid.gov/what-we-do/global-health/maternal-and-child-health (accessed March 10, 2017).

USGCRP (U.S. Global Change Research Program). 2016. *The impacts of climate change on human health in the United States: A scientific assessment.* Edited by A. Crimmins, J. Balbus, J. L. Gamble, C. B. Beard, J. E. Bell, D. Dodgen, R. J. Eisen, N. Fann, M. D. Hawkins, S. C. Herring, L. Jantarasmi, D. M. Mills, S. Saha, M. C. Sarofim, J. Trtanj, and L. Ziska. Washington, DC: U.S. Global Change Research Program.

Vigo, D., G. Thornicroft, and R. Atun. 2016. Estimating the true global burden of mental illness. *The Lancet Psychiatry* 3(2):171-178.

Wang, H., M. Naghavi, C. Allen, R. M. Barber, Z. A. Bhutta, A. Carter, D. C. Casey, et al. 2016. Global, regional, and national life expectancy, all-cause mortality, and cause-specific mortality for 249 causes of death, 1980-2015: A systematic analysis for the Global Burden of Disease Study 2015. *The Lancet* 388(10053):1459-1544.

WEF (World Economic Forum). 2017. *The global risks report 2017*. Geneva, Switzerland: World Economic Forum.

WHO (World Health Organization). 2013. *Global health workforce shortage to reach 12.9 million in coming decades*. http://www.who.int/mediacentre/news/releases/2013/health-workforce-shortage/en (accessed January 10, 2017).

2

Investing in Global Health for America

"When we try to pick out anything by itself, we find it hitched to everything else in the universse."

—John Muir

Over the past several decades, there has been marked progress in the alleviation of poverty and suffering. Life expectancy has risen worldwide, child survival has almost doubled, and the global community has turned the tide of deadly diseases. Yet, at the same time, the spread of urbanization, the speed of global travel and the movement of goods, increased consumption of animal protein, and climate change have facilitated the emergence and rapid spread of infectious diseases, such as severe acute respiratory syndrome (SARS), Middle East respiratory syndrome coronavirus (MERS-CoV), pandemic influenza, Ebola virus, and Zika virus (Burkle, 2017). Additionally, drought, famine, war, and country conflicts have led to international humanitarian and refugee crises, creating unstable conditions in which radical ideologies and diseases can thrive (WEF, 2017). Historically, the United States has made major investments in global platforms and initiatives that have largely enabled containment of threats such as infectious diseases before they reach the United States and promoted global security, stability, and prosperity. Examples of such investments include human immunodeficiency virus/acquired immunodeficiency syndrome (HIV/AIDS) treatment, infectious disease surveillance and response, vaccine development, and maternal and child health improvement. These investments have also benefited U.S. businesses both in terms of enabling a growing base of healthy, prosperous customers, as well as ensuring the safety of U.S. multinational operations around the world, and facilitated the continued leadership of the United States in research and development in biomedical sciences and technologies (Daschle and Frist, 2015; Lima et al., 2013; Wagner et al., 2015).

However, competing priorities and demands on government funding create an imperative for the United States to examine the economic benefits of investments in global health for the economy, national security, innovation, and global standing. Shifts in global economies and private-sector engagement are changing the nature of these investments (Sturchio and Goel, 2012). In the past decade, many countries that have historically received foreign aid have begun experiencing economic growth and rising middle classes. This growth has allowed traditional aid recipient countries to expand their tax base. In fact, through taxation and mobilization of domestic resources, the funds collected between 2000 and 2014 in sub-Saharan Africa rose from $100 billion to $461 billion (Runde and Savoy, 2016). The growth of many multinational businesses has also forced business executives to adopt a more global perspective regarding long-term planning, workforce development, and safety. As a country plans for both its own future and that of the world, a prudent step is to assess current investments and adapt them to reflect these global changes. Although great progress has been achieved toward the completion of the Millennium Development Goals (MDGs)[1] since their launch in 2000, there are still unfinished agendas. The transition in 2016 to the multidisciplinary Sustainable Development Goals (SDGs) illustrates the continued commitment to end poverty, save the planet, and ensure prosperity for all. There is a chance to save the lives of millions of children and adults by investing in global health over the next 20 years (Jamison et al., 2013). Furthermore, investing in health has benefits beyond saving lives and is considered to have made the largest contribution to sustainable development (Jamison et al., 2016). According to the *Lancet* Commission on Investing in Health, achieving a grand convergence in global health by 2035[2]—reducing infectious disease, maternal, and child deaths down to universally low levels within a generation—is estimated to produce benefits that would exceed the costs

---

[1] The Millennium Development Goals are "The world's time-bound and quantified targets for addressing extreme poverty in its many dimensions-income poverty, hunger, disease, lack of adequate shelter, and exclusion-while promoting gender equality, education, and environmental sustainability. They are also basic human rights-the rights of each person on the planet to health, education, shelter, and security" (Millennium Project, 2006).

[2] Achieving convergence would require significant increases in health spending in low- and lower-middle-income countries—$30 billion in low-income countries and $61 billion in lower-middle-income countries in 2035. Expected economic growth, together with other sources of revenue, such as taxes on tobacco and removal of subsidies on fossil fuels, will enable low-income countries to finance most of this agenda on their own, while middle-income countries will easily be able to leverage resources domestically (Summers and Jamison, 2013).

of investment between 9 and 20 times for low- and lower-middle-income countries, respectively[3] (Jamison et al., 2013; Yamey et al., 2016).

This chapter identifies the benefits of global health investment for the United States, discusses the current spending of the United States on global health programs, and explores opportunities for future investment based on trends affecting health such as globalization, the SDG agenda, and private-sector involvement.

WHY GLOBAL HEALTH FUNDING PROTECTS U.S. INTERESTS

There will likely always be a demand for U.S. support when it comes to disaster relief and humanitarian efforts because the U.S. response system excels at logistics and operations. But disaster response must be complemented by investment in programs and countries during steady state times—acknowledging the public health mantra of "An ounce of prevention is worth a pound of cure." Money spent on improvements to infrastructure, workforce training, and response systems—both in the United States and abroad—protects Americans from threats such as emerging infectious diseases or bioterror attacks. Such investments help to build everyday resilience so communities are prepared for all types of disasters, whether they take the form of a bus crash, an active shooter event, or an Ebola outbreak. Similarly, investing in the development of countries around the world through partnerships and capacity building can help foster stable economies with sufficient opportunities for their citizens, discouraging them from feeling forced to flee their country. Stable countries with growing middle class populations are more likely to become trading partners and to purchase U.S. goods; 11 of the top 15 U.S. trading partners are former recipients of U.S. foreign assistance programs (InterAction, 2011). Moreover, beyond just trading partners, the shared burden of noncommunicable diseases (NCDs) around the world is a strong justification for health and scientific partnerships that can lead to shared solutions to common problems. Many aid-recipient countries suffer from similar health burdens to those in the United States, such as hypertension, cancer, poor maternal health, or depression.

The reasons for U.S. investment in global health are numerous, but with so many competing priorities, limited resources dictate prioritization. However, providing foreign assistance through overseas development aid (ODA), and acting in the best interest of the United States can often be

---

[3] This estimate was found using a full income approach, where income growth plus the value of life years gained in that period results in a change in a country's full income over a time period. This accounts for the omission of reduced mortality risk in typical gross domestic product (GDP) measures to give a more complete picture (Summers and Jamison, 2013).

accomplished simultaneously. The recent change in administration in the U.S. political system is a chance to pause and take a more holistic view of each of the elements of current global health investments as part of an interconnected system. In this process, it is critical to consider the longer-term consequences that will arise from near-term decisions on the future of investments in global health.

EXISTING U.S. GLOBAL HEALTH SPENDING

U.S. funding for global health grew from $1.7 billion in 2000 to $8.47 billion in 2009 (Salaam-Blyther, 2013), increasing on an average of 19.53 percent per year. The 2009 Institute of Medicine (IOM) report *U.S. Commitment to Global Health* called for an increase in the budget for global health programs, urging the U.S. government to invest $15 billion annually in global health by 2012, of which $13 billion should be directed toward the MDGs and $2 billion toward NCDs and injuries. Unfortunately, the timing of the Great Recession of 2008 likely impacted this call for action, and while funding did increase slightly, annual U.S. global health funding continued to hover around $10 billion from 2009 to 2015 (Valentine et al., 2016), with approximately $6.5 billion dedicated to global HIV/AIDS efforts (KFF, 2012).[4] Compared to prior years, annual growth in global health spending has only been 1.6 percent between 2010 and 2016 (IHME, 2017).

The most recent budget request from President Obama for FY2017 included $10.3 billion in total funding for global health programs (Valentine et al., 2016). According to Valentine and colleagues, within the international affairs budget, most of the global health funding ($8.6 billion) in the FY2017 request is provided through the global health programs (GHP) account at the U.S. Agency for International Development (USAID) and the U.S. Department of State, including funding for The U.S. President's Emergency Plan for AIDS Relief (PEPFAR) and the President's Malaria Initiative. For a full breakdown of the GHP account, which does not include global health money spent by the U.S. Department of Health and Human Services (HHS) or the U.S. Department of Defense, see Figure 2-1. In its analysis of the global health budget, the Kaiser Family Foundation noted that Congress has approved higher funding levels for global health than those in the President's budget request for each of the past 4 fiscal years. However, whether that trend will continue is unclear.

---

[4] Appropriated U.S. funding for global health between 2009 and 2016 fluctuated: $8.46 billion in 2009, $9.016 billion in 2010, $8.86 billion in 2011 (Salaam-Blyther, 2013), $9.8 billion in 2012, $9.6 billion in 2013, $10.2 billion in 2014, $10.2 billion in 2015, and 10.2 billion in 2016 (Valentine et al., 2016).

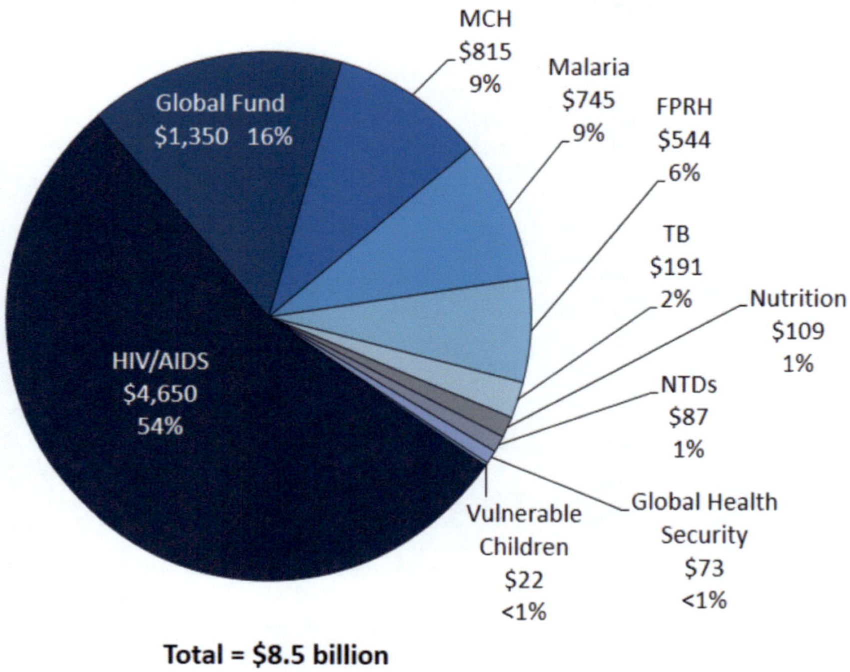

FIGURE 2-1 Global health programs (GHP) account, by program FY2017 (in USD millions).
NOTE: FPRH = family planning and reproductive health, HIV/AIDS = human immunodeficiency virus/acquired immunodeficiency syndrome, MCH = maternal and child health, NTD = neglected tropical disease, TB = tuberculosis.
SOURCE: Valentine, A., A. Wexler, and J. Kates. The U.S. global health budget: Analysis of the fiscal year 2017 budget request. (The Henry J. Kaiser Family Foundation, March 22, 2016) (http://kff.org/global-health-policy/issue-brief/the-u-s-global-health-budget-analysis-of-the-fiscal-year-2017-budget-request [accessed January 26, 2017]).

Table 2-1 illustrates global health spending by U.S. government agencies in the four focus areas of this report: emerging infectious diseases; HIV/AIDS, tuberculosis (TB), and malaria; maternal and child health; and cardiovascular disease (CVD) and cancers.

Perceptions of U.S. Global Health Spending

The American public approves of the United States taking a leading or major role in solving international problems, as revealed by a 2016 Kaiser Family Foundation survey of Americans on the United States's role in global

TABLE 2-1 U.S. Global Health Budgeted Spending on Priority Areas in 2016 (in $ millions)

Agency	Emerging Infectious Diseases	HIV/AIDS, TB, and Malaria	Maternal and Child Health*	Cardiovascular Disease and Cancer	TOTAL
USAID	$50.00	$1,026.00	$1,421.00	**	$2,497.00
U.S. Department of State		$4,320.00	$165.00		$4,485.00
CDC	$601.50	$128.40	$219.00	**	$948.90
FDA	$129.50		—		$129.50
U.S. Department of Defense	$712.20	$13.30	—		$725.50
NIH	$1,848.00	$602.10	—	$23.01	$2,450.10
BARDA	$522.00	—	—	—	$522.00
Total	$3,863.20	$6,089.80	$1,805.00	$23.01***	$11,758.00

NOTE: BARDA = Biomedical Advanced Research and Development Authority; CDC = U.S. Centers for Disease Control and Prevention; FDA = U.S. Food and Drug Administration; HIV/AIDS = human immunodeficiency virus/acquired immunodeficiency syndrome; NIH = National Institutes of Health; TB = tuberculosis; USAID = U.S. Agency for International Development.

* Budget estimates for Maternal and Child Health incorporates program areas of "Maternal and Child Health," "Nutrition," "Family Planning," and "Vulnerable Children."

** Cardiovascular disease (CVD) funding within USAID is folded into broader health systems strengthening projects, so itemized expenditures could not be identified. For CVD programs within CDC, philanthropic funding is used.

*** CVD and cancer funding from the NIH are identified as global grants provided by the National Heart, Lung, and Blood Institute and the National Cancer Institute.

SOURCES: Boddie et al., 2015; KFF, 2016; NIH, 2017.

health (Hamel et al., 2016). Striking though, is that half of Americans think the United States is spending too much on foreign aid, until they learn that foreign aid spending is just 1 percent of the budget (Hamel et al., 2016). Global health spending, specifically, was only about 0.26 percent[5] of the budget in 2016. On average, survey participants estimated foreign aid spending at 31 percent of the budget (Hamel et al., 2016). After being informed of true foreign aid expenditures, "7 in 10 Americans believe that the current level of U.S. foreign spending on health is too little or about right" (Hamel et al., 2016). While the United States contributes greatly

[5] Global health spending as a percent of the budget was calculated by using 2016 enacted global health funding ($10.2 billion) from Valentine et al. (2016) and total spending ($3.9 trillion) from the Congressional Budget Office (CBO, 2017).

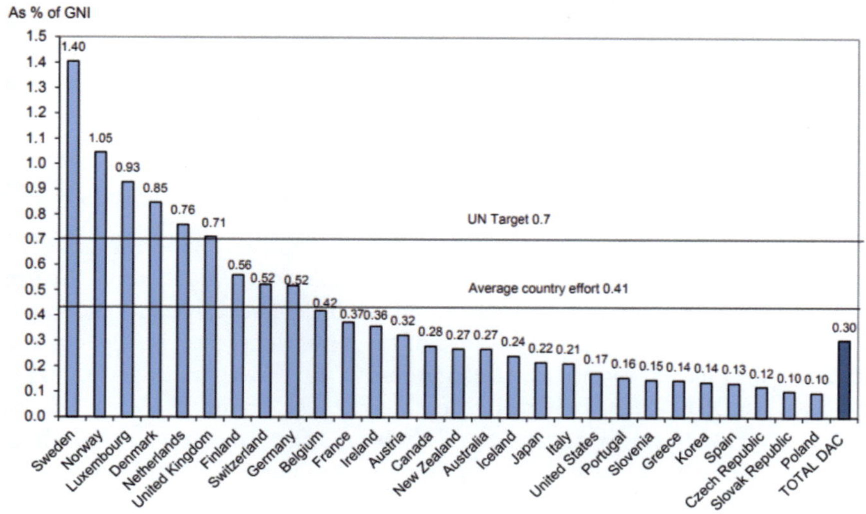

FIGURE 2-2 Net overseas development aid in 2015 as a percentage of gross national income (GNI).
NOTE: DAC = Development Assistance Committee; GNI = gross national income; ODA = overseas development aid; UN = United Nations.
SOURCE: https://www.oecd.org/dac/stats/ODA-2015-complete-data-tables.pdf (accessed January 12, 2017).

to global aid, other donor countries are just as critical to ensuring robust development assistance in health across the globe. In fact, the United States actually contributes a lower percentage of its gross national income (GNI)[6] than other high-income countries, with ODA at only 0.17 percent of GNI for the United States—below the levels of other high-income countries such as Germany, Sweden, or the United Kingdom, and well below the United Nations target of 0.7 (see Figure 2-2).

Additionally, 75 percent of Americans surveyed think the United States should give money to multilateral health organizations, such as the Global Fund to Fight AIDS, Tuberculosis and Malaria; Gavi, the Vaccine Alliance (Gavi); the United Nations; and the World Health Organization (WHO), to improve health in other countries. These findings indicate that there is broad recognition of the advantages of leveraging the different strengths of these organizations to complement the United States' strength as a bilateral donor (Hamel et al., 2016). As the role of foreign assistance in global health

[6] Gross national income is the sum of a country's gross domestic product plus net income received from overseas (OECD, 2016).

continues to shift in the coming years, it will be essential to consider the importance of other national governments and global players as partners in providing development and health aid, and the potential of synergized efforts toward shared global goals.

A CHANGING WORLD: EFFECTS OF GLOBALIZATION

In 2013, Julio Frenk and Suerie Moon argued that "globalization has intensified cross-border health threats, leading to a situation of health interdependence—the notion that no nation or organization is able to address singlehandedly the health threats it faces but instead must rely to some degree on others to mount an effective response" (Frenk and Moon, 2013, p. 936). In 2017, this societal interconnectedness, stemming largely from travel and trade, is fully apparent and shows no signs of reversal. Globalization and trade have cut poverty and global inequality, and have narrowed the gap between emerging economies and those of wealthy countries (WEF, 2017). Yet, the numerous advancements owed to globalization paradoxically pose threats to the security, well-being, and economic viability of all countries. For example, most of the food Americans eat each day comes from other parts of the world, making food defense and the prevention of foodborne illnesses a primary concern for the U.S. Food and Drug Administration. Many American businesses and their supply chains now depend on workers in foreign countries. Consequently, disease outbreaks, disasters, and poor health can diminish workforce capacity and harm business. Furthermore, industrialization often has negative effects on the environment, with mortality risk from air pollution in some locations being comparable to that of obesity (Pope et al., 2002). However, discussed in more detail in the section below, globalization also presents many opportunities for health, stemming in part from the increase in global communication and access to goods, as well as from the broader cross-disciplinary agendas that have emerged from a diverse network of global discussions.

Leveraging Globalization for Improved Global Health

Despite the increase in risks of food security, air pollution, and infectious disease outbreaks, globalization has driven innovation for the health and business sectors. Increased international trade leads to global competition, which improves the quality of products and enhances the focus on the customers, creating markets in previously inaccessible places. Similarly, sharing data and study results across countries and regions, aided by advancements in digital technology, can accelerate the elimination and eradication of global diseases and contribute to new solutions and health improvements. In November 2016, a Chinese group became the first to inject a person with cells that contained edited genes using the groundbreaking CRISPR-Cas9 technique (Cyranoski, 2016). This novel technology has the potential to revolutionize the treatment of different types of cancers, and competition between countries is expected to further fuel progress, similar to the race to the moon.

The United States is likely to benefit from such innovations that address pressing health challenges, beyond the race to master gene editing. Average body mass index and rates of homicide and child and maternal mortality are higher in the United States than in any other high-income country (Kontis et al., 2017). Moreover, life expectancy for Americans is projected to stagnate in coming years. There are opportunities to learn from other countries in order to reverse these trends; global health actors often solve problems in resource-constrained environments, so the solutions are locally appropriate and fiscally sustainable. The concept of "frugal innovation" has recently been embraced by many business leaders as they expand globally, and see resource constraints as an opportunity instead of a liability, resulting in attempts to embed frugality into the company's fundamental structure (Radjou and Prabhu, 2014). This new way of thinking could provide many opportunities for applying global health lessons to challenges faced in the United States. For example, the mobile phone–based service m-Pesa has solved the problem of limited bank account access to help Kenyans make payments through mobile phones (CBS News, 2015), which has seen extraordinary use and success since its creation. The concept has recently been specifically applied in a health context through a new program called M-Tiba that helps customers set aside money for health care needs, similar to how a health savings account works (PharmAccess Foundation, 2015). This could be adapted to certain health payment contexts in the United States to make health care payments more user-friendly. On a broader scale, the organization Global to Local, founded in 2010 in King County, Washington, identifies strategies that have been proven effective in other countries and applies them to some of King County's most diverse, underserved populations (Global to Local, 2013). Additionally, the Robert Wood Johnson Foundation created a grant program in 2015 that funds organizations to gather evidence from other countries to improve community participation and decision making in local health systems, and then bring and adapt these findings to United States (RWJF, 2015). Globalization presents the United States with many opportunities to be at the forefront of global health, with an eye for bidirectional information flow and lessons learned.

Sustainable Development Goals

Improvements in health outcomes cannot be achieved by the health sector alone. This is one of the key lessons learned through the past decade of global health efforts and progress, including the recent outbreaks of Ebola and Zika. Health is the common denominator woven through sectors such as energy, transportation, and agriculture, and only through a multidisciplinary "health in all policies" approach can there be sustainable progress toward global health goals. Reflecting the interdependence of sectors and the implications for future development, the SDGs were put forward on January 1, 2016, to supersede the MDGs ending in 2015 as a nonbinding international agreement to harmonize the three interconnected elements of economic growth, social inclusion, and environmental protection needed to promote sustainable development (UN, 2016). While the SDGs built on the MDGs created in 2000, this new era of international cooperation shifts the vision and goals beyond those simply focused on health, and toward improving the environment, energy, economic growth, and social justice.

With 17 goals and 169 targets, the Sustainable Development Agenda is too large for any one entity to successfully address and requires a multisectoral effort. To ensure success, government bodies, along with financial institutions, capital markets, and private companies, will need to be engaged in bringing the Sustainable Development Agenda to fruition. Blending funds from donor organizations, governments, and private debt and equity offers the best chance for achieving these lofty and critical development goals (Nathan, 2017). Moreover, disruptive innovation and new methods of engagement and investment will be necessary to deliver on the development agenda. But a framework for operations is lacking; although the global economy is predicted to grow to almost $100 trillion by 2021, the delivery system of goods and services is outdated and it is coming up short both in terms of protecting the planet and protecting positive social outcomes for those in need (Kharas and McArthur, 2017). Considering these factors, and the positive and negative health effects of increasing globalization, the United States must base its efforts on multidisciplinary collaboration and implementation to continue to be a leader in global health for the next decade.

LOOKING TO THE FUTURE: HOW TO BETTER INVEST U.S. FUNDS

The United States has an opportunity to think more creatively about the methods and mechanisms used to finance global health efforts, particularly as greater emphasis is placed on leveraging funding from other governments and increasing engagement of private financing. A number of approaches can be considered for optimizing limited U.S. government resources to achieve the global health goals, thereby ensuring a safe homeland and a strong trade network. In 2014, the Organisation for Economic Co-operation and Development (OECD) Development Assistance Committee reported that 17 percent of U.S. foreign aid was provided through multilateral institutions, while 83 percent was provided bilaterally (Nelson, 2015). While this trend is similar to the global allocation of resources, some donor governments conversely prefer multilateral channels. For example Sweden directed an average of 60 percent of its development assistance for health toward multilateral channels between 2010 and 2015 (Yamey et al., 2016). Congress will continually be faced with the question of whether to provide aid bilaterally or multilaterally, and although each option has its advantages and disadvantages, the global transitions under way should inform this decision. Bilateral aid gives donors more control over how their money is spent, and it allows donor countries to align development assistance with broader strategic foreign policy objectives. Conversely, multilateral channels can sometimes achieve more impact—especially in areas where problems cannot be solved by any one country alone—because of their broad reach and networks. Additionally, the methods and sources of funding for global health projects have begun to shift with the growth of middle-income countries and a burgeoning middle class, allowing greater capacity to mobilize domestic resources. Finally, the growing involvement of the private sector in health and development can be a sustainable prospect for partnership and investing in global health, which offers governments a chance to do more with current spending.

Global Public Goods

Although traditional development assistance for health (DAH) has been successful in the last several decades, in part because of large flows of philanthropic dollars, there is no room for complacency. Owing to the increasingly globalized nature of health threats, economic growth in aid-recipient countries, and the growing need of a value-for-money approach, many argue that the allocation of DAH should shift more toward support of global goods and less toward support of local- or country-specific functions. In fact, the Center for Global Development's (CGD's) White House and the World Report for 2016 stated that in the present changing landscape, government revenues—as well as remittances and foreign direct investment in countries—far exceed foreign aid in all but the poorest countries (Birdsall and Leo, 2015) (see Figure 2-3). Instead of supporting countries or their programs directly, donor governments can support efficient and effective multilateral organizations, which can shift their role to catalyze new ideas, crowd-in investment,[7] and promote global public goods.

[7] Crowding-in is an economic principle in which private investment increases as debt-financed government spending increases. This is caused by government spending boosting the demand for goods, which in turn increases private demand for new output sources.

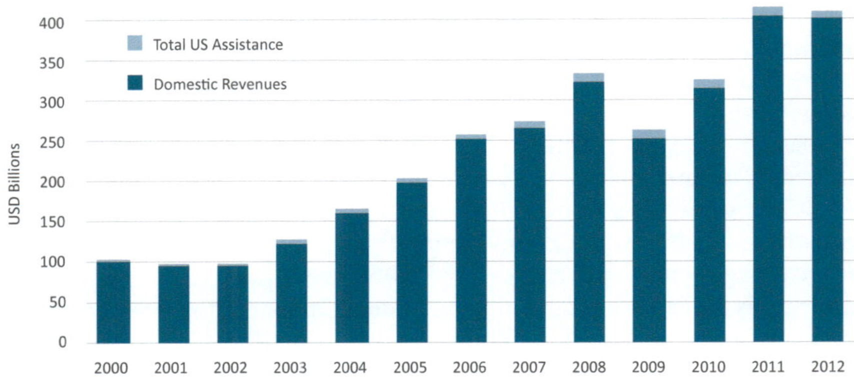

FIGURE 2-3 Domestic revenues and U.S. aid to sub-Saharan Africa.
NOTES: Aid is defined as development assistance and other official flows reported to the Organisation for Economic Co-operation and Development's Development Assistance Committee. World Bank aid figures include both concessional and non-concessional commitments by the International Development Association and the International Bank for Reconstruction and Development. USD = U.S. dollars.
SOURCES: Birdsall and Leo, 2015, and Center for Global Development (CGD), using data from the International Monetary Fund and the Development Assistance Committee of the Organisation for Economic Co-operation and Development.

Providing aid through multilateral channels allows for pooling resources, increasing purchasing power, dividing the burden, and cost sharing by donors, as well as greater coordination and aid effectiveness at the country level (Nelson, 2015).

Similarly, the World Bank and other multilateral development banks (MDBs) have typically only participated in global health in an ad hoc fashion, through provision of emergency financing during various crises in recent years. Yet, they are also uniquely positioned to meet current demands for global public goods, and through a shift in purpose, MDBs could expand their missions to encompass leadership on these issues that require a global shareholder base to respond collectively (Birdsall and Morris, 2016). In fact, a high-level panel on the future of multilateral development banking recommended that the World Bank promote global public goods critical to development as its major priority. This would be achieved through the creation of a new fund with a separate governance structure set up to disburse $10 billion annually in grant resources toward programs that cannot be easily structured as country operations (Birdsall and Morris, 2016). Thus, there are important roles for different actors, and through an overarching examination, donor countries, recipient governments, regional

MDBs, and the World Bank can identify strengths and weaknesses of different approaches.

In addition to directing funding toward multilateral channels, donor governments can help countries increase domestic financing, or domestic resource mobilization (DRM). These methodological considerations will be important to examine as the next administration reviews the current U.S. commitment toward unfished agendas such as communicable diseases including HIV/AIDS, TB, and malaria, and long-term investments in maternal and child health.

Domestic Resource Mobilization

Recent growth projections from the International Monetary Fund show an increase of 3.5 percent globally in 2017, slightly lower than previous estimates but still showing a recovery trend worldwide. Emerging market and developing economies are estimated to be slightly higher, with 4.6 percent growth in 2017 (IMF, 2016). This gross domestic product (GDP) growth is expected to continue in coming years, which will provide further support for greater DRM. Coupled with the use of sound fiscal policies, GDP growth will result in a large portion of countries graduating from DAH and beginning to fund health needs through their own domestic resources (Bhatt et al., 2015). Moreover, with the conclusion of the MDGs and creation of the SDGs in 2016, the focus is now broadening from reducing infectious disease and child mortality to the more challenging, cross-disciplinary goals of strengthening health systems and collaboration across sectors. With these trends in mind, many donors are working to support recipient governments as they transition health programs from DAH to DRM. This also reflects a shift toward even greater country ownership of their own health priorities and programs, which will inevitably translate into long-term benefits for citizens of recipient countries as they tailor the programs to their specific needs. However, many low-income and fragile-state countries will still depend on traditional sources of humanitarian aid and development assistance to support their health programs, and continued support of these programs will be critical to ensure their progress is not lost.

While this transition to DRM occurs, more DAH can be directed toward the global functions and public goods of global health. Multilateral institutions, such as the Global Fund and Gavi, are well positioned to deliver great return on investment. Directing more money toward these institutions pools global resources and leverages economies of scale that can be much more responsive to global health needs. Low- and middle-income countries (LMICs) may also stand to benefit from increased fund allocation to multilateral institutions, because such countries cannot independently produce the global public goods that those institutions can, such as research and development, knowledge sharing, market shaping, and management of cross-border externalities (Schäferhoff et al., 2015). Importantly, pursuing these elements of global public goods will be advantageous to all countries.

Leveraging the Private Sector

In addition to increasing levels of DRM with partner countries, the private sector will be a critical partner in this next stage of global health and development. An article from the 2017 World Economic Forum annual meeting argued that advancing the cross-sectoral SDGs is a business imperative and transformational change should be undertaken from an ecosystem perspective, explaining "the longevity of companies the world over is predicated on the increased access and usage of financial services by those at the bottom of the pyramid" (Nathan, 2017). The U.S. government has begun to do this in a more strategic manner, through partnerships in other sectors such as Power Africa or Feed the Future within USAID. For example, Power Africa aims to crowd-in private energy partners in LMICs and, since its inception in 2013, now has more than 130 companies involved with a projected investment of approximately $40 billion. However, through this partnership and private-sector–focused model, it has kept direct costs to the agency to only $76 million for FY2016.[8] Chapter 8 discusses financing models in more detail, but to emphasize the importance, the committee asks the reader to truly consider throughout the report, how to maximize public, private, and social sector dollars to spur economic growth and build stronger communities globally (Nathan, 2017).

THE UNITED STATES AS A GLOBAL CITIZEN

As many common global health challenges have coalesced over the past decade, including the growing burden of NCDs and potentially pandemic infectious disease outbreaks, several international agreements have been put into effect, committing political efforts and support toward improving health and life for all. As a long-time leader within the global community, the United States is a signatory on these agreements, such as the International Health Regulations (2005), the SDGs, and the Sendai Framework for Disaster Risk Reduction. Whether constituted as global action plans, frameworks, goals, or regulations, these agreements further emphasize the need and motivation for the global community to come together to advance the health and well-being of each nation's citizens. It should be the continued duty of the United States to both follow and support these global, forward-looking, collaborative efforts.

---

[8] Personal communication with Matt Rees, Power Africa, November 10, 2016.

REFERENCES

Bhatt, S., D. J. Weiss, E. Cameron, D. Bisanzio, B. Mappin, U. Dalrymple, K. E. Battle, C. L. Moyes, A. Henry, P. A. Eckhoff, E. A. Wenger, O. Briet, M. A. Penny, T. A. Smith, A. Bennett, J. Yukich, T. P. Eisele, J. T. Griffin, C. A. Fergus, M. Lynch, F. Lindgren, J. M. Cohen, C. L. J. Murray, D. L. Smith, S. I. Hay, R. E. Cibulskis, and P. W. Gething. 2015. The effect of malaria control on *Plasmodium falciparum* in Africa between 2000 and 2015. *Nature* 526(7572):207-211.

Birdsall, N., and B. Leo. 2015. *The White House and the world: Practical proposals on global development for the next US president.* Washington, DC: The Center for Global Development.

Birdsall, N., and S. Morris. 2016. *Multilateral development banking for this century's development challenges.* Washington, DC: Center for Global Development.

Boddie, C., T. K. Sell, and M. Watson. 2015. Federal funding for health security in FY2016. *Health Security* 13(3):186-206.

Burkle, F. M. 2017. The politics of global public health in fragile states and ungoverned territories. *PLOS Currents: Disasters* 1.

CBO (Congressional Budget Office). 2017. *The federal budget in 2016: An infographic.* https://www.cbo.gov/publication/52408 (accessed April 20, 2017).

CBS News. 2015. *Want to text money? Kenya's been doing it for years.* http://www.cbsnews.com/news/want-to-text-money-kenya-has-been-doing-it-for-years (accessed March 15, 2017).

Cyranoski, D. 2016. CRISPR gene-editing tested in a person: Trial could spark biomedical duel beteween China and U.S. *Nature* 539(7630).

Daschle, T., and B. Frist. 2015. *The case for strategic health diplomacy: A study of PEPFAR.* Washington, DC: Bipartisan Policy Center.

Frenk, J., and S. Moon 2013. Governance challenges in global health. *New England Journal of Medicine* 368(10):936-942.

Global to Local. 2013. *Global to Local: About us.* http://www.globaltolocal.org/overview (accessed January 26, 2017).

Hamel, L., A. Kirzinger, and M. Brodie. 2016. *2016 survey of Americans on the U.S. role in global health.* Washington, DC: The Henry J. Kaiser Family Foundation.

IHME (Institute of Health Metrics and Evaluation). 2017. *Financing Global Health 2016: Development Assistance, Public and Private Health Spending for the Pursuit of Universal Health Coverage.* Seattle, WA: IHME.

IMF (International Monetary Fund). 2016. *World economic outlook: Too slow for too long.* Washington, DC: International Monetary Fund.

InterAction. 2011. *Choose to invest in foreign assistance.* Washington, DC: InterAction. https://www.interaction.org/sites/default/files/4857/ChooseToInvest_booklet_Complete.pdf (accessed March 10, 2017).

Jamison, D., L. Summers, G. Alleyne, K. Arrow, S. Berkeley, A. Binagwaho, F. Bustreo, D. Evans, R. Feachern, J. Frenk, G. Ghosh, S. Goldie, Y. Guo, S. Gupta, R. Horton, M. Kruk, A. Mahmoud, L. Mohohlo, M. Ncube, A. Pablos-Mendez, S. Reddy, H. Saxenian, A. Soucat, K. Ulltveit-Moe, and G. Yamey. 2013. Global health 2035: A world converging within a generation. *The Lancet* 382:1898-1955.

Jamison, D., Y. Yamey, N. Beyeler., and H. Wadge. 2016. *Investing in Health: The Economic Case.* Doha, Qatar: World Innovation Summit for Health.

KFF (Kaiser Family Foundation). 2012. *U.S. federal funding for HIV/AIDS: The President's FY2013 budget request.* Washington, DC: Kaiser Family Foundation.

KFF. 2016. *U.S. global health budget tracker.* http://kff.org/interactive/budget-tracker/landing (accessed January 26, 2017).

Kharas, H., and J. W. McArthur. 2017. *We need to reset the global operating system to achieve the SDGs. Here's how*. https://www.weforum.org/agenda/2017/01/we-need-to-upgrade-the-sustainable-development-goals-here-s-how (accessed February 14, 2017).

Kontis, V., J. E. Bennett, C. D. Mathers, G. Li, K. Foreman, and M. Ezzati. 2017. Future life expectancy in 35 industrialised countries: Projections with a Bayesian model ensemble. *The Lancet* 389(10076):1323-1335.

Lima, V. D., R. Granich, P. Phillips, B. Williams, and J. S. G. Montaner. 2013. Potential impact of The U.S. President's Emergency Plan for AIDS Relief on the tuberculosis/HIV coepidemic in selected sub-Saharan African countries. *The Journal of Infectious Diseases* 208(12):2075-2084.

Millennium Project. 2006. *What they are*. Washington, D.C.: The United Nations Millennium Project. http://www.unmillenniumproject.org/goals (accessed March 10, 2017).

Nathan, T. 2017. *5 ways to make blended finance work*. https://www.weforum.org/agenda/2017/01/ways-to-make-blended-finance-work (accessed December 15, 2016).

Nelson, R. M. 2015. *Multilateral development banks: Overview and issues for Congress. CRS Report No. 7-5700*. Washington, DC: Congressional Research Service.

NIH (National Institutes of Health). 2017. *NIH reporter*. https://projectreporter.nih.gov/reporter_summary.cfm#tab2 (accessed February 8, 2017).

OECD (Organisation for Economic Co-operation and Development). 2015. *Final official development assistance figures in 2014*. Washington, DC: Organization for Economic Cooperation and Development.

OECD. 2016. *Gross national income*. https://data.oecd.org/natincome/gross-national-income.htm (accessed April 20, 2017).

PharmAccess Foundation. 2015. M-Tiba is truly leapfrogging healthcare in Kenya. *PharmAccess Foundation*, December 15.

Pope III, C. A., R. T. Burnett, M. J. Thun, E. E. Calle, D. Krewski, K. Ito, and G. D. Thurston. 2002. Lung cancer, cardiopulmonary mortality, and long-term exposure to fine particulate air pollution. *JAMA* 287(9):1132-1141.

Radjou, N., and J. Prabhu. 2014. What frugal innovaters do. *Harvard Business Review*, December 10. https://hbr.org/2014/12/what-frugal-innovators-do (accessed March 15, 2017).

Runde, D., and C. Savoy. 2016. *Domestic revenue mobilization: Tax system reform*. Washington, DC: Center for Strategic and International Studies.

RWJF (Robert Wood Johnson Foundation). 2015. *Studying promising global practices in community participation in health systems to advance adaptation in the United States*. http://www.rwjf.org/en/library/grants/2015/11/studying-promising-global-practices-in-community-participation-i.html (accessed March 7, 2017).

Salaam-Blyther, T. 2013. *U.S. global health assistance: Background issues for the 113th Congress*. Washington, DC: Congressional Research Service.

Schäferhoff, M., S. Fewer, J. Kraus, E. Richter, L. H. Summers, J. Sundewall, G. Yamey, and D. T. Jamison. 2015. How much donor financing for health is channelled to global versus country-specific aid functions? *The Lancet* 386(10011):2436-2441.

Sturchio, J. L., and A. Goel. 2012. *The private-sector role in public health: Reflections on the new global architecture in health*. Washington, DC: Center for Strategic and International Studies.

Summers, L., and D. Jamison. 2013. Policy brief #2: The returns to investing in health. *The Lancet*.

UN (United Nations). 2016. *The sustainable development agenda*. http://www.un.org/sustainabledevelopment/development-agenda (accessed January 26, 2017).

Valentine, A., A. Wexler, and J. Kates. 2016. *The U.S. global health budget: Analysis of the fiscal year 2017 budget request*. http://kff.org/global-health-policy/issue-brief/the-u-s-global-health-budget-analysis-of-the-fiscal-year-2017-budget-request (accessed January 26, 2017).

Wagner, Z., J. Barofsky, and N. Sood. 2015. PEPFAR funding associated with an increase in employment among males in ten sub-Saharan African countries. *Health Affairs (Millwood)* 34(6):946-953.

WEF (World Economic Forum). 2017. *The global risks report 2017. 12th edition*. Cologny, Switzerland: World Economic Forum. http://www3.weforum.org/docs/GRR17_Report_web.pdf (accesed March 10, 2017).

Yamey, G., J. Sundewall, H. Saxenian, R. Hecht, K. Jordan, M. Schäferhoff, C. Schrade, C. Deleye, M. Thomas, N. Blanchet, L. Summers, and D. Jamison. 2016. Reorienting health aid to meet post-2015 global health challenges: A case study of Sweden as a donor. *Oxford Review of Economic Policy* 32(1):122-146.

PART 1:

SECURING AGAINST GLOBAL THREATS

3

Infectious Diseases, Pandemic Influenza, and Antimicrobial Resistance: Global Health Security Is National Security

National security is not just about protection from state and nonstate actors, but also encompasses protection from emerging infectious diseases and other health outcomes that can threaten the nation's economic vitality and its very way of life. This point is demonstrated by the Director of National Intelligence's inclusion of the threat of pandemics and other health hazards in the U.S. intelligence community's worldwide threat assessment every year since 2009,[1] including 2016, the most recent year in which that report was available (Clapper, 2016). The U.S. Army recently estimated that if a severe infectious disease pandemic were to occur today, the number of U.S. fatalities could be nearly double the total number of battlefield fatalities sustained in all U.S. wars since the American Revolution (GAO, 2017). In the last 13 years alone, the world has seen many infectious disease outbreaks—such as sudden acute respiratory syndrome (SARS), influenza A virus subtype H1N1, Middle East respiratory syndrome coronavirus (MERS-CoV), Ebola, and Zika virus—all of which presented serious risks to the health security of countries around the world. Yet when such public health emergencies occur, funds to combat them are released in a sporadic and disjointed manner, in amounts far greater than would have been needed for prevention and preparedness. In response to the Ebola outbreak in 2014, for example, Congress appropriated $5.4 billion (Kates et al., 2015), $1.1 billion of which was spent domestically (Epstein et al.,

[1] Intelligence reports for each year can be found in the archives, located here: https://www.dni.gov/index.php/newsroom/testimonies/179-congressional-testimonies-2009 (accessed March 15, 2017).

2015), representing 120 percent of the approximately $900 million in total annual appropriations for building public health and health care preparedness capacity.[2]

As of the release of this report, both MERS-CoV and Zika continue to smolder beneath the surface with small-scale outbreaks, but there is no vaccine or treatment available should either erupt into a full-fledged epidemic in a populated area. The potential for the use of man-made biological weapons in acts of terrorism is an ongoing threat as well. While global crises have largely been avoided to date, the lack of a strategic approach to these threats could have grave consequences. If the system for responding to such threats remains reactionary, the world will not always be so lucky. Instead, strong public health infrastructure and preparedness systems are needed, along with a clear commitment from the U.S. government to drug and vaccine development. Yet in the face of competing priorities, funding for these purposes is often the first to be cut because of a failure to appreciate these threats and their potential consequences. Swift and proactive strategic action is needed now, before one or more of these threats rise to the surface and outpace the world's ability to respond.

This chapter begins by describing in detail the various dimensions of the threats to and vulnerabilities of global health security. It then outlines the human and economic costs of failing to take action to address these security challenges. The third section describes current global health programs and commitments, and why they are inadequate to meet these challenges. The chapter then presents the committee's vision of a new approach to global health security, focused on building preparedness capacity in the United States and abroad, ensuring sustainable funding for these efforts, and creating an environment for proactive research and development aimed at enhancing the nation's preparedness and response capacity. The final section presents a summary and recommendations.

THE GLOBAL HEALTH SECURITY IMPERATIVE

The World Health Organization (WHO) defines global health security as the "activities required . . . to reduce the vulnerability of people around the world to new, acute, or rapidly spreading risks to health, particularly those that threaten to cross international borders" (CDC, 2016d). To adequately address the risks to global health security, however, it is necessary to understand the inherent vulnerabilities encompassed by this definition. Today's domestic and regional health crises are increasingly influenced by

---

[2] This percentage was calculated by using fiscal year 2016 amounts of Public Health Emergency Preparedness program funding ($660 million) and Hospital Preparedness Program funding ($255 million) as the preparedness amounts.

widely interrelated global changes and forces defined by climate change; loss of biodiversity; rapid unsustainable urbanization; and scarcities of water, food, and energy (Burkle, 2017). More precise threats include zoonotic spillover or the emergence of new infectious diseases, pandemic influenza, and growing antimicrobial resistance. Exacerbating the risks resulting from these threats are vulnerabilities such as degraded public health infrastructure, vulnerable supply chains for health and medical products, and fragile nation states. This section reviews these various threats and vulnerabilities, which are summarized in Table 3-1.

Rapid Urbanization and Loss of Biodiversity: Zoonotic Spillover

The trend toward urbanization is accelerating as individuals leave less prosperous agrarian jobs in rural regions to pursue better opportunities in cities. While this rural-to-urban migration is not a new phenomenon, it has been accelerated by globalization: In 1950, only 30 percent of people worldwide lived in urban areas, but this proportion had risen to 54 percent by 2014, and it is expected to grow to 66 percent by 2050 (UN, 2014). The number of megacities (cities with populations of 10 million or more), most of which are in low- and middle-income countries (LMICs), is also projected to grow, from 28 to 41 in the next 15 years (UN, 2014). And as highlighted in the U.S. intelligence community's worldwide threat assessment, Asia and Africa are urbanizing more rapidly than any other regions (Clapper, 2016).

While urbanization is an indication of economic growth and opportunity, it also reduces biodiversity through habitat loss, fragmentation, and biological homogenization (McKinney, 2002; Pauchard et al., 2006). Since 2000, the global community has witnessed numerous outbreaks of diseases such as SARS, Ebola, Marburg, hantavirus, and avian influenza, as a result of human impacts on biodiversity (COHAB Initiative, 2010). Almost of all of these outbreaks were due to infectious disease spillover, which occurs when an immunologically naïve population comes in contact with a reservoir population that has a high pathogen prevalence. In addition to loss of biodiversity, urbanization and high population density can create an environment in which infections such as tuberculosis (TB) can thrive; more virulent strains of pathogens can evolve (Pongsiri et al., 2009); antimicrobial resistance occurs (Allen et al., 2010); and the rapid spread of disease becomes possible.

While the majority of the disease burden in past outbreaks has fallen on developing countries, increases in human mobility have increased the distances and accelerated the speed over which microbes can travel (Labonte et al., 2011). Thus, despite the global community's efforts to conquer communicable diseases in the poorest regions of the world, it has witnessed the

TABLE 3-1 Health Threats and Vulnerabilities Associated with Globalization

Threat	Global Impact	U.S. Impact
Zoonotic diseases and spillover	From 2000 to 2010, zoonotic diseases caused $200 billion in indirect economic losses (World Bank, 2010). Additionally, more than 2.5 billion cases and 2.7 million deaths can be attributed to the top 56 zoonoses (Gebreyes et al., 2014).	Since 1999, West Nile virus (WNV) has infected an estimated 3 million people (Petersen et al., 2013), resulting in approximately 43,000 illnesses due to its asymptomatic nature (Cahill et al., 2017). Costs of WNV in the United States are estimated to be $56 million per year (Barrett, 2014).
Antimicrobial resistance (AMR)	At the current rate of development of drug resistance, losses of 10 million lives per year and a cumulative loss of $100 trillion in global economic output by 2050 are projected (Review on Antimicrobial Resistance, 2016).	In the United States, AMR results in 23,000 deaths and $55–$70 billion in economic losses annually (PCAST, 2014)
Pandemic influenza	A moderately severe influenza pandemic[a] would result annually in 700,000 deaths and a cost of $570 billion (due to income loss and mortality) globally (Fan et al., 2016).	An influenza pandemic in the United States would result in 89,000–207,000 deaths and an economic loss of $71.3–$166.5 billion (Meltzer et al., 1999).
Weak public health infrastructure and protections[b]	The Zika virus, spread by *Aedes* mosquitoes,[c] emerged in Brazil in 2014 and spread rapidly to 26 neighboring countries, infecting up to 1 million people (Petersen et al., 2016). Zika's estimated cost to Latin America and the Caribbean was $3.5 billion in 2016 (World Bank, 2016c). Once eradicated from 18 countries in 1962, *Aedes aegeypti* saw a resurgence due to public health complacency and failed vector control (Whitman, 2016).	*Aedes aegeypti* is found in the southern region of the United States, meaning these states are also at risk for Zika. Mosquito surveillance and control efforts in the United States are implemented in a patchwork manner at the state and county levels (Schmidt, 2016). The urgency of combating Zika led to a $1.89 billion request by President Obama, yet appropriations were delayed by 7 months (Wexler et al., 2016). Unfortunately, the delay led to more Zika cases, and as of March 1, 2017, 5,074 cases of Zika had been confirmed in the continental United States (CDC, 2017a).

TABLE 3-1 Continued

Threat	Global Impact	U.S. Impact
Supply chain vulnerabilities	During the 2014 Ebola outbreak, high demand for personal protective equipment (PPE) was met with low inventory and capacity, and manufacturers struggled to meet the need. As a result, many countries in West Africa had to consider splitting deliveries over time (UNICEF, 2014).	A shortage of saline solution, an essential product for U.S. hospitals, occurred in 2014 as a result of recalls from the few U.S. manufacturers and weather issues. The U.S. Food and Drug Administration (FDA) had to begin importing the solution from Germany, Norway, and Spain to alleviate the need (FDA, 2016), as the lack of access to saline can be a death sentence for dialysis patients (Dembosky, 2014).
Fragile states/ conflict zones	Although Nigeria had been declared polio free in 2015, conflict with Boko Haram in its northern region prevented the establishment of proper surveillance programs, and four types of wild polio viruses were found in 2016. Because polio is highly contagious, public health officials had to initiate a massive campaign to vaccinate millions of children across West and Central Africa (Beaubien, 2016). Costs of this campaign have yet to be estimated.	The U.S. government is currently the largest donor to the Global Polio Eradication Initiative (GPEI), with a commitment of $228 million in fiscal year 2016. This funding has contributed to significant gains in reducing polio endemicity (KFF, 2016). However, state fragility is a barrier to polio eradication, and results in a need for continuous U.S. investment due to the ongoing threat.

[a] Defined as having a mortality rate of less than 10 standardized mortality units (SMUs), where 1 SMU corresponds to 735,000 deaths (Fan et al., 2016). For perspective, seasonal influenza causes 250–500,000 deaths per year (WHO, 2016c).

[b] Public health infrastructure is considered to include safe water and sanitation, as well as community preventive programs (e.g., vector control, vaccines).

[c] *Aedes* mosquitos are widespread throughout the tropics and transmit other arboviruses, such as chikungunya, dengue, and yellow fever. The principal vector for Zika, *Aedes aegypti*, is widely distributed throughout the Americas (Petersen et al., 2016). Zika has also been found to be spread by mother-to-child transmission, sexual activity, and blood transfusions (Schmidt, 2016).

reemergence of known and the emergence of new diseases. SARS is the most notable recent example of the amplification of the spread of disease enabled by today's increased interconnectedness. The first case of SARS was identified in the Guandong province, China, in November 2002 (CDC, 2013b), and by May 2003, the disease had spread to 30 countries on 6 continents (WHO, 2017b).

Pandemic Influenza

A persistent theme of the health security conversation is the threat of an influenza pandemic. Unlike seasonal influenza, a pandemic influenza virus results from a dramatic mutation in the virus. In the 20th century, three major influenza pandemics occurred—in 1918, 1957, and 1968—causing millions of deaths and wide-scale economic disruption. The 1918 pandemic alone resulted in approximately 50–100 million deaths (3–5 percent of the global population at the time) (Jeffery and David, 2006), and is cited as the most devastating epidemic in recorded history (see Annex 3-1 at the end of this chapter). However, even less severe pandemics could pose a threat to the global community, as evidenced by the two multicountry influenza pandemics that have occurred since 2000 (the 2005 H5N1 pandemic and the 2009 H1N1 pandemic). The 2009 H1N1 pandemic resulted in approximately 284,000 deaths worldwide (Viboud and Simonsen, 2012). The frequency with which influenza pandemics have occurred in the past suggests that an influenza pandemic is likely to occur again (see Box 3-1 for a description of China's current H7N9 outbreak).

Regardless of severity, the scale of morbidity and mortality for any influenza outbreak is unpredictable. Thus, any potential outbreak poses a continued national security threat and necessitates a strong public health approach (including immunization infrastructure and surveillance) in addition to continued research into vaccines and other medical tools that can mitigate their impacts from the outset. Yet progress on a universal influenza vaccine has been a hope for years (The Energy and Commerce Committee: Subcommittee on Oversight and Investigations, 2013; Vergano and Szabo, 2011), and it is increasingly difficult to maintain private-sector interest in the development of annual seasonal influenza vaccines (Ridley et al., 2016), as well as to foster high vaccination rates. For example, only 10 states vaccinated at least half of their population against the seasonal flu during the 2015–2016 flu season (Segal et al., 2016). Yet even as robust seasonal flu vaccination remains out of reach, direct medical costs of seasonal flu for the U.S. population are estimated at $10.4 billion annually, with projected annual lost earnings estimated even higher at $16.3 billion (Molinari et al., 2007).

BOX 3-1
Case Study: H7N9 Outbreak in China

First detected in 2013, a new wave of H7N9 infections began in October 2016 in provinces of China, signaling a surge exceeding that of previous years, with 555 cases and 179 deaths reported as of March 31, 2017. While the disease in birds had previously been a low-pathogenic strain, making it difficult to detect sick birds, China's agriculture ministry has said that a highly pathogenic form of the virus has been detected at live-bird markets in Guangdong province for the first time. In addition, a virus sample that could be resistant to Tamiflu has been identified.

Among the most recent surge of 304 patients, 144 (or 47 percent) had been exposed to poultry or live-poultry markets, but 11 had experienced no clear exposure, and investigations are still in progress to understand transmission routes for those cases. While WHO still believes common exposure to poultry is likely, human-to-human transmission in certain clusters has not been ruled out. Since 2013, there have been a total of 1,222 laboratory-confirmed cases of H7N9.

SOURCES: Schnirring, 2017a,b.

Antimicrobial Resistance

Antimicrobial resistance (AMR) refers to the phenomenon whereby pathogens stop responding to the drugs customarily used to combat them, making the drugs ineffective. AMR is usually attributed to overuse and inappropriate use of antimicrobial drugs, in addition to the growing issue of substandard or counterfeit drugs (Kelesidis et al., 2007). Regardless of its cause, resistance inevitably arises when pathogens become exposed to the drugs used against them. This means that use of antibiotics in livestock feed and agriculture can also contribute to the development of resistance (Littmann and Viens, 2015). As resistant microbes are found in people, animals, food, and water, they can spread from animal to person and from person to person. Globalization and increased migration, travel, and trade have substantially increased the risk of AMR around the world, as signified by the fact that resistance is found in every country (WHO, 2016a). Multidrug-resistant tuberculosis, for example, a particularly vexing public health issue, has been seen in South America, Eastern Europe, and across the African and Asian continents (WHO, 2016b). Likewise, at the Médecins sans Frontières hospital in Amman, Jordan, half of all wound infections among patients arriving from the war in Iraq and Syria are resistant to antibiotics (MSF, 2014). Each year in the United States, 2 million people experience infections that are resistant to the antimicrobials commonly used to treat them, and 23,000 people die as a result of such infections (CDC, 2013a) (see a recent example in Box 3-2). Globally, 700,000 annual deaths are attributed to drug-resistant infections (Review on Antimicrobial Resistance, 2014).

In addition to its human costs, the occurrence of resistance has major economic implications at the community, country, regional, and global levels (World Bank, 2016b). For example, AMR not only directly affects health care systems by draining workforce capacity and increasing the costs of hospital stays and second-line drugs (Long et al., 2010), but also compromises the progress achieved in reducing the burden of critical infectious diseases, such as human immunodeficiency virus (HIV), TB, and malaria (as

BOX 3-2
Case Study: A "Nightmare" Bacterium in Nevada

A female patient in her 70s in Washoe County, Nevada, arrived in the United States in early August 2016 after an extended visit to India. She was admitted to an acute care hospital on August 18 with a primary diagnosis of systemic inflammatory response syndrome, likely resulting from an infected right hip seroma likely due to a previous procedure performed outside of the United States. Investigators say the infection was caused by carbapenem-resistant Enterobacteriaceae (CRE), a multidrug-resistant organism associated with high mortality. While CRE infections are not new to Nevada or the United States, what was new in this case was that the infection was resistant to all available antimicrobial drugs. Further testing of the resistance mechanism identified the presence of New Delhi metallo-beta-lactamase (NDM-1), an enzyme that directly breaks down a powerful class of antibiotics and is also highly mobile, meaning that it is transferred easily between bacteria.

Doctors tried 14 different types of antibiotics to treat the infection, but none were successful. Further testing of the organism showed it was resistant to 26 different antibiotics, including many last-resort options, leaving the doctors with no treatment possibilities. The patient developed septic shock and died in early September 2016. While NDM-1 CRE infections are rare in the United States, this patient had been in India for 2 years previously and had been hospitalized there multiple times. This was also the case with a Swedish patient in whom NDM-1 was discovered in 2009, who had also been hospitalized in India.

The U.S. Centers for Disease Control and Prevention (CDC) estimates that more than 9,000 health care–associated CRE infections occur each year in the United States, and agency labs have confirmed at least one type of CRE in health care facilities in 44 states.

SOURCES: Chen et al., 2017; CIDRAP, 2017.

explored more in Chapter 4). Furthermore, according to the World Bank, failing to contain AMR would jeopardize achievement of the Sustainable Development Goals by 2030, as well as reverse the poverty reduction and economic growth attained through the effective use of antimicrobials (World Bank, 2016b).

The global health challenge of AMR, like many others emphasized throughout this report, cannot be solved by governments alone; private-sector involvement will be critical to achieving success. In January 2016, the pharmaceutical, biotechnology, and diagnostics industries signed a declaration on combating AMR, committing to investing in research and development aimed at meeting public health needs and to improving access to high-quality and new antibiotics for all (IFPMA, 2016). Support from all country governments in creating a sustainable market for the products of these efforts and in implementing measures to prevent further development of resistance will also be crucial. Yet unless the United States can mobilize resources and action to address this problem internationally as well as domestically, success will not be realized. Having reviewed some of the priority emerging global health threats, the section will now continue by articulating underlying vulnerabilities that can exacerbate the threats for the United States.

Public Health Infrastructure

To prevent threats such as those described in the previous sections, the United States and the global community need to support appropriate public health measures, including access to clean water and sanitation, food safety, and robust immunizations campaigns. Given that not all health security events can be prevented, however, there is also a need for preparedness and response capacity in the event of an outbreak.

Well-built and -maintained public health infrastructure geared toward both prevention and preparedness is the first line of defense against health threats. Furthermore, activities related to prevention, epidemic investigation, and control require a sophisticated level of decision making and resource coordination (Burkle, 2006). Yet, nations across the world, including the United States, have failed to invest in the necessary infrastructure and capacities. By sacrificing prevention and preparedness, nations have inevitably compromised the ability of public health systems to respond rapidly to health threats. These globally shared deficiencies became evident during the 2002–2003 SARS outbreak and the 2003–2004 H5N1 outbreak, and again during the 2014 Ebola outbreak (GHRF Commission, 2016).

Over the past decade, public health funding in the United States has remained flat at the federal level, but has been cut at drastic rates at the state and local levels (Levi et al., 2015a). During 2012, 48 percent of all local health departments reduced or eliminated services, with immunization, maternal and child health, and emergency preparedness being the program areas most affected (Levi et al., 2015a). Similarly, dedicated public health and health care emergency funding has been steadily decreasing during the last decade (see Figure 3-1).

Recent memoranda on health security from the Johns Hopkins Center for Health Security to the new administration and Congress stress the importance of building sufficient surge capacity in the U.S. health care system to provide clinical care during epidemics and catastrophes. The memoranda also emphasize building public health infrastructure with the expertise and technology to provide earlier warning of outbreaks and disasters (Inglesby and Cicero, 2017). While the implementation of such a system can be resource-intensive, it also can reap crucial rewards. Uganda, for example, was able to respond effectively to three outbreaks of Ebola (between 2007 and 2013) and one outbreak of Marburg (in 2014) because of the public health infrastructure it built after experiencing an Ebola outbreak in 2000, the largest in global history until 2014 (CDC, 2014, 2016f; GHRF Commission, 2016). Likewise, Nigeria was able to respond rapidly to its 2014 Ebola outbreak because of a preexisting polio surveillance structure and

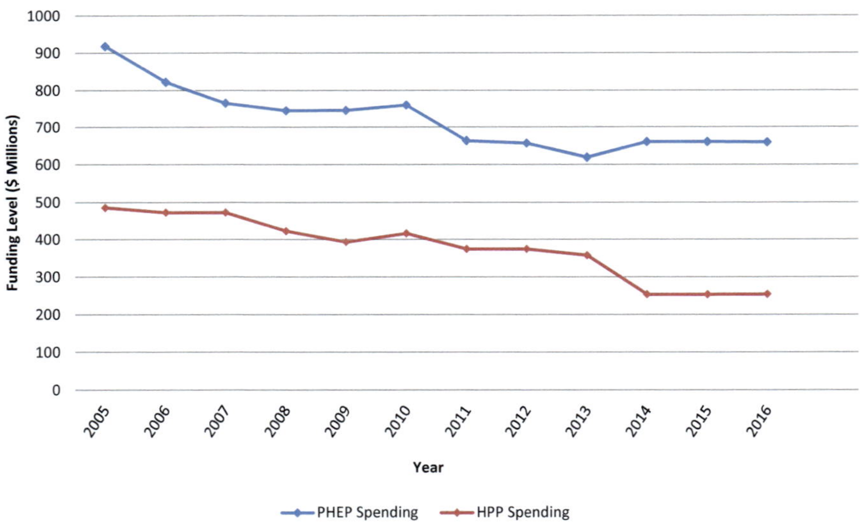

FIGURE 3-1 Public Health Emergency Preparedness and Hospital Preparedness Program funding by year, 2005–2016.
NOTE: HPP = Hospital Preparedness Program; PHEP = Public Health Emergency Preparedness.
SOURCES: Boddie et al., 2015; Levi et al., 2015b; Segal et al., 2016.

emergency operations center, as well as trained field epidemiologists. The country was able to rapidly shift the target of these capabilities from polio to contain the Ebola outbreak in Lagos, a city of 21 million people, to just 19 cases and 7 deaths (WHO, 2014b).

To ensure a strong health system, it is essential to continually support key public health programs. Public health suffers from the "out of sight, out of mind" phenomenon; consequently, success often goes unnoticed and results in complacency. When this happens, funding is cut and programs are scaled back, which often results in the resurgence of an infectious disease that was previously under control. Until resurgence occurs, however, gaps in prevention draw little attention. To illustrate this cycle, Box 3-3 describes the examples of dengue and yellow fever resurgence in Brazil, malaria resurgence in Venezuela, and polio resurgence in conflict zones.

The Supply Chain System

The current supply chain system that supports the deployment of medical products is not well matched to the demands that a health security threat would create—a gap that represents a significant vulnerability. For everyday needs, the medical and public health sectors have come to rely on a just-in-time delivery system. Less a delivery system than an inventory strategy, such a system aims to supply a small amount of products as needed. The resulting limited stockpiles of medical products are the most notable aspect of this vulnerability, and the supply chains for these stockpiles only contribute to the problem. The United States, for example, currently imports 75–80 percent of the raw materials for drugs meant for the U.S. domestic market (GAO, 2007), which increases susceptibility to the effects of a public health emergency should an outbreak occur in an exporting country. Supply chain issues are not limited to raw materials, but also apply to widely used medications themselves. A 2009 study, for example, found that 100 percent of 30 identified essential generic life-saving medicines[3] were manufactured overseas—mainly in India or China—with long supply chains and no significant stockpiles. In the event of a pandemic in these countries or a disruption at any point along these supply chains, U.S. hospitals would lose the ability to provide these drugs to patients (Osterholm and Olshaker, 2017). Similarly, according to a 2016 report by the Trust for America's Health (TFAH), 40 percent of states lack backup medical supplies to cope with a pandemic influenza or other major outbreak should their supplies be low (Segal et al., 2016). Because of the just-in-

[3] The list of 30 drugs was based on responses from hospital pharmacists about what drugs were absolutely needed in their specialty. These included albuterol, heparin, insulin, nitroglycerine, and various other drugs and antibiotics (Osterholm and Olshaker, 2017).

BOX 3-3
Case Studies of Infectious Disease Resurgence

Dengue and yellow fever resurgence in Brazil: Brazil spent much of the 20th century trying to eradicate the *Aedes aegypti* mosquito, responsible for carrying dengue fever, yellow fever, and now the Zika virus, understanding that the threat of multiple diseases could thereby be addressed. Brazil declared success in 1958 and again in 1973, but given the regional territory of the mosquito, long-term eradication was not possible without concurrent effort in all of the Americas, and Brazil's success did not last. Mosquito control services were drastically reduced in the 1990s, and in 2002 Brazil suffered the worst outbreaks of dengue fever in its history. Eventually, the Zika virus followed. Furthermore, as the result of a combination of relaxed mosquito control, low immunization rates for yellow fever (only 46 percent in 2015), and other factors, Brazil saw a resurgence of yellow fever in February 2017, which has become one of the worst outbreaks the country has seen since the 1940s. Many are now concerned that the outbreak could spread to cities and become an urban phenomenon, possibly spreading to other countries in the region.

Malaria resurgence in Venezuela: In 1961, Venezuela was certified by the World Health Organization (WHO) as having eliminated malaria, 9 years ahead of the United States. However, economic turmoil in Venezuela led to a resurgence of the disease not just in remote wooded areas but across the entire nation. Because of this economic turmoil, people resorted to working at gold mines (where mosquitos and malaria thrive) and then returned to urban areas after being infected. This pattern was compounded by shortages of medicines and cessation of preventive interventions, such as spraying, in the cities, allowing malaria to be passed from infected individuals to others. While this represents a daunting problem for Venezuela, it also poses a threat to neighboring countries.

Polio resurgence: WHO launched the Global Polio Eradication Initiative in 1988, with the goal of achieving eradication by 2000. By 2003, most of the 126 polio-endemic countries (the exceptions being Afghanistan, Egypt, India, Niger, Nigeria, and Pakistan) had been able to eradicate the disease. Sadly, the breakdown of interventions in Nigeria resulted in the resurgence of polio there, which eventually spread to 21 other countries, 13 of which were reinfected after previous elimination of the disease. Continued spread was eventually contained because of immunization efforts. Now, polio remains endemic in only three countries: Afghanistan, Nigeria, and Pakistan. While polio eradication is still technically feasible, budgetary constraints and fatigue can endanger success. Most important, efforts in these three countries are threatened by conflict.

SOURCES: Akil and Ahmad, 2016; Atchon, 2016; Beaubien, 2017; Casey, 2016; Ghafoor and Sheikh, 2016; GPEI, n.d.; Lowy, 2017; Rey and Girard, 2008; Simpson et al., 2014; WHO, 2016d.

time delivery system, many health care systems can be one local supply breakdown away from an emergency for their patients. Box 3-4 provides examples of the effects of these limitations in supply chains during previous public health emergencies.

As evidenced by the examples in Box 3-4, the supply chain systems currently in place are not always capable of meeting a surge in demand. Because ensuring surge capacity and adequate stockpiles will likely result in financial losses for manufacturers, governments must incentivize them to do so. For example, Canada purchases flu vaccines from manufacturers annually—10.4 million in 2013 (The Canadian Press, 2014)—to ensure the production of a reserve supply (Public Health Agency of Canada, 2017). The U.S. Office of the Assistant Secretary for Preparedness and Response (ASPR) has begun to take similar action through its partnership with the Centers for Innovation in Advanced Development and Manufacturing, focused on assisting in addressing the shift in vaccine production capabilities overseas by the biopharmaceutical industry (see Chapter 7). However, this vaccine initiative addresses just one part of the problem; and additional solutions are needed even for such items as saline, gloves, masks, and other routine health supplies.

BOX 3-4
Examples of Stockpile Shortages and Supply Chain Breakdowns

2003 severe acute respiratory syndrome (SARS) outbreak: Nurses in Canada experienced shortages of N95 masks, most of which had been shipped to Asia. As the main manufacturers of the masks (3M and Kimberly-Clark) lacked existing stockpiles, nurses instead had to use less-protective masks.

2014 Ebola outbreak and personal protective equipment (PPE): The need for highly robust PPE, the thousands of cases, and high levels of panic as every hospital tried to prepare for incoming patients caused the demand for adequate PPE to outpace the supply. While Dupont, Kimberly-Clark, and 3M increased their production in an effort to keep pace with the demand, the capacity to meet the need was lacking. Furthermore, the U.S. Centers for Disease Control and Prevention spent $2.7 million on PPE supplies for the United States, even though there were only a handful of cases in the country, exacerbating shortages for those fighting the outbreak in West Africa.

SOURCES: Hinshaw and Bunge, 2014; Northam, 2014; Wysocki and Lueck, 2006.

Fragile States Threatening Global Successes

Despite the political and public health progress achieved in many countries, the governments of some LMICs have become so ineffective that these countries are considered failed states. Violence and war threaten the stability of their region and the world, including the progress of global health successes such as immunization and infectious disease control. The 2017 World Economic Forum Annual Risks Report identifies involuntary large-scale migration as the second most likely global risk of concern. The nature of this risk has been demonstrated in Syria, where conflict has driven migration to neighboring countries, transferring pressures to already weakened economies, fueling radicalization and violence, and demonstrating the consequences of ignoring such challenges (WEF, 2017).

Of particular relevance in the present context, the occurrence of conflict and war often results in the destruction of a health system and its public health interventions, creating an ideal environment for diseases to spread unchecked (Michelle et al., 2007).[4] Prior to the current civil war in Syria, for example, its vaccination rates were among the highest in the Mediterranean region—at above 90 percent (Alwan, 2015). In 2014, however, polio, measles, and pertussis resurged in Syria and spread to Iraq, threatening public health in both countries. When such resurgence occurs, it can require drastic responses, since as long as cases exist anywhere in the world, such diseases will constantly be a threat to everyone. Even those who have been vaccinated are at risk given the need for herd immunity for vaccinations to be fully effective (Fine et al., 2011). As another example, as a result of recent conflict and war in Yemen, that country launched a major polio vaccination campaign in February 2017 because of fears that the disease would reappear, even though the country was declared polio-free in 2009.

Given the real dangers posed by state fragility and conflicts, the global community has an imperative to take action. However, a response all too often is launched after an emergency has occurred—a pattern that needs to end. According to Frederick Burkle of the Harvard Humanitarian Initiative,

> If one accepts that disasters keep us honest by defining the public health and exposing its vulnerabilities, the global community must emphasize prevention and preparedness and re-legitimize it under international law to ensure protective strategies that intercede in fragile states before they deteriorate to the point of no return. (Burkle, 2017, p. 2)

---

[4] Regions of the world that have been particularly affected by conflict in recent years are the Lake Chad region in Africa and the WHO Mediterranean Region. Conflict caused by Boko Haram near Lake Chad has raised concerns by officials about polio resurgence. Countries in the WHO Mediterranean Region, which consists of the Middle East and North Africa, have been struck by conflict and wars, but most of those affected are inaccessible to aid and medical supplies, leading to disease resurgence and a state of emergency (Alwan, 2015).

U.S. leadership plays an important role in supporting healthy societies abroad. However, the effects of state fragility on security and progress in global health warrant early and swift intervention. The costs of failing to support global health, especially in terms of basic public health protections, can be high.

Finding: Wide-ranging threats to global health security influenced by resource scarcity, rapid urbanization, and inadequacies in stewardship of medications are poised to exploit the vulnerability of all countries, including the United States. These threats range from infectious disease spillover to pandemic influenza, to antimicrobial resistance, and are exacerbated by such vulnerabilities as degrading public health infrastructure, weak medical supply chains, and fragile states.

THE COSTS OF INACTION

Failure to act to address the threats and vulnerabilities detailed above has severe human and economic costs, many of which have been demonstrated throughout previous outbreaks and emergencies.

Human Costs

Since 2009, the world has witnessed multiple regional and global outbreaks of diseases whose effects could have been mitigated had better prevention and preparedness measures been in place. Following the H1N1 outbreak in 2009, the U.S. Centers for Disease Control and Prevention (CDC) led an international research team that examined the global death toll from the pandemic; the team's estimate was 284,000 deaths worldwide due to H1N1 directly. In addition, the virus indirectly caused 201,200 respiratory deaths and another 83,300 deaths due to cardiovascular disease (Roos, 2012). In another example, as of April 2016, 11,325 people had died in the 2014 Ebola outbreak in West Africa (CDC, 2016a), and if the outbreak had unfolded in any nearby megacity, the death toll would have been far higher. Moreover, an additional 10,623 people were estimated to have died from other causes in the three Ebola-affected countries during the outbreak, simply as a result of the chaos and reduced availability of services (Parpia et al., 2016). This latter figure represents an almost 100 percent increase in deaths that occurred simply because the health system had to halt or reduce all other services to focus its attention on Ebola, reversing progress on many diseases and health issues because of the lack of surge capacity. Looking to future threats, according to the National Bureau of Economic Research, even a moderately severe influenza pandemic could lead to 2 million or more excess deaths worldwide (Fan et al., 2016).

Economic Costs

Past outbreaks have illustrated that the economic losses they cause can far exceed the costs of preventing them. For example, the eradication of smallpox worldwide led to benefits outweighing costs at a ratio of 159:1 globally (Barrett, 2013). The costs of infectious disease outbreaks are likely to rise, moreover, as such outbreaks become more frequent as a result of expanding travel and trade, as well as environmental changes (Pike et al., 2014). The costs are only partially attributable to treating and controlling the disease itself; additional costs result from panic and the "worried well" flooding hospitals and stripping pharmacies of medical supplies. Indeed, panic can have more of a negative effect on an economy than an outbreak itself, as evidenced by the discourse in the United States during the Ebola outbreak. Once an Ebola patient had been diagnosed in the United States and $5.4 billion in response funds had been allocated, $1.1 billion was spent on domestic response, including public health studies, state and local laboratory capacity, state and local preparedness, and domestic migration activities (Epstein et al., 2015). Of this amount, $119 million was spent just on domestic quarantine activities, including screening at five major U.S. airports, medical consultations, investigations of potentially sick travelers, and follow-up (CDC, 2015a). And while commendable efforts were made by thousands of federal, state, and local government workers (White House, 2015), it is important to keep in mind that this domestically focused $1.1 billion was disbursed in response to only four cases nationwide.[5] The amount spent likely would have increased greatly if the number of cases had risen even to 10 or 20.

Following the SARS outbreak in 2003, which lasted less than 1 year, global costs of the pandemic were assessed to be $40–$54 billion (Jonas, 2014a; McKibbin, 2004). According to a World Bank policy research paper, the four most affected economies in East Asia (China, Hong Kong, Taiwan, and Singapore) experienced estimated gross domestic product (GDP) losses of $13 billion (Brahmbhatt and Dutta, 2008). Similarly, Guinea, Liberia, and Sierra Leone together were projected to suffer a crippling loss in foregone economic growth in 2015 as a result of the Ebola epidemic. After positive GDP growth in 2013 in all three countries, 2014 saw Guinea's GDP growth drop from 4 percent to 0.1 percent and Liberia's from 8.7 percent to 0.7 percent, while Sierra Leone's GDP growth declined from

[5] This number does not include cases of patients who became sick while working in West Africa and returned to the United States for treatment.

4.6 percent in 2014 to –21.5 percent in 2015 (World Bank, 2016a). Many of these economic losses could have been prevented had a more resilient health system capable of preventing and detecting outbreaks been in place (World Bank, 2015).

In addition to determining the cost of past outbreaks, it is important to examine models of future outbreaks to better inform policy and planning. The projected economic impact of an influenza pandemic ranges from $570 billion per year, including the intrinsic value of lives lost prematurely and illness suffered (Fan et al., 2016),[6] to $2 trillion[7] in direct costs, worker absenteeism, and disruptions in business (Burns et al., 2008).

The Bottom Line

Infectious disease outbreaks clearly impose terrible costs in terms of human suffering and mortality, as well as economic costs that threaten progress and stability in countries around the world, and that greatly exceed the costs of prevention and preparedness measures (GHRF Commission, 2016; Jonas, 2014b). Given the human and economic toll repeated time and again, the question then arises of how many more such outbreaks must occur before the global community acknowledges this as a threat that warrants taking sustainable action and musters the collective will to do so.

Finding: The committee believes that these threats will only become more prevalent, due to global changes such as urbanization, resource scarcity, population growth, and environmental changes, resulting in high human and economic costs.

THE CURRENT GLOBAL COMMITMENT

Even as increasing globalization is making the world ever more vulnerable to infectious disease outbreaks—whether due to natural, accidental, or intentional causes—thereby threatening national and global security, methods of distributing global aid are changing. While U.S. development policy has remained focused on U.S. aid as a way to build prosperous nations, it has become increasingly clear that, to achieve better health for their people, recipient countries no longer want to be considered beneficiaries of

[6] This study, conducted by the National Bureau of Economic Research, estimated the effect of a moderately severe pandemic (one with a mortality rate of less than 10 SMUs, where 1 SMU corresponds to 735,000 deaths). The costs include expected income losses and the intrinsic value of lives lost and illness suffered (Fan et al., 2016).

[7] This study, conducted by the World Bank, estimated the cost of a moderate influenza pandemic (one that would reduce global output by more than 2 percent). The costs included are direct costs, worker absenteeism, and disruptions in business (Burns et al., 2008).

bilateral aid, but rather partners in multilateral groups (Birdsall and Leo, 2016). Given that no single nation can be protected if other nations remain unprepared to counter biological threats,[8] the United States has a unique opportunity to capitalize on this shift in the nature of desired relations. It should move to encourage partnerships and cross-sector coordination focused on achieving the shared goal of security from infectious disease threats for all people. To fully understand the importance of this commitment, one must first know the history that contributed to the need for such investment of U.S. resources abroad.

The International Health Regulations

The International Health Regulations (IHR), which replaced the International Sanitary Regulations in 1969, were updated in 2005 following the global SARS outbreak to reflect the rapid expansion of international trade and tourism. While WHO had developed the vision for this update in the late 1990s, the 2003 SARS pandemic brought increased attention to the need to shift from halting diseases at national borders to finding and halting them at their source. This revision helped strengthen capacity and cooperation in many countries. However, the 2009 H1N1 pandemic, which served as the first true test of the revised IHR, revealed continued vulnerabilities in public health capacities at all levels, limitations in scientific knowledge concerning response, difficulties in decision making under uncertain conditions, complexities in international cooperation, challenges in communication among experts and with the public, and shortcomings of WHO decision making (WHO, 2011a).

Unfortunately, as of 2014, only about 33 percent of the 196 WHO member countries were in compliance with IHR core capacities (Katz, 2016). Thus, there exists an imperative for robust information sharing, monitoring, and response capacities both in the United States and abroad—where most infectious disease outbreaks originate—to enable proper preparation for the next and perhaps more dangerous outbreak. Many experts have recommended working toward an international consensus framework to fulfill the obligation of Article 44 of the IHR. Such a framework would guide best practices in collecting and sharing research and surveillance data in a timely and accurate manner across countries and with the public and private sectors to inform the management of any type of infectious disease event (Nuzzo and Shearer, 2017).

---

[8] Executive Order 13747, Advancing the Global Health Security Agenda to Achieve a World Safe and Secure from Infectious Disease Threats, 3 C.F.R. 13747.

The Global Health Security Agenda

To ensure that countries around the world would meet IHR core capacity requirements for public health emergencies, the U.S. government, along with international partners, launched the Global Health Security Agenda (GHSA) in February 2014. Originally a 2-year, $85 million commitment (Morrison, 2014), support for the GHSA increased as a result of the Ebola outbreak. Now supported by one-time supplemental funding[9] (Frieden, 2016) of $1 billion (GHSA, 2017), the GHSA seeks to improve national-level capacity to prevent, detect, and respond to infectious disease threats, and it has established 11 action packages[10] to achieve these goals (CDC, 2016c). Rather than creating a new strategy aimed at health security, the GHSA builds on existing U.S. strategies that provide for capacity building, technical assistance, and commodity support. Where the GHSA is novel, however, is in its coordination of these strategies and its elevation of global health security to senior-level attention (Holgate, 2014).

Building Epidemiological Capacity

In line with the GHSA's mandate of building workforce capacity, fostering the development of a cohort of public health experts with knowledge of the salient science and policy can help with early detection of and response to outbreaks. If this capacity building is done in a sustainable manner, a full transfer of U.S., Canadian, and European public health responders will not be necessary whenever an outbreak occurs. During the 2014 Ebola outbreak, the strong public health capacity in Nigeria—encompassing trained field epidemiologists and an active and functioning emergency operations center (previously supporting polio surveillance)—managed to successfully monitor 900 people through deployment of the country's established team of field epidemiologists while also engaging community leaders and members (Courage, 2014; Frieden, 2014). The Field Epidemiology and Training Program (FETP) within CDC develops expertise in detecting diseases locally and preventing them from spread-

[9] The GHSA is partially funded by leftover Ebola emergency funds in the fiscal year (FY) 2015 Omnibus Package (Consolidated and Further Continuing Appropriations Act, 2015, Public Law 113-235, Title VI, 113th Congress), which became redirected but expire in FY2019 (Segal et al., 2016).

[10] The GHSA's Action Packages are categorized into three domains: Prevent, Detect, and Respond. Under the Prevent Domain are the Action Packages for Antimicrobial Resistance, Zoonotic Disease, Biosafety and Biosecurity, and Immunization. Under the Detect Domain are the Action Packages for National Laboratory Systems, Real Time Surveillance, International Reporting, and Workforce Development. Under the Response Domain are the Action Packages for Emergency Operation Centers, Multisector Rapid Response, and Medical Countermeasures/Personnel Deployment (CDC, 2016c).

ing globally. The program has trained more than 3,100 epidemiologists in more than 70 countries since 1980 (CDC, 2016e), and has been based in Nigeria since 2008. In 2013–2014 alone, African FETP graduates responded to more than 100 outbreaks, including Lassa fever in Nigeria, polio in Cameroon and Nigeria, and monkeypox in The Democratic Republic of the Congo (CDC, 2015b). This program is also supported by the GHSA, which, through its action package on workforce development, saw the establishment, expansion, or participation of 17 countries in FETP programs to increase the number of disease detectives (GHSA, 2017) (see Box 3-5). Continued support of epidemiology training improves surveillance and detection capabilities abroad, and provides another opportunity for more robust institutional pathways for bidirectional information sharing, allowing for faster detection of new diseases and outbreaks and changes in protocols that may be necessary.

BOX 3-5
Country Examples of Field Epidemiology Training Program (FETP) Deployment Since the Launch of the Global Health Security Agenda (GHSA)

Pakistan: Outbreaks of such childhood diseases as measles, diphtheria, and pertussis can be prevented with vaccines but remain common in parts of Pakistan. When outbreaks occur, they are particularly dangerous to children. Between January and March 2016, Pakistan's Field Epidemiology Training Program graduates responded to four distinct outbreaks of vaccine-preventable diseases across five provinces. Disease detectives investigated the reasons for low vaccination coverage and initiated a campaign that provided vaccinations and health awareness sessions, helping to contain the outbreaks and protect thousands of people, including children.

Uganda: The United States has been strengthening Uganda's public health laboratory and surveillance systems; training disease detectives; and supporting Uganda's Public Health Emergency Operations Center (PHEOC), first established in 2013 for outbreak preparedness and response. In March 2016, the quick activation of the PHEOC, enhanced laboratory and diagnostic capacities, and disease detectives from the FETP helped the Ministry of Health contain a yellow fever outbreak and rapidly establish a surveillance and specimen referral system to identify potential new cases. The response efforts were substantially improved relative to the 2010 yellow fever outbreak, when it took more than 40 days just to diagnose the disease correctly.

SOURCE: GHSA, 2017.

Concerns for the Future of the GHSA

The GHSA is financed by one-time supplemental funding, which will run out by 2017 (Frieden, 2016), and there is concern about what will happen thereafter. In information-gathering requests administered to CDC country directors and comments made by high-ranking government officials (GU GHSS and HGI, 2017), strong support for the continuation of the GHSA has been expressed. Although an executive order signed by President Obama in November 2016 called for GHSA's advancement and established long-term policy objectives for the United States to build on its achievements (Rice, 2016), there is no guarantee as to its future direction.

Global health security requires stable support systems for preparedness and response capacity in LMICs. Sustained funding by the global community is imperative to support this capacity and prevent the reversal of the progress that has been achieved. Following the West Africa Ebola outbreak, multiple high-level panels and commissions were charged with identifying needed WHO reforms (described further in Chapter 9). These groups also highlighted the need for countries to partner with WHO to ensure that they can implement the core capacities necessary to comply with the IHR, with the goal of having every government develop and publish concrete plans by 2020 (Gostin et al., 2016). Meeting this need will require continued participation by the United States. The GHSA is a valuable initiative that has been able not only to coordinate the vast array of U.S. programs in global health security but also to create transparent and mutually accountable means for countries around the world to assess their own capacities. While it is hoped that capacity-building efforts will eventually be assumed by national governments, until then, the umbrella of programs supported by the GHSA and the focus of global health security itself requires continuous funding. Absent this concerted effort to ensure the development of resilient health systems in LMICs, capable of preventing and responding to emergencies, the risk of another Ebola-like epidemic remains a very real threat to all countries around the world.

Efforts to Combat Antimicrobial Resistance

In 2014, recognizing the growing threat of AMR and its national and global implications, President Obama signed an executive order on combating antibiotic-resistance bacteria.[11] This executive order formed the basis of the National Strategy for Combating Antibiotic-Resistant Bacteria (White House, 2014b) and established a federal interagency task force for Combat-

[11] Executive Order 13676. Combating Antibiotic-Resistant Bacteria. 3 C.F.R. 13676.

ing Antibiotic-Resistant Bacteria.[12] Among its functions, the task force was asked to submit a 5-year National Action Plan incorporating the recommendations of the report on combating antibiotic resistance of the President's Council of Advisors on Science and Technology (PCAST) (PCAST, 2014). In addition, the task force co-chairs were charged with establishing the Presidential Advisory Council on Combating Antibiotic-Resistant Bacteria (PACCARB) to provide advice and guidance for their work.

While the PACCARB acknowledged that important steps have been taken to achieve the milestones outlined in the National Action Plan, its initial assessment identified overarching issues and generated recommendations for further improvement. Goal 5 of the plan—"Improve international collaboration and capacities for antibiotic-resistance prevention, surveillance, control, and antibiotic research and development"—has particular relevance to global partnerships (PACCARB, 2016), and PACCARB therefore made recommendations for improving international collaboration and capacity that include

- improving measures of effectiveness by identifying outcome indicators,
- ensuring resources commensurate with supporting the goals,
- expanding the number of countries involved,
- leveraging the expertise of nongovernmental organization (NGO) assets,
- broadening the scope of One Health, and
- expanding engagement around research and development.

Up to 30 percent of drugs sold in LMICs have been found to be counterfeit, an issue that represents a significant risk for the development of AMR (Cockburn et al., 2005). The U.S. government has made efforts to stem the flow of substandard and counterfeit pharmaceuticals by engaging with NGOs and nonprofits, efforts that could help combat AMR. The U.S. Agency for International Development (USAID) has entered into a number of partnerships in hopes of reducing the number and availability of counterfeit drugs. Perhaps the most important of these is with the U.S. Pharmacopeial Convention—the Promoting the Quality of Medicines Program. This program operates in 28 countries and has been able to assist 17 countries

[12] The task force is co-chaired by the secretaries of defense, agriculture, and health and human services and made up of representatives from the U.S. Departments of State, Justice, Veterans Affairs, and Homeland Security, as well as the U.S. Environmental Protection Agency, the U.S. Agency for International Development, the Office of Management and Budget, the Domestic Policy Council, the National Security Council, the Office of Science and Technology Policy, and the National Science Foundation. Executive Order 13676, Combating Antibiotic-Resistant Bacteria, 3 C.F.R. 13676.

with quality monitoring and surveillance (USP, 2017a,b). Building on such partnerships could help combat the significant threat to the supply chain of pharmaceuticals posed by counterfeit drugs.

Additionally, embracing the One Health approach across sectors can help not only in optimizing the use of resources but also in improving the effectiveness of interventions aimed at promoting health in humans, animals, and the environment. The One Health approach recognizes that human health is closely related to the health of the environment and of animals. Given that 6 of every 10 infectious diseases in humans are spread from animals, the One Health approach aims to encourage collaborative efforts of multiple disciplines working locally, nationally, and globally to achieve the best health for people, animals, and the environment (CDC, 2017b). This approach is implemented in global activities such as the GHSA and the use of animal–human interface officers at CDC's Global Disease Detection sites (CDC, 2016b).

While there has been progress toward Goal 5 of the National Action Plan, there remain challenges that hinder its full realization, including difficulties in providing incentives for the development of diagnostics and therapeutics. However, a particularly critical barrier is the lack of sufficient funds to advance the AMR agenda. Although Congress appropriated $1 billion in FY2016 for combating AMR, the overwhelming majority of that funding was earmarked for domestic spending, with approximately $835 million being allocated to the U.S. Department of Health and Human Services (HHS) (Cabezas, 2016). U.S. hospitals certainly deserve and demand high levels of proper stewardship and infection control, but unless preparedness and surveillance capacities are built and sustained internationally, AMR will continue to threaten U.S. citizens regardless of how prepared U.S. hospitals may be. The example presented previously in Box 3-2 highlights how rapidly bacterial pathogens can spread and how important it is to invest in these capacities globally.

World leaders committed to uniting in the fight against AMR at a high-level meeting on AMR held at the United Nations (UN) in September 2016, only the fourth time that the UN General Assembly has met to discuss a health issue. This high level of political commitment provides a unique opportunity to develop and implement a coordinated global strategy for addressing the problem (UN, 2016). The committee concurs with the initial assessment of PACCARB and underscores the critical need to accelerate this work to ensure that milestones and deliverables of the National Action Plan are realized. Annex 3-2 provides additional detail on efforts to combat AMR and the National Action Plan.

Finding: The growing threat of antimicrobial resistance resulting from poor stewardship, weak surveillance systems, and a lack of

potential new therapeutics will be a major threat to the entire global community—in terms of both lives lost and impacts on the global economy—in the next 10 years.

A NEW APPROACH TO MEETING THE CHALLENGES OF GLOBAL HEALTH SECURITY

Despite many efforts at the global, regional, national, and community levels, the world is no safer now from infectious diseases than it was 20 years ago when the Institute of Medicine report *America's Vital Interest in Global Health* was written. By virtue of their unpredictability and global effect, infectious diseases remain a perpetual challenge for the global community (Fauci and Morens, 2012). Since 1997, each U.S. presidential administration has been faced with an emerging or reemerging infectious disease that assumed high political priority, including HIV/AIDS, H5N1 influenza, SARS, MERS-CoV, Ebola, and Zika (Fauci, 2017). More recently, AMR received high-level attention from the UN as a global crisis (UN, 2016), and, as described earlier in Box 3-1, the largest outbreak of influenza A (H7N9) to date is currently occurring in China (Iuliano, 2017). Whether the challenge is attributable to limitations of the design and methods employed or the vision and funding for programs being too short-sighted and ad hoc, the United States needs to reorient programs and platforms to truly protect U.S. citizens, at home and abroad, from threats to their health and safety and the corresponding economic consequences. This reorientation needs to focus on preparing to prevent and preparing to respond, both of which require strong coordination and innovation while building resilience across all sectors.

Preparedness and Disaster Risk Reduction

The first need is for intentional stewardship of a true preparedness agenda. Building strong public health systems becomes more difficult each year with declining funding. The United States needs to take a more proactive approach to being prepared and reducing the risk of public health emergencies.

Mitigation Through Building Capacity

Parallel to this shift of focus on adequate and forward-looking funding, capacity building and outbreak prevention need to be prioritized. Since the Ebola outbreak, numerous reports have been written that advocate for building country capacity and creating resilient health systems in developing countries to enable better responses in the future. Domestically, the

Federal Emergency Management Agency (FEMA) began shifting its priorities from disaster response to mitigation and prevention, finding that for every $1 it invests in mitigation, it saves $4 in response (MMC, 2005). The agency now has begun incorporating incentives into its frameworks and funding for localities that can demonstrate investment in mitigation. This same concept can be applied to investments in global health security through a lens of disaster risk reduction (see Box 3-6). Effective strategies for comprehensively building resilient health systems in low-resource settings remain elusive. However, disaster risk reduction (DRR) can make it possible to address the challenge incrementally through such goals as increasing health workforce capacity and building resilience.

The 2015 Sendai Framework for Disaster Risk Reduction calls for investing in DRR for resilience through cost-effective measures that can save lives, reduce losses, and enhance economic and social well-being (UNISDR, 2015). Such measures include strengthening the design and implementation of inclusive policies through engagement with the community, such as by improving access to basic health care, food security, housing, and education, with the goal of eradicating poverty (UNISDR, 2015). Also necessary is coherence across systems and cooperation among the academic, scientific, governmental, and private sectors to promote capacity building. Viewing these efforts through a lens of DRR can synergize existing programs, create opportunities for partnership, and lead to greater systems capacity in a country. Through such partnerships as the GHSA, it is more cost-effective

BOX 3-6
Disaster Risk Reduction

Disasters often follow natural hazards. A disaster's severity depends on how much impact a hazard has on society and the environment. The scale of the impact in turn depends on the choices people make for their lives and for the environment. These choices relate to how food is grown, where and how homes are built, what kind of government the nation has, how its financial system works, and even what is taught in schools. Each decision and action either makes people more vulnerable or more resilient to disasters.

Disaster risk reduction (DRR) is the concept and practice of reducing disaster risks through systematic efforts to analyze and reduce the causal factors of disasters. Reducing exposure to hazards, lessening the vulnerability of people and property, wisely managing land and the environment, and improving preparedness and early warning for adverse events are all examples of DRR.

SOURCE: UNISDR, 2016.

to invest in building resilience and preventing outbreaks than to respond once an epidemic is out of control (World Bank, 2012). Supporting this concept, an international commission released a report in 2016 calling for building health system core capacities in developing countries and aligning them with the SDGs to better respond to health emergencies (GHRF Commission, 2016).

At Home and Abroad

In addition to building capacity at the source of an outbreak, achieving global health security for the United States will require a robust U.S. infrastructure to detect and respond to biological threats, whether naturally occurring, accidental, or intentional. Yet, a 2016 report issued by TFAH states that over the past 15 years, one-third of funds for health security and one-half of funds for health care system preparedness have been cut. In 2002, for example, health emergency preparedness funding was $940 million, and by FY2016 it had decreased to $660 million (Segal et al., 2016)—this despite the constant emergence of threats that the U.S. health infrastructure has often just barely avoided. Similarly, annual funding for health care system preparedness has been reduced to just $255 million nationally, an amount intended to support every hospital in the country in being prepared for disasters. As noted earlier, these preparedness amounts are moderate, yet whenever public health emergency or outbreak occurs, large amounts of funding are directed toward response. Indeed, the money the United States has spent on just five outbreak responses since 2005 exceeds the combined spending on public health and health care preparedness capacity building efforts in that same time period (see Figure 3-2).

A report from the Blue Ribbon Study Panel on Biodefense recommends that Public Health Emergency Preparedness cooperative agreements for state and local infrastructure be funded to authorized levels or the president's request, whichever is higher (Blue Ribbon Study Panel on Biodefense, 2015). Although this recommendation was implemented through the Consolidated Appropriations Act of 2016, neither President Obama nor Congress returned funding to levels that existed following the 2001 anthrax attacks (Blue Ribbon Study Panel on Biodefense, 2016). The committee believes that now more than ever, sustainable and adequate funding is needed to build readiness into public health and health care infrastructure, and that appropriate funding levels for this purpose are those that were in place in the initial years of the Public Health Security and Bioterrorism Response Act of 2002. This assessment is supported by those of other experts who call for funding levels to return to FY2006 levels, or roughly $1 billion (Watson et al., 2017).

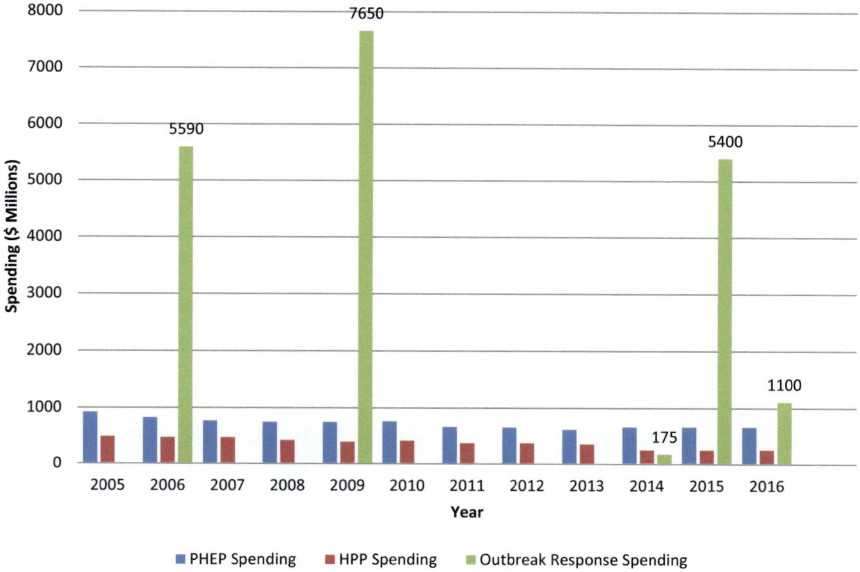

FIGURE 3-2 Public Health Emergency Preparedness and Hospital Preparedness Program funding versus outbreak response spending by year, 2005–2016.
NOTE: HPP = Hospital Preparedness Program; PHEP = Public Health Emergency Preparedness.
SOURCES: Appropriations Committee, 2016; BARDA, 2007; Kates et al., 2015; Levi et al., 2015b; Segal et al., 2016; White House, 2009, 2014a.

Finding: Funding for preparedness has decreased dramatically since the Public Health Security and Bioterrorism Response Act was enacted in 2002. In fiscal year 2016, funding for the Public Health Emergency Preparedness program decreased from its initial level of $1.03 billion to $660 million, and funding for the Hospital Preparedness Program decreased from an initial level of $515 million to $255 million.

A Well-Coordinated Response

Although strong and prepared health systems, both in the United States and abroad, are of paramount importance for identifying and containing the next outbreak, some level of response capability will always be necessary. As discussed above, however, the funding needed for response can be reduced by investments in prevention and preparedness. The direct costs of treating just two Ebola patients in the United States at the specialty center in Nebraska, for example, were estimated at more than $1 million (Gold, 2014). If mitigation and prevention efforts can halt an outbreak at the source, before it extends beyond a region, these costs are less likely to be incurred. For the United States, the current approach to organizing response is inadequate, and a better system for disbursing response funds is long overdue.

U.S. Interagency Coordination

During the Ebola outbreak, the United States contributed key resources and critical global leadership in a time of crisis. However, many suggestions have been made since then for how to better execute such a massive response. First, no response framework currently exists to guide agencies during this type of international event (similar to FEMA's domestic National Response Framework); thus, there is no clear leader for the United States in an international health emergency. Creation of an international response framework would provide a command structure and an awareness of roles and responsibilities for the agencies involved, including the blending of international and domestic responses. The success of a U.S. response is dependent on the strengths of each agency working in parallel—the logistics of the U.S. Department of Defense (DoD); the policy of HHS; the coordination and international authorities of the U.S. Department of State; the country-level knowledge of USAID and CDC; and the wealth of expertise from the private sector, NGOs, and academia. The Ebola response initially was chaotic and lacking in coordination until the White House appointed a czar to direct it. Although this was a step in the right direction, there were pitfalls that could have been avoided from the beginning. Moreover, simply selecting a czar every time a new outbreak occurs prevents the development of a longitudinal knowledge base that can be drawn on in future public health emergencies.

The 2016 report of the Blue Ribbon Study Panel on Biodefense also identifies this problem with the overall U.S. strategy, and calls for a Biodefense Coordination Council in the office of the vice president (Blue Ribbon Study Panel on Biodefense, 2016). As of the release of this report, that recommendation has yet to be implemented. Echoing this need for high-level coordination, other experts have recommended a dedicated leadership position and office to lead health security efforts (Watson and Watson, 2017). Options to this end include creating a department or office in one of the agencies involved in a response or creating an interagency working group. However, challenges arise with respect to the politics of such a coordinating role and the authority needed to drive a massive, multifaceted response. USAID's Office of Foreign Disaster Assistance (OFDA) assumes this coordinating role for the U.S. response during nonhealth emergencies, such as earthquakes and famines in other countries, but typically is not activated for health emergencies (although a disaster assistance response team [DART] was deployed during the 2014 West Africa Ebola outbreak) (Gavi, 2014). Expanding the mandate of OFDA and the DART capability could be a mechanism for the necessary coordination. Yet given the breadth of expertise needed during a complex health emergency and the difficulties of coordinating so many agencies, the committee believes a strong coordinating body is needed for health emergencies that has appropriate authority, logistics, and subject matter expertise, as well as a dedicated budget.

Finding: Although multiple agencies bring unique expertise to a U.S. government–led response, it is difficult to coordinate an urgent plan during a crisis without strong leadership, a well-defined chain of command, and an adequate budget.

Sustainable Funding

Though preparedness has proven a difficult agenda for which to compel resources, once an emergency does occur, funding, often in large amounts, is directed retroactively to that issue. By this point, most of the damage has already been done, and clinicians, epidemiologists, researchers, and other stakeholders are scrambling to catch up with the emergency. The nation simply cannot afford to stand by while critical funds to fight these outbreaks are held back. After 7 months of disagreement and delay in approving President Obama's request for $1.9 billion in Zika funding, for example, Congress finally approved $1.1 billion with the passage of the Zika Response Appropriations Act of 2016[13] (Wexler et al., 2016). Until then, agencies were forced to shift funds from other accounts for Zika-related activities, including borrowing from the Ebola supplemental funding and from CDC's state-level emergency public health care preparedness account (Epstein and Lister, 2016; Kodjak, 2016).

Many experts have called for a standing public health emergency fund. The committee agrees with this recommendation; however, it is important to understand that this funding would be reserved for response activities only. Multiple respondents from the information gathering conducted by the committee (explained in Chapter 1) reported that global budgets for fighting diseases such as TB and malaria can lapse when large-scale outbreaks occur because money is redirected. A lack of secure funding for outbreak response prevents—and, the committee believes, sometimes reverses—progress in other global health arenas. Money to address an outbreak once the United States is in response mode is important and nec-

[13] Zika Response Appropriations Act, H.R. 5243. 2016.

essary, but carving it out of existing pools of funds dedicated to important ongoing health issues would be imprudent, and could even seed the risk for a separate future outbreak. In a 2016 letter, PCAST recommended that Congress establish a public health emergency response fund[14] of at least $2 billion, modeled after the U.S. Disaster Relief Fund for FEMA (PCAST, 2016). FEMA's Disaster Relief Fund is funded annually, and unused funds from the previous fiscal year are carried over to the next. The recommended public health emergency response fund would likewise consist of funds that would carry over across years and could be replenished by routine and emergency appropriations. Access to the funds would be contingent on the express authorization of the President or the joint agreement of the secretaries of HHS and the U.S. Department of Homeland Security (DHS) (PCAST, 2016). The committee, along with other stakeholders (Watson et al., 2017), concurs with this recommendation, supporting the rapid mobilization of federal responses across the interagency community that plays a leading role in these events.

Finding: When an emergency does occur, funding for response is mired in bureaucratic processes, so that the funds are not available in a timely manner, but are often eventually released in amounts that far outweigh what is requested to prevent the emergency.

Innovation Agenda: Getting Ahead of the Pathogens

Budget caps and annual appropriations have challenged global health research and development funding, which in turn can compromise agencies' ongoing efforts when they are forced to plan the development of critical medical products just 1 year at a time. Additionally, for such diseases as Ebola and Zika and other emerging threats, funding for research and development of critical medical products, including vaccines and therapeutics, is highly reactionary. Unless money is invested up front, researchers and agencies will constantly be scrambling to get ahead of an outbreak, and industry will always consider the risks of becoming involved. Like the challenge of antimicrobial resistance, these problems cannot be solved after a threat has emerged.

[14] According to the PCAST letter, "There is a Public Health Emergency Fund that was authorized in 1983 and placed at the disposal of HHS, but it has not been replenished since 1993, despite repeated national level infectious disease emergencies. In addition to being moribund, it is specific to HHS and therefore more narrow than what we propose here. There is also a Public Health and Social Services Emergency Fund. This fund is used by the Assistant Secretary for Preparedness and Response to fund some preparedness activities, but it has not been used as a contingency or reserve fund" (PCAST, 2016).

The Public Health Emergency Medical Countermeasure Enterprise

Successfully developing and procuring vaccines and drugs that are needed during an outbreak will require forward thinking and exploration of unique solutions that may not be risk-free. To help coordinate the efforts of the federal government, in 2006 HHS established the Public Health Emergency Medical Countermeasure Enterprise (PHEMCE). Its mission is to coordinate efforts related to medical countermeasures with all interagency partners. Led by the Office of the Assistant Secretary for Preparedness and Response, core members include CDC, the National Institutes of Health (NIH), the U.S. Food and Drug Administration (FDA), the U.S. Department of Veterans Affairs (VA), DoD, DHS, and the U.S. Department of Agriculture (USDA). The PHEMCE has made much progress since its inception, but because of its focus on preparedness, its scope does not encompass all global health research and development. Thus, questions remain around information sharing related to rare or noncommunicable diseases (global health research and development is explored further in Chapter 7). Additionally, opportunities remain for improved communication and coordination even within the focus on medical countermeasures. The 2016 letter from PCAST calls in the near term for a new interagency entity charged with planning, coordination, and oversight of national biodefense activities, including development of a national biodefense strategy (PCAST, 2016). Creation of this entity would further encourage information sharing related to research priorities and areas of synergy for agencies involved in the development of medical countermeasures.

Leveraging Assets from the U.S. Department of Defense

A 2016 analysis led by Duke Global Health Institute found opportunities for using what works well more effectively and identified DoD's medical research capabilities as having greatly underutilized potential for global health research and development (Yamey et al., 2016). In particular, DoD has both Army and Navy overseas laboratories in key strategic locations that facilitate international research collaboration, laboratory diagnostics, and surveillance. Because of their focus on locally relevant diseases and their reliance on locally hired research personnel, these laboratories have become integrated into public health efforts of the host nations, and can be assets in capacity building in those countries (Peake et al., 2011). To realize this potential, some have called for longer tours of duty at these laboratories and better communication with the academic and private sectors (Peake et al., 2011). The increase in defense spending pledged by the current administration—perhaps as much as $500 billion (Tiefer, 2016)—presents an opportunity to leverage DoD's research capacity to improve global health research and development. This idea was echoed at a 2015 workshop held by the National Academies of Sciences, Engineering, and Medicine on rapid medical countermeasures response (NASEM. 2016b), and further highlighted by DoD's involvement in the development of an Ebola diagnostic test that became the first to receive emergency use authorization for use with U.S. citizens (BioFire Defense, 2014). While DoD's mission is to protect military personnel, many of its research and development efforts can be leveraged to protect the civilian population, both domestic and international.

The Importance of Proactive Partnerships

The U.S. government plays a key role in promoting research and development for global health. While funding from the National Institutes of Health (NIH) and DoD is critical for research on the basic science of emerging infectious diseases, Biomedical Advanced Research and Development Authority (BARDA) funding is filling a vital gap. In addition, FDA ensures safety and efficacy throughout the research and development process. However, governments alone cannot be responsible for driving the global health research and development agenda forward, as the vast amounts of money required for the development of vaccine and therapeutics far outstrip the available government resources (see Table 3-2 for funding levels).

Partnerships are vital; the private sector is and will continue to be a key player, but it needs to be included from the initial design stage of projects and be viewed as a partner, not just a source of funds. The newly launched Coalition for Epidemic Preparedness Innovations (CEPI), for example, supported by the governments of Germany, Japan, and Norway plus the Bill & Melinda Gates Foundation and the Wellcome Trust, is investing $540 million to finance and coordinate the development of new vaccines to protect against infectious diseases, and views industry partnerships as a cornerstone operating principle (CEPI, 2017). Chapter 7 explores market incentives for accelerating research and development for medical product development in more detail, but these types of public–private partnerships and alternative business models are critical to making progress in many of these complex global health areas that lack a clear market.

Finding: Sufficient progress has not been made on the development of vaccines and diagnostics to successfully prevent, detect, and respond to these threats. No system exists to support this development beyond the interagency Public Health Emergency Medical Countermeasures Enterprise and the goodwill of industry partners, which is not a sustainable model.

TABLE 3-2 Federal Spending on Research and Development for Emerging Infectious Diseases 2010–2016, by Agency ($ millions)

	2010	2011	2012	2013	2014	2015	2016
NIH							
NIAID	$4,818.28	$4,775.97	$4,490.71	$4,256.33	$4,401.20	$4,417.56	$4,715.70
FIC	$69.98	$69.32	$69.49	$65.55	$67.58	$67.58	$70.12
General Influenza Funding	$308.00	$272.00	$251.00	$304.00	$262.00	$263.00	$284.00
BARDA	$32.00	$378.00	$415.00	$415.00	$413.05	$473.00	$522.00
FDA							
Pandemic Influenza	$46.70	$43.60	$30.00	$32.10	$38.30	$38.30	$40.00
Antimicrobial Resistance	$30.20	$27.70	$44.10	$25.90	$26.80	$32.50	$47.30
Advancing Medical Countermeasures Initiative	$0	$170.00	$20.00	$21.80	$24.60	$24.50	$24.50
Life Sciences Biodefense Lab	$0	$0	$0	$0	$17.70	$17.70	$17.70
TOTAL	$5,305.16	$5,736.59	$5,320.30	$5,120.68	$5,251.22	$5,334.13	$5,721.31

NOTE: BARDA = Biomedical Advanced Research and Development Authority; FDA = U.S. Food and Drug Administration; FIC = John E. Fogarty International Center for Advanced Study in the Health Sciences; NIAID = National Institute of Allergy and Infectious Diseases; NIH = National Institutes of Health.

SOURCES: Boddie et al., 2015; NIAID, 2015.

Reducing Impacts of Disaster Through Emergency Response Capacity in Low- and Middle-Income Countries

For LMICs, simple and cost-effective intervention strategies can reduce the effects of acute disasters. Emergency response capacity may appear to be a secondary priority in LMICs, but there are simple interventions that can build their resilience as well as their capabilities for emergency response. The implementation of the previously explained DRR principles, aimed at enhancing capabilities to minimize the impacts of mass casualty events and natural disasters, is a crucial need in all of these countries. In fact, more than 5 million people die each year as a result of injuries worldwide—1.7 times the number of fatalities that result from malaria, TB, and HIV/AIDS combined (WHO, 2014a). More than one-quarter of these deaths are road fatalities (WHO, 2017c), which occur predominantly in LMICs (Ning et al., 2016; WHO, 2009). Thus, these countries have a great unmet need for building trauma response capacity. Meeting this need will require the combined efforts and capabilities of research funding organizations, professional societies, NGOs, ministries of health, and governments. Regardless of whether injuries are caused by traffic crashes, earthquakes, or terrorist attacks, there are low-cost opportunities for increasing emergency response capacity to all hazards. While equipping these countries with functional modern trauma hospitals may not be feasible, providing basic training in essential surgical skills, expanding the workforce with the capacity to respond to trauma, and enabling more robust and rapid information sharing are cost-effective options that can help reduce the burden of injury and reduce mortality during a disaster (Acerra et al., 2009; King et al., 2015; Mock et al., 2012).

Increasing Trauma Capacity Through Training

Close to 2 million lost lives—one-third of all deaths due to injury—in LMICs could have been saved in 2008 by training a workforce to implement inexpensive, basic trauma care (Mock et al., 2012). Training nonphysicians in prehospital triage, for example, allows for the appropriate allocation of health care resources to respond to injuries as well as emergent diseases. Improving and standardizing care at the prehospital level has the potential to significantly decrease mortality at the earliest stages of disaster response.

These basic needs can be met by educating the workforce and disseminating guidelines and standardized protocols of care to create elementary but cost-effective systems of emergency and trauma care. The WHO Essential Trauma Care Project could be used to provide first responders with minimal training in simple life-saving care (Acerra et al., 2009; Mock et al., 2006). LMICs, in collaboration with such institutions and agencies as

DoD, NIH, and USAID, are poised to design and implement programmatic interventions and capacity-building programs tailored to the local and regional needs of poor communities and thereby develop more resilient health systems.

A Role for the U.S. Department of Defense

DoD recognizes the logistical impossibility of maintaining force readiness entailing continuously deployed medical facilities in all vulnerable regions of the world. Understanding this limitation, DoD has achieved tremendous gains in trauma care on the battlefield over the last decade that have had a dramatic impact on survival rates among warfighters (Mabry, 2015). Deployed medics and physicians often are depended upon to operate outside of their areas of expertise (NASEM, 2016a), a task-shifting approach that can be applied in low- and middle-income settings. Thus, with the ultimate goal of saving every injured warfighter on the battlefield, DoD has developed a rapid and nimble learning health system. Through an approach termed "focused empiricism,"[15] it has identified interventions that work, and then adapts its clinical protocols to rapidly implement this new evidence.

This knowledge, however, does not always translate back to civilian health systems. Accordingly, a 2016 National Academies report was commissioned to advise the United States on how better to integrate the expertise and evidence from DoD into HHS and civilian hospitals. The authoring committee of that report found that prehospital military trauma care is often more advanced than what U.S. civilian emergency medical services protocols allow (Elster et al., 2013; NASEM, 2016a). Just as that committee identified an opportunity for disseminating DoD knowledge to the U.S. civilian health system, there is also an opportunity for knowledge gained from operating in austere conditions to be shared and implemented around the world.

Some key lessons from military health operations include using pain medications, such as ketamine, in the prehospital stage to minimize pain and postinjury mental health sequelae (NASEM, 2016a). Ketamine has

---

[15] As defined by a recent National Academies report (NASEM, 2016a, p. 6), "Focused empiricism is a concept embraced by U.S. military medical leadership to capture its approach to process improvement under circumstances in which (1) high-quality data are not available to inform clinical practice changes, (2) there is extreme urgency to improve outcomes because of high morbidity and mortality rates, and (3) data collection is possible (Elster et al., 2013). A key principle of focused empiricism is using the best data available in combination with experience to develop clinical practice guidelines that, through an iterative process, continue to be refined until high-quality data can be generated to further inform clinical practice and standards of care."

been found to be an extremely useful anesthetic in the global south because of its applicability in low-resource settings without access to electricity for ventilators or oxygen and its ease of administration by nonanesthetists. As shown by the military, it is also often used off-label as an analgesic and makes surgeries such as cesarean sections possible in many austere environments, leading WHO to designate it as an essential medicine. Combat gauze, a clotting agent used to stop blood loss more quickly, is another important life-saving advance used in the military, which has been found to be associated with a 93 percent survival rate (Ran et al., 2010). An easy and cost-effective intervention, combat gauze could be adopted by responders in LMICs. Inspiring the Stop the Bleed campaign in the United States, military first responders also carry proper tourniquets for hemorrhage control when assessing for evacuation to a higher-level facility. A study following the 2013 Boston Marathon bombing found that prehospital response to extremity exsanguination was inadequate, and that better transfer of information on techniques and tools from the battlefield is needed (King et al., 2015), which could be accomplished through proper use and administration of tourniquets. This same observation applies to global health programs and platforms.

The lessons learned from the battlefield about injury assessment, triage, and emergency care can be used to dramatically improve trauma care in LMICs. Building this capacity in U.S. partner countries would be beneficial not only for citizens of those countries but also for U.S. citizens traveling abroad. It also would support DoD interests abroad, as maintaining a civilian trauma system—especially during conflict—is an obligation of the military that helps it achieve its own strategic objectives. The better such a system functions, the fewer injured civilians will require treatment in military field hospitals. These efforts already occur, as the military understands the benefits of engaging with partner nations and building and supporting their health system capabilities (DHA, n.d.). In a recent example, U.S. Navy sailors provided Kenyan soldiers tactical combat medical training, including basic cardiopulmonary resuscitation; first aid; techniques for stopping massive bleeding; and the use of tourniquets, splints, and compression (DeNault, 2016). Similar training was provided to Ugandan soldiers as well (McDonald, 2015). Conducting workshops for local communities that provide such training can improve their ability to mitigate their burden of injury and trauma, as well as increase their readiness for disaster and build resilience. These types of training opportunities and information exchanges could become more prevalent through increased communication between DoD, the U.S. Department of State, and countries' militaries or ministries of health, or through USAID in health systems–building activities.

Finding: An emergency response workforce can be developed through traditional public health training programs; rapid and nimble implementation of emerging evidence and best practices for providing effective and efficient health care; and leveraging the knowledge base developed in other networks, such as the U.S. military.

SUMMARY AND RECOMMENDATIONS

Wide-ranging threats to global health security influenced by resource scarcity, rapid urbanization, and inadequacies in stewardship of medications are poised to exploit the vulnerability of all countries, including the United States (Clapper, 2016; GAO, 2017; WHO, 2016a). These threats range from infectious disease spillover to pandemic influenza, to antimicrobial resistance, and are exacerbated by such vulnerabilities as degrading public health infrastructure, weak medical supply chains, and fragile states. It is critical for the United States to realize the severity of these threats and to take proactive measures to combat them by building capabilities and protections in a sustainable and cost-effective manner.

However, health preparedness systems and infrastructure (in the United States and abroad) are drastically underresourced (Boddie et al., 2015; Levi et al., 2015b). As a result, levels of preparedness are decades behind where they should be, making it difficult to meet the massive needs that arise when an emergency occurs. Funding for preparedness has decreased dramatically since the Public Health Security and Bioterrorism Response Act was enacted in 2002. In fiscal year 2016, funding for the Public Health Emergency Preparedness program decreased from an initial level of $1.03 billion in 2003 to $660 million (Levi et al., 2015b; Segal et al., 2016) and funding for the Hospital Preparedness Program decreased from an initial level of $515 million in 2004 to $255 million (Segal et al., 2016). Yet, once an emergency does occur, large amounts of funding are released, but typically not in a timely or systematic manner. For example, during the Ebola outbreak in 2014, which involved just four U.S. cases, the United States spent $1.1 billion on domestic response (Epstein et al., 2015), more than 120 percent of the nation's entire annual budget for capacity building for health preparedness systems. Airport screening and follow-up of potentially sick passengers alone incurred costs totaling $119 million (CDC, 2015a). However, in response to the Zika virus the following year, the funding response was much different. After 7 months of disagreement and delay in approving President Obama's request for $1.9 billion in Zika funding, Congress finally approved $1.1 billion with the passage of H.R. 5243[16]

---

[16] Zika Response Appropriations Act, H.R. 5243. 2016.

(Wexler et al., 2016). Until then, agencies were forced to shift funds from other accounts for Zika-related activities, including borrowing from the Ebola supplemental funding and from CDC's state-level emergency public health care preparedness account (Epstein and Lister, 2016; Kodjak, 2016). Moreover, although multiple agencies bring unique expertise to a U.S. government–led response, it is difficult to coordinate an urgent plan during a crisis without strong leadership, a well-defined chain of command, and an adequate budget.

Finally, sufficient progress has not been made on the development of vaccines and diagnostics to successfully prevent, detect, and respond to these threats. No system exists to support this development beyond the interagency Public Health Emergency Medical Countermeasures Enterprise and the goodwill of industry partners, which is not a sustainable model. Adequately protecting U.S. citizens requires strong capabilities to detect the potential for a pandemic, ensure the availability of needed medical products, and provide the necessary capacity in the nation's hospitals and health departments.

Conclusion: The current system for addressing health security threats described in this report is inadequate. A proactive, comprehensive approach would be more cost-effective and generate higher returns than ad hoc reactionary responses to individual events as they occur. The former approach can be enabled through the development of cross-cutting platforms, and a targeted systematic investment strategy (discussed in Recommendations 12 and 13 in Chapter 8) can enable this needed approach. Simultaneously, there is a need for improved coordination during an international public health emergency that combines the knowledge, networks, and assets of domestic and international health emergency response within the relevant U.S. government agencies and empowers action and decision-making through dedicated leadership and funding.

Conclusion: Health preparedness systems and infrastructure (in the United States and abroad) are drastically underresourced. As a result, levels of preparedness for health departments and hospitals are decades behind where they should be, making it difficult to meet the massive needs that arise when an emergency occurs. Addressing these inadequate funding levels is a critical priority.

Conclusion: An important positive step to improve rapid response capacity would be to implement the recommendation of the President's Council of Advisors on Science and Technology to establish a public health emergency response fund, with adequate funding in place, to be used only for response activities in declared public health emergencies.

Conclusion: To ensure that the drugs, vaccines, diagnostics, and devices critically needed to address health security threats are developed and available, a critical medical product development fund is required. This fund would support long-term, stable research and development to engage industry, academia, and other partners in the development of medical products for high-priority threats (based on the listing of the Public Health Emergency Medical Countermeasures Enterprise).

Recommendation 1: Improve International Emergency Response Coordination

The administration should create a coordinating body for international public health emergency response that is accountable for international and domestic actions and oversee preparedness for and responses to global health security threats. This body should have its own budget, experience with handling logistics, and the authority necessary to coordinate players across the government at the deputy secretary level. This coordinating body should do the following:

- **Oversee the creation of an International Response Framework to guide the U.S. response to an international health emergency. Through this framework, this body would coordinate and direct activities involved in international response and preparedness, but would not duplicate functions already established in the Office of the Assistant Secretary for Preparedness and Response, the U.S. Centers for Disease Control and Prevention, the U.S. Agency for International Development, or the U.S. Department of Defense.**
- **Oversee three separate funding streams, dedicated to investments in preparedness, emergency response, and critical medical product development. The Office of Management and Budget should conduct an analysis to determine the appropriate levels for these three funding streams, commensurate with the associated risk, understanding that predictable and timely funds for these three purposes are critical.**
- **Align and coordinate efforts with effective multilateral organizations to reduce duplication and promote efficiency in building capacity and resilience in other countries.**

The growing threat of antimicrobial resistance resulting from poor stewardship, weak surveillance systems, and a lack of potential new therapeutics will be a major threat to the entire global community—in terms of both lives lost and impacts on the global economy—in the next 10 years. While there has been progress toward Goal 5 of the National Action Plan, there remain challenges that hinder its full realization, including difficulties in providing incentives for the development of diagnostics and therapeutics. However, a particularly critical barrier is the lack of sufficient funds to advance the AMR agenda. While funds have been appropriated in recent years toward domestic efforts, there is very little money for international activities focused on AMR. Yet, with up to 30 percent of drugs being sold in LMICs found to be counterfeit (Cockburn et al., 2005; WHO, 2011b), there is a need for focused attention on safeguarding legitimate pharmaceutical supply chains that can complement a "One Health" approach to ensure proper stewardship of antibiotics and robust communication across the human and animal health sectors (CDC, 2017b), thereby reducing the spread of AMR.

Conclusion: A coordinated and dedicated global effort to address the threat of antimicrobial resistance is needed, with a focus on countries experiencing a high incidence.

Conclusion: It is essential to remain engaged and coordinated with domestic and international stakeholders, including the World Health Organization, the United Nations Secretary-General's Committee on Antimicrobial Resistance, and the Global Health Security Agenda.

Recommendation 2: Combat Antimicrobial Resistance

The U.S. Department of Health and Human Services, the U.S. Department of Defense, the U.S. Department of Agriculture, and the U.S. Agency for International Development (USAID) should continue to invest in national capabilities and accelerate the development of international capabilities to detect, monitor, report, and combat antibiotic resistance. Efforts to this end should include the following:

- **Enhance surveillance systems to ensure that new resistant microbial strains are identified as soon as they emerge.**
- **Assist low-income countries in improving infection control and antimicrobial stewardship.**

- **USAID should leverage current supply chain partnerships with other countries to strengthen antibiotic supply chains, thus reducing the use of illegitimate antimicrobials and improving drug quality.**
- **Incentivize the development of therapeutics (including alternatives to antibiotics), vaccines, and diagnostics for use in humans and animals.**

While many low- and middle-income countries function in low-resource settings during steady-state times, disasters can plunge these countries into even more challenging and austere circumstances. While modern infrastructure often is not feasible in these countries because of high costs, smaller-scale steps entailing process innovation can be taken in communities to improve their ability to respond to disasters. Whether responding to more slowly evolving public health emergencies such as disease outbreaks or more immediate injury events such as road traffic accidents, earthquakes, or terror attacks, having a properly trained workforce in accordance with the principles of disaster risk reduction can lead to safer and more resilient communities. Such a workforce can be developed through traditional public health training programs; rapid and more nimble implementation of emerging evidence and best practices for providing effective and efficient health care; and leveraging of the knowledge base developed in other networks, such as the U.S. military. Enabling the right systems capacity to reduce risk, respond, and then iterate and innovate can allow for greater progress in a shorter period of time. After many years of insufficient siloed and ad hoc investments, this type of systems approach, information exchange, and country coinvestment and partnership would be a welcome change.

Conclusion: Simple yet effective strategies exist for reducing the risk of disaster for communities around the world. Employing the principles of disaster risk reduction when developing capacity for health care preparedness and response provides a framework for continuous learning and its iterative application to health care delivery systems.

Recommendation 3: Build Public Health Capacity in Low- and Middle-Income Countries

The U.S. Centers for Disease Control and Prevention, the National Institutes of Health, the U.S. Department of Defense, and the U.S. Agency for International Development should expand training and information exchange efforts to increase the capacity of

low- and middle-income countries to respond to both public health emergencies and acute mass casualty disasters. This training and information exchange should encompass core capacities such as surveillance, epidemiology, and disaster and injury care response, as well as enhanced capabilities to improve communication and information pathways for the dissemination of innovative findings.

ANNEX 3-1

THE 1918–1919 INFLUENZA PANDEMIC

The 1918–1919 influenza pandemic occurred toward the final years of World War I and infected up to 500 million people (one-third of the global population at the time), resulting in 50–100 million deaths (3–5 percent of the global population) (Jeffery and David, 2006). The war and the influenza pandemic were closely intertwined, and as a result, the disease spread globally and affected almost every country involved in the war. In addition to its global reach, the pandemic had a number of unique characteristics. Rather than appearing in the familiar annual pattern of influenza, the 1918–1919 pandemic took place in three waves that occurred in quick succession, the first of which was in the spring of 1918.

While identifying a point of origin for the pandemic is difficult given that it appeared to spread simultaneously throughout Europe, Asia, and North America, evidence suggests that it emerged in the United States (Barry, 2004) and spread to Europe when the United States entered the war (Byerly, 2010). During the first wave, illness rates were high, but death rates were close to normal. The second wave, occurring in the fall of 1918, spread the disease globally and was highly fatal, likely a result of the crowded conditions in training camps and trench warfare that enabled the virus to evolve. The third phase occurred in early 1919, and although less deadly, continued to spread the disease.

The occurrence of three pandemic waves in such quick succession was unprecedented, as was the age group the pandemic uniquely affected: young adults. Typically, the highest influenza mortality rates occur among the very young and the very old. However, the 1918–1919 pandemic also heavily affected those aged 20–40, an age group in which half of the deaths during the pandemic occurred.

Although 675,000 Americans were among the dead, the legacy of the 1918–1919 influenza pandemic has receded from memory in the United States, such that historians call it "America's forgotten pandemic" (Garrett, 2007). This fading from memory is dangerous considering that learning from the past is instrumental in adequately preparing for the future. That the pandemic likely originated in the United States, moreover, serves as a reminder that such threats can emerge anywhere.

ANNEX 3-2

COMBATING ANTIMICROBIAL RESISTANCE

Global Community Efforts

The global community has given increased attention to the threat of antimicrobial resistance (AMR) in recent years as a result of multigovernment and multistakeholder declarations calling for immediate concerted global action to address this issue. The 2009 US-EU Summit Declaration established a Transatlantic Taskforce on AMR to strengthen collaboration between the United States and the EU in promoting the adequate use of antimicrobials for animal and human health, implementing prevention strategies in hospital and community settings, and developing new antimicrobials (TATFAR, 2014).

In 2014, the 67th World Health Assembly (WHA) requested that the World Health Organization (WHO) director general develop a global action plan to address the growing threat of AMR. In a tripartite collaboration with the World Organisation for Animal Health (OIE) and the Food and Agriculture Organization (FAO) of the United Nations (UN), and embracing the One Health approach, the World Health Organization (WHO) developed the Global Action Plan on AMR with the technical support of its Strategic and Technical Advisory Group on AMR (STAG-AMR) (WHO, 2015). This global action plan outlines five strategic objectives with corresponding actions for Member States, the Secretariat (composed of WHO, OIE, and FAO), and international organizations and other partners. The five objectives are

1. to improve awareness and understanding of AMR through effective communication, education, and training;
2. to strengthen the knowledge and evidence base through surveillance and research;
3. to reduce the incidence of infection through effective sanitation, hygiene, and infection prevention measures;
4. to optimize the use of antimicrobial medicines in human and animal health; and
5. to develop the economic case for sustainable investment that takes account of the needs of all countries and to increase investment in new medicines, diagnostic tools, vaccines, and other interventions.

WHO called on Member States to develop national action plans aligned with these global plan objectives within 2 years of the plan's endorsement by the WHA in May 2015. WHO, in collaboration with FAO and OIE, prepared a manual to guide the development or refinement of these national plans and a monitoring and evaluation framework to help countries track the progress of the implementation of their national plans. As of the release of this report, only 31 countries had shared their national action plans for AMR with the WHO library, with only a few months remaining until the deadline in May 2017 (WHO, 2017a).

The U.S. National Action Plan

The U.S. National Action Plan for Combating Antibiotic-Resistant Bacteria was released in March 2015 (CDC, 2015c). The plan outlines in detail objectives; subobjectives; Year 1, Year 3, and Year 5 milestones; performance metrics; and implementation timelines for each goal in the National Strategy. These goals include the following:

1. Slow the Emergence of Resistant Bacteria and Prevent the Spread of Resistant Infections.
2. Strengthen National One-Health Surveillance Efforts to Combat Resistance.
3. Advance Development and Use of Rapid and Innovative Diagnostic Tests for Identification and Characterization of Resistant Bacteria.
4. Accelerate Basic and Applied Research and Development for New Antibiotics, Other Therapeutics, and Vaccines.
5. Improve International Collaboration and Capacities for Antibiotic-Resistance Prevention, Surveillance, Control, and Antibiotic Research and Development.

As required by executive order, the Task Force for Combating Antibiotic-Resistant Bacteria submitted a report (PACCARB, 2016) assessing the progress made toward the proposed milestones for each of the National Action Plan goals after the first 180 days of the plan's release. That report identified key actions taken to advance each of the five goals.

For goal 1, the report noted that both human and animal health stewardship efforts were under way: the Centers for Medicaid & Medicare Services revised the participation requirements for inpatient and long-term care facilities to include antibiotic stewardship programs, and the U.S. Food and Drug Administration (FDA) amended the veterinary feed directive (VFD) regulations to allow the use of a VFD drug only under the supervision of a licensed veterinarian. For goal 2, the U.S. Centers for Disease Control and Prevention (CDC), in collaboration with FDA, launched the AR Isolate Bank, a repository of samples of well-characterized resistance bacteria profiles. This repository will serve as a data source for industry and academia for the development of new diagnostics and treatment. For goal 3, the National Institutes of Health (NIH) invested more than $11 million to support the first year of research for nine projects aimed at developing rapid diagnostic tools for resistant bacteria. Goal 4 proved to be one of the most challenging, as the pipeline for antibiotic development is quite small, with very limited incentives for industry. Nevertheless, the U.S. government continues to support discovery and early-stage development of new drugs. Finally, for goal 5, the U.S. government worked closely with international partners to support implementation of WHO's Global Action Plan on AMR through its work with the Global Health Security Agenda (GHSA) AMR Action Package. Specifically, the GHSA AMR Action Package supports the development of national action plans; the development and strengthening of surveillance and laboratory capacity; and the development of new treatments, diagnostics, preventive measures, and systems to prolong the effective use of current therapies.

REFERENCES

Acerra, J. R., K. Iskyan, Z. A. Qureshi, and R. K. Sharma. 2009. Rebuilding the health care system in Afghanistan: An overview of primary care and emergency services. *International Journal of Emergency Medicine* 2(2):77-82.

Akil, L., and H. A. Ahmad. 2016. The recent outbreaks and reemergence of poliovirus in war and conflict-affected areas. *International Journal of Infectious Diseases* 49:40-46.

Allen, H. K., J. Donato, H. H. Wang, K. A. Cloud-Hansen, J. Davies, and J. Handelsman. 2010. Call of the wild: Antibiotic resistance genes in natural environments. *Nature Reviews Microbiology* 8(4):251-259.

Alwan, A. 2015. *The cost of war*. http://www.who.int/mediacentre/commentaries/war-cost/en (accessed December 15, 2016).

Appropriations Committee. 2016. *Division B: Zika response and preparedness*. https://www.appropriations.senate.gov/imo/media/doc/092216-CR-Zika%20Supplemental%20Summary.pdf (accessed February 19, 2017).

Atchon, K. 2016. Resurgence of poliomyelitis in Nigeria: A big blow to the world eradication efforts? *MOJ Public Health* 4(6).

BARDA (Biomedical Advanced Research and Development Authority). 2007. *Report to Congress: Pandemic preparedness spending*. Prepared in Response to Request in Conference Report 109-359.

Barrett, A. D. T. 2014. Economic burden of West Nile virus in the United States. *The American Journal of Tropical Medicine and Hygiene* 90(3):389-390.

Barrett, S. 2013. Economic considerations for the eradication endgame. *Philosophical Transactions of the Royal Society B: Biological Sciences* 368(1623):20120149.

Barry, J. M. 2004. The site of origin of the 1918 influenza pandemic and its public health implications. *Journal of Translational Medicine* 2(1):3.

Beaubien, J. 2016. *How Boko Haram is keeping polio alive in Nigeria*. http://www.npr.org/sections/goatsandsoda/2016/09/14/493755014/nigeria-has-to-wipe-out-polio-again (accessed February 14, 2017).

Beaubien, J. 2017. *Brazil's expanding yellow fever outbreak started with monkeys*. http://www.npr.org/sections/goatsandsoda/2017/02/17/515444290/brazils-expanding-yellow-fever-outbreak-started-with-monkeys?utm_content=buffer23e6e&utm_medium=social&utm_source=twitter.com&utm_campaign=buffer (accessed February 23, 2017).

BioFire Defense. 2014. *Biofire defense receives emergency use authorization of FilmArray Ebola tests*. Salt Lake City, UT.

Birdsall, N., and B. Leo. 2016. The White House and the world—practical proposals on gloabl development for the next U.S. President. Washington, DC: The Center for Global Development.

Blue Ribbon Study Panel on Biodefense. 2015. *A national blueprint for biodefense: Leadership and major reform needed to optimize efforts*. Washington, DC: Hudson Institute and Inter-University Center for Terrorism Studies.

Blue Ribbon Study Panel on Biodefense. 2016. *Biodefense indicators: One year later, events outpacing federal efforts to defend the nation*. Washington, DC: Hudson Institute, Potomac Institute for Policy Studies, and Inter-University Center for Terrorism Studies.

Boddie, C., T. K. Sell, and M. Watson. 2015. Federal funding for health security in FY2016. *Health Security* 13(3):186-206.

Brahmbhatt, M., and A. Dutta. 2008. *On SARS type economic effects during infectious disease outbreaks*. Washington, DC: World Bank.

Burkle, F. M. 2006. Globalization and disasters: Issues of public health, state capacity and political action. *Journal of International Affairs* 59(2):231-265.

Burkle, F. M. 2017. The politics of global public health in fragile states and ungoverned territories. *PLOS Currents: Disasters* 1.

Burns, A., D. van der Mensbrugge, and H. Timmer. 2008. *Evaluating the economic consequences of avian influenza*. Washington, DC: World Bank.

Byerly, C. R. 2010. The U.S. military and the influenza pandemic of 1918–1919. *Public Health Reports* 125(Suppl 3):82-91.

Cabezas, M. 2016. *U.S. government budgets dedicated to combating antibiotic-resistant bacteria activities*. Washington, DC: U.S. Department of Health and Human Services Office of Budget.

Cahill, M., Y. Yao, D. Nock, P. Armstrong, T. Andreadis, M. Diuk-Wasser, and R. Montgomery. 2017. West Nile virus seroprevalence, Connecticut, USA, 2000–2014. *Emerging Infectious Disease Journal* 23(4).

Casey, N. 2016. Hard times in Venezuela breed malaria as desperate flock to mines. *New York Times*. August 15.

CDC (U.S. Centers for Disease Control and Prevention). 2013a. *Antibiotic resistance threats*. Washington, DC: Centers for Disease Control and Prevention, HHS.

CDC. 2013b. *CDC SARS response timeline*. https://www.cdc.gov/about/history/sars/timeline.htm (accessed February 22, 2017).

CDC. 2014. *Marburg hemorrhagic fever outbreak in Uganda*. https://www.cdc.gov/vhf/marburg/outbreaks/uganda/2014-oct.html (accessed February 27, 2017).

CDC. 2015a. *CDC's Ebola response in the United States and abroad*. https://www.cdc.gov/budget/documents/ebola/2015-ebola-and-gh-security-activities-factsheet.pdf (accessed December 15, 2016).

CDC. 2015b. *Infographic: Field Epidemeology Training Programs in Africa*. https://www.cdc.gov/globalhealth/infographics/fetp_africa.htm (accessed February 14, 2017).

CDC. 2015c. *National Action Plan for Combating Antibiotic-Resistant Bacteria*. Atlanta, GA: U.S. Centers for Disease Control and Prevention.

CDC. 2016a. *2014-2016 Ebola outbreak in West Africa*. https://www.cdc.gov/vhf/ebola/outbreaks/2014-west-africa (accessed December 15, 2016).

CDC. 2016b. *Global activities*. https://www.cdc.gov/onehealth/global-activities/index.html (accessed March 15, 2017).

CDC. 2016c. *Global Health Security Agenda: Action packages*. https://www.cdc.gov/globalhealth/security/actionpackages (accessed December 10, 2016).

CDC. 2016d. *Global Health Security Agenda: Frequently asked questions*. https://www.cdc.gov/globalhealth/healthprotection/ghs/faqs.htm#one (accessed December 15, 2016).

CDC. 2016e. How CDC invests in people: Developing disease detectives. *Updates from the field* Spring 2016(21).

CDC. 2016f. *Outbreaks chronology: Ebola virus disease*. https://www.cdc.gov/vhf/ebola/outbreaks/history/chronology.html (accessed February 22, 2017).

CDC. 2017a. *Case counts in the US*. https://www.cdc.gov/zika/geo/united-states.html (accessed March 6, 2017).

CDC. 2017b. *One Health*. https://www.cdc.gov/onehealth (accessed March 15, 2017).

Cegielski, J. P. 2010. Extensively drug-resistant tuberculosis: "There must be some kind of way out of here." *Clinical Infectious Diseases* 50(Supplement 3):S195-S200.

CEPI (Coalition for Epidemic Preparedness Innovations). 2017. *New vaccines for a safer world*. http://cepi.net/sites/default/files/CEPI_2pager_03_Feb_17.pdf (accessed February 14, 2017).

Chen, L., R. Todd, J. Kiehlbauch, M. Walters, and A. Kallen. 2017. Notes from the field: Pan-resistant New Delhi metallo-beta-lactamase-producing *Klebsiella pneumoniae*—Washoe County, Nevada, 2016. *Morbitity and Mortality Weekly Report* 66:33.

CIDRAP (Center for Infectious Disease Research and Policy). 2017. *Pan-resistant CRE reported in Nevada.* http://www.cidrap.umn.edu/news-perspective/2017/01/pan-resistant-cre-reported-nevada (accessed February 14, 2017).

Clapper, J. 2016. Statement of James R. Clapper, Director of National Intelligence before the House Permanent Select Committee on Intelligence. Hearing on Worldwide Threat Assessment of the U.S. Intelligence Community. February 25, 2016.

Cockburn, R., P. N. Newton, E. K. Agyarko, D. Akunyili, and N. J. White. 2005. The global threat of counterfeit drugs: Why industry and governments must communicate the dangers. *PLOS Medicine* 2(4):e100.

COHAB (Co-operation on Health and Biodiversity Initiative). 2010. *The importance of biodiversity on human health.* https://www.cbd.int/doc/health/cohab-policy-brief1-en.pdf (accessed December 15, 2016).

Courage, K. 2014. How did Nigeria quash its Ebola outbreak so quickly? *Scientific American,* October 18.

Dembosky, A. 2014. *Shortage of saline solution has hospitals on edge.* http://www.npr.org/sections/health-shots/2014/06/22/323679204/shortage-of-saline-solution-has-hospitals-on-edge (accessed March 3, 2017).

DeNault, T. 2016. *U.S. sailors hold medical training with Kenyan defense forces.* http://www.health.mil/News/Articles/2016/10/12/US-Sailors-hold-medical-training-with-Kenyan-Defense-Forces (accessed February 14, 2017).

DHA (Defense Health Agency). n.d. *Building partner capacity and interoperability.* http://www.health.mil/Military-Health-Topics/Health-Readiness/Global-Health-Engagement/Building-Partner-Capacity-and-Interoperability (accessed February 14, 2017).

Elster, E. A., F. K. Butler, and T. E. Rasmussen. 2013. Implications of combat casualty care for mass casualty events. *Journal of the American Medical Association* 310(5):475-476.

Epstein, S. B., and S. A. Lister. 2016. *Zika response funding: Request and congressional action.* Washington, DC: Congressional Research Service.

Epstein, S. B., S. A. Lister, A. Belasco, and D. J. Jansen. 2015. *FY2015 funding to counter Ebola and the Islamic State (IS).* Washington, DC: Congressional Research Service.

Fan, V. Y., D. T. Jamison, and L. H. Summers. 2016. *The inclusive cost of pandemic influenza risk.* Cambridge, MA: National Bureau of Economic Research.

Fauci, A. S. 2017. Keynote address. In *Pandemic Preparedness in the Next Administration*: Georgetown University Center for Global Health Science and Security and Harvard Global Health Institute.

Fauci, A. S., and D. M. Morens. 2012. The perpetual challenge of infectious diseases. *New England Journal of Medicine* 366(5):454-461.

FDA (U.S. Food and Drug Administration). 2016. *FDA updates on saline drug shortage.* http://www.fda.gov/Drugs/DrugSafety/ucm382255.htm (accessed February 14, 2017).

Fine, P., K. Eames, and D. L. Heymann. 2011. "Herd immunity": A rough guide. *Clinical Infectious Diseases* 52(7).

Frieden, T. R. 2014. CDC telebriefing: CDC update on first Ebola case diagnosed in the United States, October 5, Atlanta, Georgia.

Frieden, T. R. 2016. Presentation by Dr. Thomas Frieden (CDC director). In *Global Security Forum 2016: The Global Health Security Agenda–Its First Years and the Way Forward.* Center for Strategic and International Studies.

GAO (U.S. Government Accountability Office). 2007. *Drug safety: Preliminary findings suggest weakness in FDA's program for inspecting foreign drug manufacturers.* Washington, DC: Government Accountability Office.

GAO. 2017. *Defense civil support: DOD, HHS, and DHS should use existing coordination mechanisms to improve their pandemic preparedness.* Washington, DC: Government Accountability Office.

Garrett, T. A. 2007. *Economic effects of the 1918 influenza pandemic: Implications for a modern-day pandemic.* St. Louis, MO: Federal Reserve of St. Louis.

Gavi (Gavi, the Vaccine Alliance). 2014. *Co-financing policy evaluation.* http://www.gavi.org/results/evaluations/co-financing-policy-evaluation (accessed February 13, 2017).

Gebreyes, W. A., J. Dupouy-Camet, M. J. Newport, C. J. B. Oliveira, L. S. Schlesinger, Y. M. Saif, S. Kariuki, L. J. Saif, W. Saville, T. Wittum, A. Hoet, S. Quessy, R. Kazwala, B. Tekola, T. Shryock, M. Bisesi, P. Patchanee, S. Boonmar, and L. J. King. 2014. The global One Health paradigm: Challenges and opportunities for tackling infectious diseases at the human, animal, and environment interface in low-resource settings. *PLOS Neglected Tropical Diseases* 8(11):e3257.

Ghafoor, S., and N. Sheikh. 2016. Eradication and current status of poliomyelitis in Pakistan: Ground realities. *Journal of Immunology Research* V.2016, article no. 6837824.

GHRF Commission (Commission on a Global Health Risk Framework for the Future). 2016. *The neglected dimension of global security: A framework to counter infectious disease crises.* doi: https://doi.org/10.17226/21891.

GHSA (Global Health Security Agenda). 2017. *Advancing the global health security agenda: Progress and early impact from U.S. investment.* Washington, DC: Global Health Security Agenda.

Gold, J. 2014. *Statement of Chancellor Jeff Gold, M.D. University of Nebraska Medical Center, Omaha, Nebraska before the Committee on Energy and Commerce Subcommittee on Oversight & Investigations* (Date: 11/18/2014). Hearing on *Update on the U.S. Public Health Response to the Ebola Outbreak.* https://energycommerce.house.gov/hearings-and-votes/hearings/update-us-public-health-response-ebola-outbreak (accessed January 15, 2017).

Gostin, L. O., O. Tomori, S. Wibulpolprasert, A. K. Jha, J. Frenk, S. Moon, J. Phumaphi, P. Piot, B. Stocking, V. J. Dzau, and G. M. Leung. 2016. Toward a common secure future: Four global commissions in the wake of Ebola. *PLOS Medicine* 13(5):e1002042.

GPEI (Global Poliomyelitis Eradication Initaitive). n.d. *Endemic countries.* http://polioeradication.org/where-we-work/polio-endemic-countries (accessed March 3, 2017).

GU GHSS and HGHI (Georgetown University Center for Global Health Science and Security and Harvard Global Health Institute). 2017. Pandemic preparedness in the next administration. Georgetown University Center for Global Health Science and Security and Harvard Global Health Institute.

Hinshaw, D., and J. Bunge. 2014. U.S. buys up Ebola gear, leaving little for Africa. *The Wall Street Journal,* November 24.

Holgate, L. 2014. Presentation by NSC. In *The Launch of the Global Health Security Agenda.* Center for Strategic and International Studies.

IFPMA (International Federation of Pharmaceutical Manufacturers & Associations). 2016. *Declaration by the pharmaceutical, biotechnology and diagnostics industries on combating antimicrobial resistance.* Davos, Switzerland: International Federation of Pharmaceutical Manufacturers & Associations.

Inglesby, T., and A. Cicero. 2017. Protecting the nation from health security threats. *Health Security* 15(1):1-5.

Iuliano, A. D. 2017. Increase in human infections with avian influenza A (H7N9) virus during the fifth epidemic—China, October 2016–February 2017. *Morbidity and Mortality Weekly Report* 66.

Jeffery, K. T., and M. M. David. 2006. 1918 influenza: The mother of all pandemics. *Emerging Infectious Diseases* 12(1):15-22.

Jonas, O. 2014a. Global health threats of the 21st century. *Finance and Development* 51(4).

Jonas, O. 2014b. *Pandemic Risk.* Washington, DC: World Bank.

Kates, J., J. Michaud, A. Wexler, and A. Valentine. 2015. *The U.S. response to Ebola: Status of the FY2015 emergency Ebola appropriation*. Washington, DC: The Henry J. Kaiser Family Foundation.

Katz, R. 2016. Presentation for the National Academies of Sciences, Engineering, and Medicine. Paper read at Global Health and the Future of the United States: A Changing Landscape of Global Health, September 29, Washington, DC.

Kelesidis, T., I. Kelesidis, P. I. Rafailidis, and M. E. Falagas. 2007. Counterfeit or substandard antimicrobial drugs: A review of the scientific evidence. *Journal of Antimicrobial Chemotherapy* 60(2):214-236.

KFF (Kaiser Family Foundation). 2016. *The U.S. government and global polio efforts*. http://www.kff.org/global-health-policy/fact-sheet/the-u-s-government-and-global-polio-efforts (accessed March 10, 2017).

King, D. R., A. Larentzakis, and E. P. Ramly. 2015. Tourniquet use at the Boston marathon bombing: Lost in translation. *Journal of Trauma and Acute Care Surgery* 78(3):594-599.

Kodjak, A. 2016. *Congress ends spat, agrees to fund $1.1 billion to combat Zika*. http://www.npr.org/sections/health-shots/2016/09/28/495806979/congress-ends-spat-over-zika-funding-approves-1-1-billion (accessed December 15, 2016).

Labonte, R., K. Mohindra, and T. Schrecker. 2011. The growing impact of globalization for health and public health practice. *Annual Review of Public Health* 32:263-283.

Levi, J., L. M. Segal, R. Gougelet, and R. St. Laurant. 2015a. *Investing in America's health: A state-by-state look at public health funding and key health facts*. Washington, DC: Trust For America's Health.

Levi, J., L. M. Segal, D. A. Lieberman, K. May, and R. St. Laurant. 2015b. *Outbreaks: Protecting Americans from infectious diseases*. Washington, DC: Trust For America's Health.

Littmann, J., and A. M. Viens. 2015. The ethical significance of antimicrobial resistance. *Public Health Ethics* 8(3):209-224.

Long, L., M. Fox, I. Sanne, and S. Rosen. 2010. The high cost of second-line antiretroviral therapy for HIV/AIDS in South Africa. *AIDS* 24(6):915-919.

Lowy, I. 2017. Leaking containers: Success and failure in controlling the mosquito *Aedes aegypti* in Brazil. *American Journal of Public Health* 107(4):517-524.

Mabry, R. 2015. Challenges to improving combat casualty survival on the battlefield. *Military Medicine* 179(5):477.

McDonald, O. 2015. *Navy corpsmen, Ugandans work together to save lives*. http://www.health.mil/News/Articles/2015/12/17/Navy-corpsmen-Ugandans-work-together-to-save-lives (accessed February 14, 2017).

McKibbin, W. J. 2004. *Economic modeling of SARS: The G-Cubed approach*. Sydney, Australia: The Lowy Institute for International Policy.

McKinney, M. L. 2002. Urbanization, biodiversity, and conservation: The impacts of urbanization on native species are poorly studied, but educating a highly urbanized human population about these impacts can greatly improve species conservation in all ecosystems. *BioScience* 52(10):883-890.

Meltzer, M. I., N. J. Cox, and K. Fukuda. 1999. The economic impact of pandemic influenza in the United States: Priorities for intervention. *Emerging Infectious Diseases* 5(5):659-671.

Michelle, G., L. Dominique, F. Pierre, and A. C. Maire. 2007. Conflict and emerging infectious diseases. *Emerging Infectious Diseases* 13(11):1625.

MMC (Multihazard Mitigation Council). 2005. *Natural hazard mitigation saves: An independent study to assess the future savings from mitigation activities*. Washington, DC: National Institute of Building Sciences, The Multihazard Mitigation Council.

Mock, C., M. Joshipura, J. Goosen, and R. Maier. 2006. Overview of the essential trauma care project. *World Journal of Surgery* 30(6):919-929.

Mock, C., M. Joshipura, C. Arreola-Risa, and R. Quansah. 2012. An estimate of the number of lives that could be saved through improvements in trauma care globally. *World Journal of Surgery* 36(5):959-963.

Molinari, N. A., I. R. Ortega-Sanchez, M. L. Messonnier, W. W. Thompson, P. M. Wortley, E. Weintraub, and C. B. Bridges. 2007. The annual impact of seasonal influenza in the US: Measuring disease burden and costs. *Vaccine* 25(27):5086-5096.

Morrison, J. S. 2014. Introduction. In *The Launch of the Global Health Security Agenda.* Washington, DC: Center for Strategic and International Studies.

MSF (Médecins Sans Frontières). 2014. *The fight against antibiotic resistance.* http://www.doctorswithoutborders.org/article/fight-against-antibiotic-resistance (accessed February 14, 2017).

NASEM (National Academies of Sciences, Engineering, and Medicine). 2016a. *A national trauma care system: Integrating military and civilian trauma systems to acheive zero preventable deaths after injury.* Washington, DC: The National Academies Press.

NASEM. 2016b. *Rapid medical countermeasure response to infectious diseases: Enabling sustainable capabilities through ongoing public and private-sector partnerships: Workshop summary.* Washington, DC: The National Academies Press.

NIAID (National Institute of Allergy and Infectious Diseases). 2015. *Fiscal year 2015 fact book.* Bethesda, USA: National Institute of Allergy and Infectious Diseases.

Ning, P., D. C. Schwebel, H. Huang, L. Li, J. Li, and G. Hu. 2016. Global progress in road injury mortality since 2010. *PLOS ONE* 11(10):e0164560.

Northam, J. 2014. *Ebola protective suits are in short supply.* http://www.npr.org/2014/10/07/354230895/ebola-protective-suits-are-in-short-supply (accessed December 15, 2016).

Nuzzo, J. B., and M. P. Shearer. 2017. International engagement is critical to fighting epidemics. *Health Security* 15(1):33-35.

Osterholm, M. T., and M. Olshaker. 2017. *Deadliest enemy: Our war against killer germs.* New York: Little Brown and Company.

PACCARB (President's Advisory Council on Combating Antibiotic-Resistant Bacteria). 2016. *Initial assessments of the national action plan for combating antibiotic-resistant bacteria.* Washington, DC: U.S. Department of Health and Human Services.

Parpia, A. S., L. Ndeffo-Mbah Martial, N. S. Wenzel, and A. P. Galvani. 2016. Effects of response to 2014–2015 Ebola outbreak on deaths from malaria, HIV/AIDS, and tuberculosis, West Africa. *Emerging Infectious Diseases* 22(3):433-441.

Pauchard, A., M. Aguayo, E. Pena, and R. Urritia. 2006. Multiple effects of urbanization on the biodeversity of developing countries: The case of a fast-growing metropolitan city (Concepción, Chile). *Biological Conservation* 127:272-281.

PCAST (President's Council of Advisors on Science and Technology). 2014. *Report to the president on combating antibiotic resistance.* Executive Office of the President, President's Council of Advisors on Science and Technology.

PCAST. 2016. *Biodefense letter to President Obama.* Executive Office of the President, President's Council of Advisors on Science and Technology.

Peake, J. B., J. S. Morrison, M. M. Ledgerwood, and S. E. Gannon. 2011. *The Defense Department's enduring contributions to global health.* Washington, DC: Center for Strategic & International Studies.

Petersen, E., M. E. Wilson, S. Touch, B. McCloskey, P. Mwaba, M. Bates, O. Dar, F. Mattes, M. Kidd, G. Ippolito, E. I. Azhar, and A. Zumla. 2016. Rapid spread of Zika virus in the Americas—implications for public health preparedness for mass gatherings at the 2016 Brazil Olympic Games. *International Journal of Infectious Diseases* 44:11-15.

Petersen, L. R., P. J. Carson, B. J. Biggerstaff, B. Custer, S. M. Borchardt, and M. P. Busch. 2013. Estimated cumulative incidence of West Nile virus infection in US adults, 1999-2010. *Epidemiology & Infection* 141(3):591-595.

Pike, J., T. Bogich, S. Elwood, D. C. Finnoff, and P. Daszak. 2014. Economic optimization of a global strategy to address the pandemic threat. *Proceedings of the National Academy of Sciences of the United States of America* 111(52):18519-18523.

Pongsiri, M. J., J. Roman, V. O. Ezenwa, T. L. Goldberg, H. S. Koren, S. C. Newbold, R. S. Ostfeld, S. K. Pattanayak, and D. J. Salkeld. 2009. Biodiversity loss affects global disease ecology. *BioScience* 59(11):945-954.

Public Health Agency of Canada. 2017. *Supply and distribution of flu vaccine in Canada.* http://www.phac-aspc.gc.ca/im/supply-approvisionment-eng.php (accessed February 27, 2017).

Ran, Y., E. Hadad, S. Daher, O. Ganor, J. Kohn, Y. Yegorov, C. Bartal, N. Ash, and G. Hirschhorn. 2010. QuikClot Combat Gauze use for hemorrhage control in military trauma: January 2009 Israel defense force experience in the Gaza strip—a preliminary report of 14 cases. *Prehospital and Disaster Medicine* 25(06):584-588.

Review on Antimicrobial Resistance. 2014. *Antimicrobial resistance: Tackling a crisis for the health and wealth of nations.* London, UK: Review on Antimicrobial Resistance.

Review on Antimicrobial Resistance. 2016. *Tackling drug-resistant infections globally: Final report and recommendations.* London, UK: Wellcome Trust and UK Government.

Rey, M., and M. P. Girard. 2008. The global eradication of poliomyelitis: Progress and problems. *Comparative Immunology, Microbiology, & Infectious Diseases* 31(2-3):317-325.

Rice, S. E. 2016. *Statement by National Security Advisor Susan E. Rice on the executive order on advancing the global health security agenda.* The White House.

Ridley, D. B., X. Bei, and E. B. Liebman. 2016. No shot: US vaccine prices and shortages. *Health Affairs (Millwood)* 35(2):235-241.

Roos, R. 2012. *CDC estimate of global H1N1 pandemic deaths: 284,000.* http://www.cidrap.umn.edu/news-perspective/2012/06/cdc-estimate-global-h1n1-pandemic-deaths-284000 (accessed December 15, 2016).

Schmidt, C. W. 2016. Zika in the United States: How are we preparing? *Environmental Health Perspectives* 124(9):A157-A165.

Schnirring, L. 2017a. *China confirms high-path H7N9 in market poultry.* http://www.cidrap.umn.edu/news-perspective/2017/02/china-confirms-high-path-h7n9-market-poultry (accessed March 5, 2017).

Schnirring, L. 2017b. H7N9 analyses hint at genetic mutations, drug resistance. *Center for Infectious Disease Research and Policy*, February 20.

Segal, L. M., D. A. Lieberman, and K. May. 2016. *Ready or not: Protecting the public's health from diseases, disasters, and bioterorrism.* Washington, DC: Trust For America's Health.

Simpson, D. M., N. Sadr-Azodi, T. Mashal, W. Sabawoon, A. Pardis, A. Quddus, C. Garrigos, S. Guirguis, S. S. Zahoor Zaidi, S. Shaukat, S. Sharif, H. Asghar, and S. C. Hadler. 2014. Polio eradication initiative in Afghanistan, 1997-2013. *Journal of Infectious Diseases* 210 (Suppl 1):S162-S172.

TATFAR (Transatlantic Task Force on Antimicrobial Resistance). 2014. *Progress report.* Atlanta, GA: Transatlantic Taskforce on Antimicrobial Resistance (U.S. Department of Health and Human Services and European Commission).

The Canadian Press. 2014. *Flu vaccine supply could be boosted by half-million doses.* http://www.cbc.ca/news/health/flu-vaccine-supply-could-be-boosted-by-half-million-doses-1.2491983 (accessed February 27, 2017).

The Energy and Commerce Committee: Subcommittee on Oversight and Investigations (113th Congress). *Influenza: Perspective on current season and update on preparedness.* February 6, 2013.

Tiefer, C. 2016. President Trump is likely to boost U.S. military spending by $500 billion to $1 trillion. *Forbes*, November 9.

UN (United Nations). 2014. *World urbanization prospects.* New York: United Nations Department of Economic and Social Affairs, Population Division.

UN. 2016. *Draft political declaration of the high-level meeting of the General Assembly on antimicrobial resistance.* New York: United Nations.

UNICEF (United Nations International Children's Emergency Fund). 2014. *Ebola virus disease: Personal protective equipment and other Ebola-related supplies.* Washington, DC: United Nations International Children's Emergency Fund.

UNISDR (United Nations International Strategy for Disaster Reduction). 2015. *Sendai Framework for Disaster Risk Reduction.* Geneva, Switzerland: United Nations Office for Disaster Risk Reduction.

UNISDR. 2016. *What is disaster risk reduction?* https://www.unisdr.org/who-we-are/what-is-drr (accessed March 17, 2017).

USP (U.S. Pharmacoepial Convention). 2017a. *2017.* http://www.usp-pqm.org/results/pqm-in-numbers (accessed March 15, 2017).

USP. 2017b. *Where we work.* http://www.usp-pqm.org/where-we-work (accessed March 15, 2017).

Vergano, D., and L. Szabo. 2011. *Long-term, universal flu shot on horizon. USA Today,* July 26.

Viboud, C., and L. Simonsen. 2012. Global mortality of 2009 pandemic influenza A H1N1. *The Lancet Infectious Diseases* 12(9):651-653.

Watson, C. R., and M. Watson. 2017. Funding and organization of US federal biosecurity programs. *Health Security* 15(1):6-7.

Watson, M., J. B. Nuzzo, M. P. Shearer, and D. Meyer. 2017. Strengthening U.S. public health prepardness and response operations. *Health Security* 15(1):20-21.

WEF (World Economic Forum). 2017. *The global risks report 2017.* Geneva, Switzerland: World Economic Forum.

Wexler, A., S. Oum, and J. Kates. 2016. *The status of funding for Zika: The President's request, congressional proposals, and final funding.* http://kff.org/global-health-policy/issue-brief/the-status-of-funding-for-zika-the-presidents-request-congressional-proposals-final-funding (accessed March 6, 2017).

White House. 2009. Letter from the President regarding H1N1. Washington, DC: The White House. https://obamawhitehouse.archives.gov/the-press-office/letter-president-regarding-h1n1 (accessed March 10, 2017).

White House. 2014a. Fact sheet: U.S. response to the Ebola epidemic in West Africa. Washington, DC. https://obamawhitehouse.archives.gov/the-press-office/2014/09/16/fact-sheet-us-response-ebola-epidemic-west-africa (accessed March 6, 2017).

White House. 2014b. *National Strategy for Combating Antibiotic Resistant Bacteria.* The White House.

White House. 2015. Fact sheet: Progress in our Ebola response at home and abroad. Washington, DC: Office of the Press Secretary.

Whitman, E. 2016. *How Zika virus–carrying Aedes aegypti mosquitos were eradicated, and then returned.* http://www.ibtimes.com/how-zika-virus-carrying-aedes-aegypti-mosquitoes-were-eradicated-then-returned-2309666 (accessed March 6, 2017).

WHO (World Health Organization). 2009. *Global status report on road safety: Time for action.* Geneva, Switzerland: World Health Organization.

WHO. 2011a. *Strengthening response to pandemics and other public-health emergencies: Report of the review committee on the functioning of the International Health Regulations (2005) and on pandemic influenza (H1N1) 2009.* Geneva, Switzerland: World Health Organization.

WHO. 2011b. *Survey of the quality of selected antimalarial medicines circulating in six countries of sub-Saharan Africa.* Geneva, Switzerland: World Health Organization.
WHO. 2014a. *Injuries and violence: The facts.* Geneva, Switzerland: World Health Organization.
WHO. 2014b. *WHO declares end of Ebola outbreak in Nigeria.* http://www.who.int/mediacentre/news/statements/2014/nigeria-ends-ebola/en (accessed December 15, 2016).
WHO. 2015. *Global Action Plan on Antimicrobial Resistance.* Geneva, Switzerland: World Health Organization.
WHO. 2016a. *Antimicrobial resistance.* http://www.who.int/mediacentre/factsheets/fs194/en (accessed February 14, 2017).
WHO. 2016b. *Global tuberculosis report.* Geneva, Switzerland: World Health Organization.
WHO. 2016c. *Influenza (seasonal) fact sheet.* http://www.who.int/mediacentre/factsheets/fs211/en (accessed February 15, 2017).
WHO. 2016d. *WHO vaccine-preventable diseases: Monitoring system. 2016 global summary.* http://apps.who.int/immunization_monitoring/globalsummary/estimates?c=BRA (accessed February 23, 2017).
WHO. 2017a. *Antimicrobial resistance: Library of national action plans.* Geneva, Switzerland: World Health Organization.
WHO. 2017b. *Cumulative number of reported probable cases of severe acute resiratory syndrome (SARS).* http://www.who.int/csr/sars/country/en (accessed February 27, 2017).
WHO. 2017c. *Top 10 causes of death.* http://www.who.int/mediacentre/factsheets/fs310/en/index1.html (accessed March 18, 2017).
World Bank. 2010. *People, pathogens and our planet: Volume 1—towards a One Health approach for controlling zoonotic diseases.* Washington, DC: World Bank.
World Bank. 2012. *People, pathogens and our planet: Volume 2—the economics of One Health.* Washington, DC: World Bank.
World Bank. 2015. *Ebola: Most African countries avoid major economic loss but impact on Guinea, Liberia, Sierra Leone remains crippling.* http://www.worldbank.org/en/news/press-release/2015/01/20/ebola-most-african-countries-avoid-major-economic-loss-but-impact-on-guinea-liberia-sierra-leone-remains-crippling (accessed February 27, 2017).
World Bank. 2016a. *2014–2015 West Africa Ebola crisis: Impact update.* Washington, DC: World Bank Group.
World Bank. 2016b. *Drug-resistant infection: A threat to our economic future (discussion draft).* Washington, DC: World Bank.
World Bank. 2016c. *The short-term economic costs of Zika in Latin America and the Caribbean.* http://pubdocs.worldbank.org/en/410321455758564708/The-short-term-economic-costs-of-Zika-in-LCR-final-doc-autores-feb-18.pdf (accessed March 6, 2017).
Wysocki, B. J., and S. Lueck. 2006. Just-in-time inventories make U.S. vulnerable in a pandemic: Low stockpiles at hospitals boost efficiency but leave no extras for flu outbreak. *The Wall Street Journal,* January 12.
Yamey, G., A. Thoumi, J. Gonzalez-Smith, C. Binanay, I. Bharali, Z. Johar, D. Ridley, and N. Chapman. 2016. *Strengthening the United States government's role in product development for global health.* Durham, NC: Duke Global Health Institute and Duke Margolis Center for Health Policy.

4

Addressing Continuous Threats: HIV/AIDS, Tuberculosis, and Malaria

Although emerging and immediate infectious diseases often dominate media attention and captivate much of the dialogue around global health threats, the global community must not forget the continuing, persistent global health priorities the world has been addressing for several decades: human immunodeficiency virus/acquired immunodeficiency syndrome (HIV/AIDS), tuberculosis (TB), and malaria. In 2002, AIDS was the leading cause of death worldwide among people ages 15–59, and more than 30 million people worldwide were infected (UNAIDS, 2016a). Although HIV/AIDS is no longer necessarily a death sentence, and people living with HIV/AIDS are able to treat it as a chronic disease, there is still no vaccine and no cure. With 2 million new infections, 1.1 million deaths, and 36.7 million people living with HIV in 2015, there is a clear need for heightened attention (UNAIDS, 2015d). TB, often an overlooked danger, saw 10.4 million new cases in 2015 and 1.4 million deaths[1] worldwide (WHO, 2016c). In the United States alone, 9,557 cases of TB occurred in 2015. Although this was a 64.2 percent decrease from 1992, it was a 1.6 percent increase from 2014 (CDC, 2016a). Multiple strains of TB are resistant to one or more medications, with very few new drugs under development to address them. Finally, malaria continues to plague many countries, with 212 million new cases causing 429,000 deaths globally in 2015 (WHO, 2016d). Although

[1] There were 1.8 million TB deaths worldwide in 2015, but 0.39 million of these occurred among people with an HIV infection. When an HIV-positive person dies from TB, the underlying cause is classified as HIV in the *International Classification of Disease Systems* (ICD-10th Revision) (WHO, 2016c).

malaria is rarely carried by mosquitoes in the United States, it is a constant threat to many U.S. travelers, international employees, and military members visiting and working in other countries. HIV/AIDS, TB, and malaria have a huge detrimental effect on the afflicted countries, making it difficult to foster growing economies and progressive societies.

This chapter begins by exploring the disease burden of HIV/AIDS and the progress made on reducing that burden in recent decades through bilateral and multilateral programs. It then provides future opportunities for programs and focus areas given the characteristics of the disease and patient populations now understood. Next, this chapter reviews the historic lack of funding toward tuberculosis and the danger it presents as many resistant strains continue to circulate. It also discusses the favorable reductions in malaria incidence and prevalence over the past 20 years, thanks to many dedicated programs. However, though much success has been achieved in all three disease areas, the chapter closes by cautioning against complacency—as all of these diseases are capable of resistance and resurgence.

HIV/AIDS

Beginning in the early 2000s, the HIV/AIDS pandemic and the global attention it received resulted in a great deal of funding and research toward finding drugs and other treatments and helping those with HIV improve their quality of life. Because of these concerted efforts by the global community, about 18.2 million people living with HIV now have access to antiretroviral therapy—a major feat, considering that just 16 years ago, fewer than 1 million people had access (HHS, 2016). This increased access is a testament to the power of collective action, as the global target of 15 million people receiving HIV treatment by 2015 was reached 9 months ahead of schedule (UNAIDS, 2015c). As a result of these efforts, new infections decreased globally by 35 percent between 2000 and 2015, and AIDS-related deaths decreased by 42 percent between 2005 and 2015 (UNAIDS, 2015a). Such an accomplishment is due in large part to the availability of sustainable funding, which is infrequently accessible for infectious disease efforts.

The story of the HIV/AIDS pandemic is still fraught with tragedy. Despite this success, people in sub-Saharan Africa continue to face the highest burden of disease worldwide, with 69.5 percent[2] of people living with HIV and 65.2 percent[3] of new infections occurring in that region in

[2] In 2015, 36.7 million people were living with HIV globally, 25.5 million of whom were in sub-Saharan Africa. These figures were obtained by selecting "People living with HIV" as an indicator (UNAIDS, 2016a).

[3] In 2015, 2.1 million new HIV infections occurred globally, 1.37 million of which were in sub-Saharan Africa. These figures were obtained by selecting "New HIV infections" as an indicator (UNAIDS, 2016a).

2015 (UNAIDS, 2016a). Additionally, progress within vulnerable populations has been slower in sub-Saharan Africa than other parts of the world, with adolescent girls and young women at disproportionate risk: AIDS is the leading cause of death among women of reproductive age (UNAIDS, 2015c). Global progress is also precariously at risk, as only 60 percent of people with HIV know their status, and the remaining 40 percent still need access to HIV testing services (HHS, 2016). That people under the age of 25 frequently do not know their HIV status and that there are now 200 million people between 15 and 24 years of age in sub-Saharan Africa creates the potential for the pandemic to surge out of control again (PEPFAR, 2016a).

The global community and U.S. government's enthusiasm to end the AIDS pandemic has led to the establishment of lofty targets. Current global strategy is guided by the 90-90-90 agenda of the Joint United Nations Programme on HIV/AIDS, which, by 2020 aims to have 90 percent of people living with HIV knowing their status; 90 percent of people with diagnosed HIV infection receiving sustained antiretroviral treatment; and 90 percent of all people on antiretroviral treatment having viral suppression (UNAIDS, 2014a). To support these goals, funders have crafted their own strategies. For example, the Global Fund to Fight AIDS, Tuberculosis and Malaria Strategy 2017–2022 to End Epidemics aims to maximize the impact of its investments through finding differentiated approaches for diverse country contexts, increased alignment, and planning for sustainability of programs that tackle the disease (Global Fund, 2016).

The global monetary support for HIV/AIDS programs now totals about $19 billion annually, dwarfing funding provided for any other single disease. In 2015, $10.9 billion—57 percent of the total—came from domestic, in-country sources (AVERT, 2017; UNAIDS, 2016b). However, donor sources contribute in a variety of ways, especially for low-income countries that still heavily rely on external aid to finance their HIV response, with 44 countries relying on 75 percent or more of international assistance in 2014 (AVERT, 2017). Private funding accounted for $618 million in fiscal year (FY) 2014 (Kates et al., 2016). The U.S. President's Emergency Plan for AIDS Relief (PEPFAR), which is responsible for the U.S. government's response to global HIV, contributed $5.22 billion in FY2016 to bilateral HIV/AIDS programs,[4] $1.35 billion to the Global Fund[5] (PEPFAR, 2016c), and $117.9 million toward TB/HIV programs (PEPFAR, 2016b). This funding has remained stagnant for several years, forcing the PEPFAR program

---

[4] Funding for bilateral HIV/AIDS programs covers funding for bilateral funding programs and regional programs in addition to contributions to the Joint United Nations Programme on HIV/AIDS, the International AIDS Vaccine Initiative, microbicides, and National Institutes of Health AIDS research (PEPFAR, 2016c).

[5] This is the total U.S. contribution to the Global Fund.

to make difficult decisions in priorities as more patients are put on lifelong treatment regimens.

PEPFAR's Progress and Potential

The PEPFAR program, began under the Bush administration in 2003, has seen tremendous success during its 13 years of existence (see Box 4-1), and has crossed through multiple phases of varying focus. Initially, it was a true emergency response at a time when entire generations in Africa were dying, leaving behind 14 million orphans and vulnerable children (PEPFAR, 2016a). One of PEPFAR's strengths from its inception has been its use of senior-level leadership to monitor and coordinate its interagency efforts to drive change.

BOX 4-1
The U.S. President's Emergency Plan for AIDS Relief (PEPFAR) Achievements to Date

The influence of PEPFAR has been profound, thanks to many years of bipartisan support from Congress. In addition to providing 11.5 million people with life-saving drugs, preventing 2 million babies from being born with human immunodeficiency virus (HIV), and halving the adult death rate in PEPFAR-supported countries within 5 years of program rollout, PEPFAR has led to a number of economic benefits for partner countries that improve the prosperity of American businesses and the safety of the American people, including

- 13 percent higher employment rates among men in PEPFAR countries than in non-PEPFAR countries;
- a three times higher development rate in PEPFAR countries as compared to non-PEPFAR countries
- an increase in positive opinion of the United States from 40 to 68 percent by people in PEPFAR countries compared to 40 to 46 percent in non-PEPFAR countries between 2007 and 2011;
- an 86 percent viral suppression among those being treated in Zimbabwe, Zambia, and Malawi, indicating these countries are on the path to controlling the epidemic;
- a 16 to 20 percent less likelihood of dying of human immunodeficiency virus/acquired immunodeficiency syndrome (HIV/AIDS) in PEPFAR countries as compared to non-PEPFAR countries;
- a positive trend toward lower tuberculosis rates for PEPFAR countries.

SOURCES: Cohen, 2016; Daschle and Frist, 2015; Lima et al., 2013; Richter, 2012; Tarnoff and Lawson, 2016; Wagner et al., 2015.

The program shifted to Phase II under the Obama administration once the crisis had abated; it maintained a focus on saving lives but placed greater emphasis on sustainability through partnership frameworks and mutual accountability. PEPFAR most recently shifted to Phase III, directing attention to what is likely to be the most challenging phase: getting the pandemic under sustainable control (PEPFAR, 2012a). As of September 30, 2015, PEPFAR has supported antiretroviral treatment for 9.5 million people and has reduced the number of new infections in its focus countries from 2.58 million in 2003 to 1.48 million in 2015 (PEPFAR, 2017a). With so many individuals dependent on the PEPFAR program for life-saving treatment and the dangerous potential for regression given the rapid youth population growth in many PEPFAR countries, there is an ethical imperative that PEPFAR be continued. Furthermore, more people are living with HIV/AIDS today than when the program started in 2003 (UNAIDS, 2016a), demonstrating the need for continued investment. The sustainability of an ongoing program like PEPFAR demands occasional realignment and shifting of priorities, as well as changes in the way it operates while maintaining its prior humanitarian commitments. Such changes should reflect the changes in the pandemic and various microepidemics (i.e., small-scale, community-level epidemics) as the disease continues to evolve.

PEPFAR has recently increased its use of data-driven programming. This change has allowed the program to report statistics on the HIV/AIDS burden in countries and on antiretroviral coverage and patients' viral loads at the district level. The data-driven focus has improved the measurement of the number of patients on treatment. Increased data collection has been accompanied by a concomitant increase in understanding the socioeconomic influences of virus transmission, which should continue to be examined and analyzed to determine the best course of action. For example, although the incidence rates of HIV in most PEPFAR countries have declined, the rates have increased for populations most at risk, such as young women. As many as 380,000 adolescent girls and young women (ages 10–24) are infected each year globally, often due to gender-based violence (GBV) and exploitation by older men (UNAIDS, 2014b). In fact, women who experience GBV are three times more likely to contract HIV than women who do not (PEPFAR, 2015). Additionally, this group of women acquires HIV 5 to 7 years earlier than men (UNAIDS, 2014b) and is three times more likely to be HIV positive than men of the same age (PEPFAR, 2015).

One of the main future challenges for the PEPFAR program will be ascertaining the amount of money it can spend on direct treatment for patients versus the amount it can spend on prevention. When the PEPFAR program was created, the initial authorization from Congress called for 55 percent of funding to be spent on treatment. That requirement was carried over in the reauthorization legislation in 2008 but was relaxed slightly in

2013, when the PEPFAR Stewardship and Oversight Act of 2013[6] called for just half of bilateral funds to be directed toward treatment and care versus 55 percent (KFF, 2017c; PEPFAR, 2017a).

Next Generation of PEPFAR

The clear returns from PEPFAR investments show that its involvement contributes to better overall health outcomes in a country. Studies have indicated that PEPFAR focus countries have higher male employment rates than similar non-PEPFAR focus countries[7] (Wagner et al., 2015) and have improved opinions of the United States (Daschle and Frist, 2015). Further enabling PEPFAR platforms to serve other country-specific health needs could increase this return on investment. Doing so is critical for driving future U.S. global health efforts and for establishing global partnerships to help build robust, broad, and efficient in-country health systems that ensure equitable access to the quality health care needed to help end the AIDS pandemic.

To look to the future in phasing down direct PEPFAR costs and incorporating health needs of countries, a priority for PEPFAR should be to continue supporting countries in their transition from bilateral aid to domestic financing by aiding in the mobilization of domestic resources for HIV/AIDS (and health more broadly). This shift would inevitably also allow more country ownership and decision making in their planning of national AIDS programs. This effort will require realistic country-specific assessments and strategies for building each national health system's capacity to assume financial and operational responsibilities for service delivery. A caveat is that domestic resource mobilization may be a more realistically viable option for middle-income countries than for many low-income countries, which may have very little fiscal space in which to maneuver. In those cases, low-income countries will continue to rely on support from donors like the United States in order to keep HIV infection rates from surging out of control. A range of opinions exists about how to best support national governments in this transition, but many emphasize the need to incentivize and encourage country-driven funding by devising innovative, creative, and flexible financing strategies (Oomman et al., 2007; PEPFAR, 2009; Resch et al., 2015). Since meeting with other partners in 2015, PEPFAR and the U.S. Treasury are working with ministries of finance in recipient countries to create HIV expenditure committees and improve coordination

---

[6] PEPFAR Stewardship and Oversight Act of 2013, Public Law 113-56.

[7] PEPFAR focus countries include Botswana, Côte d'Ivoire, Ethiopia, Guyana, Haiti, Kenya, Mozambique, Namibia, Nigeria, Rwanda, South Africa, Tanzania, Uganda, Vietnam, and Zambia (KFF, 2017c).

of funding sources to increase efficiency and use domestic resources most effectively (PEPFAR, 2016a). Under these partnerships, the U.S. Department of the Treasury may provide technical assistance to finance ministries to strengthen public financial management of health resources. Another means for decreasing recipient countries' reliance on PEPFAR for AIDS treatment is for the U.S. government to direct more of its AIDS budget to the Global Fund, which utilizes a unique e-marketplace[8] to create a competitive market for specific health products and a Pooled Procurement Mechanism by which the Global Fund negotiates favorable procurement terms for health products (Global Fund, 2017). As a way to make current taxpayer funds go further, PEPFAR should also continue to employ key partnerships with the private sector focused on prevention, treatment, and care and support. In the case of supply chain management, for example, one partnership implemented new approaches to several steps in the supply chain, ensuring inventory was used before expiration and managing costs through pooling procurement (Sturchio and Cohen, 2012). Partially because of this infrastructure, PEPFAR was able to increase its proportion of generic drugs and contribute to reducing the annual cost of treatment per patient by nearly $700 (PEPFAR, 2012b).

The committee solicited information from the U.S. Agency for International Development (USAID) and the U.S. Centers for Disease Control and Prevention (CDC) field staff in multiple countries on PEPFAR's successes and challenges.[9] Overall, respondents reported that the PEPFAR program was generally well-received in countries and was significantly increasing the number of patients on treatment and decreasing HIV infection rates. Some respondents noted that country leaders understandably appreciated the technical and financial support provided by PEPFAR but wanted a greater degree of responsibility in decision making and prioritizing. In some cases, the priority of the U.S. program did not reflect the health priority of the host government. To alleviate this mismatch, some respondents recommended a shift in focus toward health systems strengthening or capacity building.

Broadening the Approach

There has been a growing understanding—both in the United States and internationally—of the need to broaden the spectrum of health care in a country by adopting a "development lens" that addresses the social and economic vulnerabilities of families and individuals multisectorally to achieve better outcomes in health, education, and livelihood (UNAIDS,

[8] See more at http://www.wambo.org/home (accessed March 8, 2017).

[9] See Chapter 1 for the full description of the information-gathering process.

2015c). Field staff respondents supported this approach by noting that although epidemic control is important, thousands of children and adults dying from preventable causes such as lack of access to care or safe water demonstrates the program's need to broaden. Offering various types of interventions through the PEPFAR platform can ensure that patients are being viewed holistically while they are interacting with the health care system. For example, when HIV patients visit a clinic for treatment or testing, they could also be provided with education on nutrition or blood pressure screening and hypertension awareness, as some pilot projects are beginning to do through PEPFAR. Anecdotal results report that a patient with HIV who is on antiretroviral therapy can now receive care for hypertension or diabetes at the same clinic (Green, 2016). These program innovations are still somewhat limited in their design and depth, however, and funding is difficult. With all these considerations in mind, alternative methods of operation could be explored that can complement innovative financing strategies.

When considering new, broader approaches, there is a clear objective to couple PEPFAR's services with those of other U.S. agencies and non-governmental organizations (NGOs) working on nutrition efforts. People who take antiretroviral therapy often encounter food insecurity as a critical barrier to linkage to care, treatment adherence, retention in care, and viral load suppression. Malnourished people living with HIV are two to six times more likely to die within the first 6 months of treatment than similar patients who are not malnourished (UNAIDS, 2015b). Currently, nutrition assessment, counseling, and support are classified as "near core" interventions based on country context, but nutrition should be prioritized for all PEPFAR patients (PEPFAR, 2016a).[10]

Leveraging Partnerships

Although PEPFAR has had informal partnerships with host-country stakeholders (i.e., civil society), it has now begun to incorporate these relationships into all aspects of its programming in order to achieve sustainability and self-sufficiency. PEPFAR's 2017 *Annual Report to Congress* states that now more than ever it encourages full participation of civil society to ensure they "have a voice at the decision-making table" (PEPFAR, 2017a). Partner governments and civil society organizations are now keenly in-

[10] PEPFAR defines "core" interventions as activities central to HIV/AIDS that are critical to saving lives and preventing new infections and are grounded in science. "Near-core" interventions are defined as activities that directly support HIV/AIDS goals and cannot yet be done well by other partners or the host government, and "non-core" interventions are activities that do not directly affect HIV/AIDS goals and/or can be taken on by other partners or the host government (PEPFAR, 2016a).

volved in all aspects of the country operational plan process, which for the first time includes representatives from ministries of health and a large number of civil society organizations. This is a much different approach to country operational plan development than in previous years, and it has been extremely well-received by country stakeholders. The committee fully supports this new direction for PEPFAR and encourages more partnerships like the Determined, Resilient, Empowered, AIDS-free, Mentored, and Safe women (DREAMS) initiative (described in Box 4-2) and other engagements with community-level organizations to help drive sustainability, implementation, and effectiveness.

PEPFAR funding rules require that money is spent only on activities that focus on narrowly defined indicators related to scaling up treatment and decreasing HIV infection. Although the committee agrees these goals are important, addressing more general health goals through the same PEPFAR intervention would be easier if the indicators were defined a little more broadly. For example, "capacity building" could be added to the 50 percent on treatment and care allocation. Local workforce capacity is an ongoing challenge in many of these countries. The Medical Education Partnership Initiative (MEPI) and Nursing Education Partnership Initiative (NEPI) were created in response to the poor treatment outcomes resulting from the paucity of trained medical professionals in PEPFAR countries in 2010. These programs allowed PEPFAR to fund African medical institutions to increase the number of high-quality, in-country nurses and doctors (OARAC, 2015).

In their 5 years of partnerships, MEPI and NEPI have significantly improved capacity for education and research at in-country universities. For instance, at the University of Botswana, the MEPI program helped to establish and strengthen teaching sites, which led to the first-ever graduation of 80 locally trained doctors. The successes of the MEPI and NEPI partnerships mean the progress made possible by PEPFAR interventions will not be lost because there are too few medical professionals to treat patients. In FY2017, this partnership will be reinstated under a new name and, in learning from past MEPI and NEPI programs, will be more focused on medical and nursing education. Awardee institutions are encouraged to collaborate with the newly formed African Forum for Research and Education in Health, international partners that share the same goals, and successful MEPI and NEPI programs (NIH, 2016). This updated program will emphasize interdepartmental collaboration within awardee universities, as well as the development of partnerships with other universities and schools in their country to further expand the research workforce and resources. These goals advance the Fogarty International Center work by expanding research capacity among individuals, institutions, and larger networks and strengthening partnerships to advance global health research.

BOX 4-2
The Determined, Resilient, Empowered, AIDS-free, Mentored, and Safe Women (DREAMS) Initiative

DREAMS is a $385 million partnership addressing the multidisciplinary factors that contribute to disproportionately high rates of human immunodeficiency virus (HIV) infection in young women. The partnership focuses on young women in high-burden locations of Kenya, Lesotho, Malawi, Mozambique, South Africa, Tanzania, Uganda, Zambia, and Zimbabwe, with a goal of 40 percent reduction in new HIV infections among adolescent girls and young women by the end of 2017.

The multifactorial nature of a social disease such as HIV/acquired immunodeficiency syndrome (AIDS) requires changing nonhealth factors, such as increasing access to secondary education, reducing gender-based violence, building stronger parenting relationships, and changing the community norms and structures that prevent the success of young women. To make these changes in a robust and successful way, DREAMS leverages expertise from private and philanthropic partners. Johnson & Johnson is using its marketing expertise in understanding consumer behavior to target services to young girls. The Bill & Melinda Gates Foundation is funding impact evaluation and implementation research to evaluate success. Gilead is purchasing medication and funding operational expenses for pre-exposure prophylaxis (PrEP) for uninfected young women at high risk. Nike's Girl Effect is funding the use of a toolkit to help identify and target adolescent girls in the hardest-to-reach areas, develop culturally appropriate brands, and address social norm change. Finally, ViiV Healthcare is providing capacity-building support to community organizations.

The team has also launched the DREAMS Innovation Challenge, committing $85 million to test newer solutions for preventing new infections among adolescent girls and young women. The challenge was designed to infuse new thinking and high-impact approaches and to engage new partners with local understanding.

Countries are taking this partnership to a new level by direct investment. Swaziland now has close to national HIV coverage for adolescent girls and young women. South Africa created a national campaign to take DREAMS beyond the initial five districts to a national-level program leveraging existing stakeholder activities across the country.

NOTE: Girls and young women account for around three-quarters of new HIV infections among adolescents in sub-Saharan Africa.
SOURCE: PEPFAR, 2017a.

Understanding some of these broader determinants, PEPFAR's DREAMS project began in 2014 as a $385 million partnership to reduce HIV infection in young women in 10 sub-Saharan African countries. Recognizing that HIV infection vulnerabilities in this population extend far beyond the health sector, DREAMS addresses the structural drivers of HIV infection, such as poverty, gender-based violence and inequality, and education (see Box 4-2) (PEPFAR, 2017b). The program is still young and represents only 5 percent of the PEPFAR budget. The committee believes that more cross-sector and multidisciplinary programs like this should be explored not only to reduce HIV infection rates, but also to more holistically address social and development challenges and have a greater effect overall while leveraging the strengths of other stakeholders.

A Continued Focus on Data and Metrics

Despite the major progress made in addressing the HIV/AIDS pandemic, serious barriers prevent ending the pandemic. Most importantly, as noted previously, nearly half of all people living with HIV are unaware of their status, underscoring the urgency of closing the testing gap. Late diagnosis of HIV infection is the most substantial barrier to scaling up HIV treatment (UNAIDS, 2015c), but it also presents continuing challenges in keeping the epidemic under control if those who are infected are unaware. With the increase in data collection, PEPFAR has now been able to undertake public health impact assessments in 13 countries to measure progress toward epidemic control, with three completed so far (PEPFAR, 2017a). These public health impact assessments are comprehensive and measure prevalence, incidence, historic mortality, and service coverage down to the household level (PEPFAR, 2016a). Starting in FY2017, PEPFAR will also require implementing partners to provide yearly differentiated technical and direct support to sites and patients.

New infections still outpace the number of patients on treatment, so HIV prevention, and not just treatment, must be a focus of the next phase of the program. The pandemic cannot be solved through treatment alone, yet it will play a key role given the significant gains realized through using treatment as prevention. Recognizing this, PEPFAR increased funding for HIV prevention in young women in 2015 through the DREAMS initiative, expanded voluntary medical circumcision to prevent infections in young men, and in 2017 expanded Prevention for Treatment efforts to decrease transmission in young men (PEPFAR, 2017a). Additionally, with new guidelines from the World Health Organization (WHO) on antiretroviral therapy–based prevention, including pre-exposure prophylaxis (PrEP) (WHO, 2016a), PEPFAR is supporting a scale-up of PrEP in key populations, including adolescent girls and young women, which is the first time girls have had access to PrEP outside of a research setting. This scale-up is being supported by public–private partnerships such as DREAMS and through Gilead, which is financially supporting purchasing and operational expenses for PrEP for young women (PEPFAR, 2017a). However, there is still much to be done to prevent new infections. Prevention requires a comprehensive package that includes behavioral and structural interventions and condom programming in addition to PrEP, HIV testing, voluntary male circumcision for HIV-negative men, and prevention of mother-to-child transmission, necessitating a varied approach to financing (UNAIDS, 2015c).

An estimated $30 billion will be needed to meet the ambitious 90-90-90 targets by 2020 (UNAIDS, 2014a, 2015c); currently, the world is short $19 billion. Moving forward, there is an opportunity to approach the next phase of PEPFAR in a multisectoral and multifaceted manner. Because results vary by country and interventions do not have the same effectiveness in all places, continued granular-level data collection and community-level understanding of community-level epidemics will be critical. Moreover, broad prevention efforts will need to be implemented at the community level and across sectors—with the support and involvement of country and community leaders—to truly reduce HIV infection rates.

SUMMARY AND RECOMMENDATION

PEPFAR is in great part responsible for the tremendous success achieved in slowing the HIV/AIDS pandemic globally since 2003. In addition to this progress on its primary goal, studies have shown that the countries in which PEPFAR is active had better opinions of the United States (Daschle and Frist, 2015) and also saw a 13 percent increase in employment rates among men compared to non-PEPFAR countries (Wagner et al., 2015). A truly bipartisan, collaborative program that has undergone transitions and shifts throughout the past 15 years, PEPFAR has shifted its focus from responding to an emergency to sustaining care while targeting at-risk populations, reflecting corresponding changes in the pandemic. However, the successes achieved should not be taken as a rationale for downscaling PEPFAR. The need for the program remains: Approximately 9.5 million people currently receive antiretroviral treatment through PEPFAR support, while 2.1 million new HIV infections still occur each year (PEPFAR, 2017a). PEPFAR's next phase will continue to require cross-sector and data-driven efforts, as well as strong country partnerships, if the number of new HIV infections and AIDS-related deaths is to be dramatically reduced in as many countries as possible by 2030.

Conclusion: Now that the pandemic has evolved from requiring an emergency response to requiring a more sustained response, with patients needing chronic care, the PEPFAR platform needs to evolve accordingly. Given the substantial reduction in drug costs, the impact of treatment on prevention, and the ease of measurement of treatment outcomes, program ownership needs to shift to countries. At the same time, PEPFAR needs to leverage its existing structures and platforms to address patient and population health issues more comprehensively, while continuing to fulfill the ethical imperative of providing life-saving treatment to those already covered by its programming.

Recommendation 4: Envision the Next Generation of PEPFAR

With its next reauthorization, Congress should fund The U.S. President's Emergency Plan for AIDS Relief (PEPFAR) at current levels, and allow for more flexibility within the PEPFAR program by continuing to relax specific funding targets for all program areas. Continued accountability, efficiency, and measurement of results should be emphasized. In the future, moreover, PEPFAR should focus on the following key areas:

- **Ensure that national governments assume greater ownership of national HIV/AIDS programs through joint planning and decision making, and that they increase domestic funding to help cover the costs of prevention and treatment.**
- **Adapt its delivery platform to become more of a cost-effective, chronic care system that is incorporated into each country's health system and priorities.**
- **Continue to support the Global Fund to Fight AIDS, Tuberculosis and Malaria (Global Fund), and rely on it for specific functions where it has the comparative advantage. Such functions could include the Global Fund's efficient procurement of products and multipartner efforts to encourage countries to transition to domestic sources of funding.**
- **Enhance emphasis on primary prevention through multisector efforts, including strong interventions against gender-based violence, given that many new HIV infections are occurring in adolescent girls.**

TUBERCULOSIS

TB, an airborne disease, has been historically underprioritized. Although TB was placed on the international agenda after WHO declared it to be a global emergency in 1993—which only occurred after public health complacency in the 1970s and 1980s led to its resurgence (Ogden et al., 2003)—the world has struggled to reduce the global burden of TB, facing significant challenges in tackling the disease in the world's poorest regions. Although the progress made in reducing TB incidence and mortality should be celebrated (including an approximate 1.4 to 2.3 percent reduction per year between 2000 and 2015 [WHO, 2016c]), progress has nonetheless been slow. In fact, TB has now surpassed HIV/AIDS as the leading cause of death by an infectious disease worldwide. In 2015 there were 10.4 million new cases of TB and 1.4 million deaths attributed to TB (WHO, 2016c),[11] as opposed to 1.1 million deaths attributed to HIV/AIDS (UNAIDS, 2016b).

TB is truly a global disease, with the highest absolute burden during 2015 being in Southeast Asia, Africa, and the Western Pacific[12] (WHO, 2016c). The current global approach on TB is driven by WHO's End TB Strategy, which provides goals for the Sustainable Development Goal era. These goals include achieving a 95 percent reduction in TB deaths and a 90 percent reduction in TB incidence by 2035. An additional goal is reducing the percentage of TB-affected households experiencing catastrophic medical expenditures to zero by 2030 (WHO, 2016c). Meeting these goals requires an acceleration of effort, costing an estimated $8.3 billion in global resources in 2016. Unfortunately, global financing for these goals was 30 percent short of what was required. As a testament to poor international assistance for TB, 84 percent of the $6.6 billion available in 2016 for TB care and prevention in low- and middle-income countries (LMICs) came from domestic resources. Weak international support particularly affected national TB programs in low-income countries, which required foreign assistance for about 90 percent of their program funding (WHO, 2016c).

Epidemiological Complexity of Tuberculosis

This lack of support for TB control is exacerbated by the complexities of TB infection and epidemiology, which become especially problematic in low-resource settings. First, TB is difficult to diagnose, and the resulting inadequate case finding is an obstacle to global TB control (WHO, 2016c). As a bacterial infection with an especially long growth cycle, TB cannot be easily detected with rapid diagnostic tests as is done for other diseases relevant to global health. The predominant method for diagnosing TB in LMICs is direct sputum smear microscopy,[13] which is quick but limited in its ability to detect pediatric TB,[14] drug-resistant TB, and TB/HIV

[11] In 2015, an additional 0.39 millions deaths were caused by HIV/TB coinfection.

[12] A reason Southeast Asia and Africa rank so high is that China, India, Indonesia, Nigeria, Pakistan, and South Africa accounted for 60 percent of new cases in 2015 (WHO, 2016c).

[13] Direct sputum smear microscopy uses laboratory techniques to analyze a sample of sputum (a mixture of fluids coughed up from the respiratory tract) for the TB bacteria (Singhal and Myneedu, 2015). Serial samples may be required to confirm TB diagnoses, but many patients may fail to appear for a follow-up appointment, often due to an inability to afford repeat visits to a health facility (Harries et al., 1998; Kemp et al., 2007).

[14] Because of limitations of direct sputum smear microscopy among children, pediatric TB is often called a "hidden epidemic," an issue that is worsened by lack of treatment options.

coinfection (the latter two are discussed in later sections) (Desikan, 2013; Keshavjee and Farmer, 2012). Second, treatment length and complexity add to the diagnostic challenge. Due to the long growth cycle of TB, treatment can often take 6 to 9 months. Furthermore, treatment relies on combination chemotherapy, which uses multiple drugs (Laurenzi et al., 2007). Although TB drug regimens are highly effective when provided under strictly regulated clinical trial conditions (above 90 percent)[15] (Laurenzi et al., 2007), adherence outside of these settings is lower due to physical barriers to access and lengthy treatment, which results in average global success rates of about 83 percent (Laurenzi et al., 2007; WHO, 2016c).

Drug-Resistant Tuberculosis

Poor adherence to TB treatment has resulted in a rapid increase of monoresistant TB, multidrug-resistant TB (MDR-TB), and even extensively drug-resistant TB (XDR-TB).[16] First recognized in 1948, drug-resistant TB steadily grew but was more or less ignored (similar to nonresistant TB) until the early 1990s (Nachega and Chaisson, 2003). This lack of attention was partly driven by the emergence of combination chemotherapy in the mid-1900s, which led to the belief that TB would be conquered, and consequently resulted in the elimination of federal funding for TB control in the United States by 1972 (Cegielski, 2010). Similarly, funding for TB research dropped to just $514,000 in the United States in 1979 (Petrakos, 1993). Just as TB resurged during the 1970s and 1980s, so too did MDR-TB, with outbreaks in multiple U.S. states[17] (Cegielski, 2010; Petrakos, 1993) and epidemics reported across the globe (Cegielski, 2010). In 2015 alone there were approximately 480,000 new cases of MDR-TB, 9.5 percent of which were XDR-TB cases. Furthermore, 3.9 percent of all new TB cases in 2015 were MDR-TB cases (WHO, 2016c). While these numbers seem small, they may underestimate the true burden of drug-resistant bacteria as the method for determining resistance (sputum culture) can take up to 6 weeks (CDC, 2013) and requires sophisticated laboratory capacity that is lacking in many LMICs.

The rise of drug resistance is a blow to global TB control efforts, as monoresistant TB and MDR-TB also can be spread from person to person (CDC, 2016b). It was previously thought that XDR-TB only was acquired

[15] The studies referenced are clinical trials conducted in the United States and the United Kingdom, settings that do not apply to everyday circumstances in LMICs.

[16] Monoresistant TB is TB that is resistant to one TB drug. MDR-TB is TB that is resistant to at least two commonly used TB drugs. XDR-TB is TB that is resistant to two or more first-line drugs in addition to at least two second-line drugs used to treat MDR-TB (WHO, 2012a).

[17] New York City alone spent more than $1 billion to curb a TB epidemic in the early 1990s (Frieden et al., 1995).

due to repeated treatment failure. However, recent findings indicate that even XDR-TB can be spread from person to person (Shah et al., 2017). To make matters worse, length of treatment for these drug-resistant strains is even longer—up to 20 months[18]—and their success rates even lower: 52 percent for MDR-TB and 28 percent for XDR-TB (WHO, 2016c). Low treatment success rates make XDR-TB especially lethal, with the long-term chances of survival being only 15 percent (Pietersen et al., 2014). Although preventing these resistant strains is vital from a security standpoint, it is also very cost-effective. The cost to treat TB ranges from $100 to $500 per person in LMICs, yet the costs for treating MDR-TB and XDR-TB can reach up to $10,000 and $26,000, respectively (Laurence et al., 2015; Nieburg et al., 2015; Pooran et al., 2013).

TB/HIV Coinfection

The frequent coinfection of TB with HIV poses another epidemiological challenge. In fact, the risk of developing TB is 26 to 31 times greater for those who have HIV/AIDS than those who do not (WHO, 2017b). In 2015, one-third of those living with HIV were infected with TB, and of the 10.4 million new cases of TB, 1.2 million occurred in people living with HIV (WHO, 2016c). Furthermore, for those living with HIV in resource-poor settings, TB is the largest single cause of death (UNAIDS, 2016b), accounting for 34.45 percent of HIV deaths.[19] Coinfection has been found to result in a dangerous interaction in the body, with HIV being linked to the progression of a TB infection and TB being reported to worsen HIV infection (Getahun et al., 2010; Whalen et al., 1995). Further exacerbating this issue is that HIV coinfection is associated with the malabsorption of anti-TB drugs (Patel et al., 1995) and has been found to be a risk factor for acquiring MDR-TB (Suchindran et al., 2009). The extensive treatment required to care for coinfected patients exerts enormous pressure on health systems found in LMICs, where 99 percent of TB-related HIV deaths occur (Pawlowski et al., 2012).

Paradigm Shift for Tuberculosis

The complexity of TB, in terms of its epidemiology, rise in drug-resistant strains, and its interaction with HIV, poses a major problem for global efforts directed toward both TB and HIV. That these diseases frequently occur in the same country (see Figure 4-1) sheds light on the challenges that country governments, multilateral organizations, and U.S.-led

---

[18] New WHO recommendations have shortened regimens for MDR-TB to 9–12 months.

[19] This percentage is derived from dividing the number of HIV deaths due to TB (0.39 million) by the total number of HIV-related deaths (1.1 million) in 2015 (UNAIDS, 2016b).

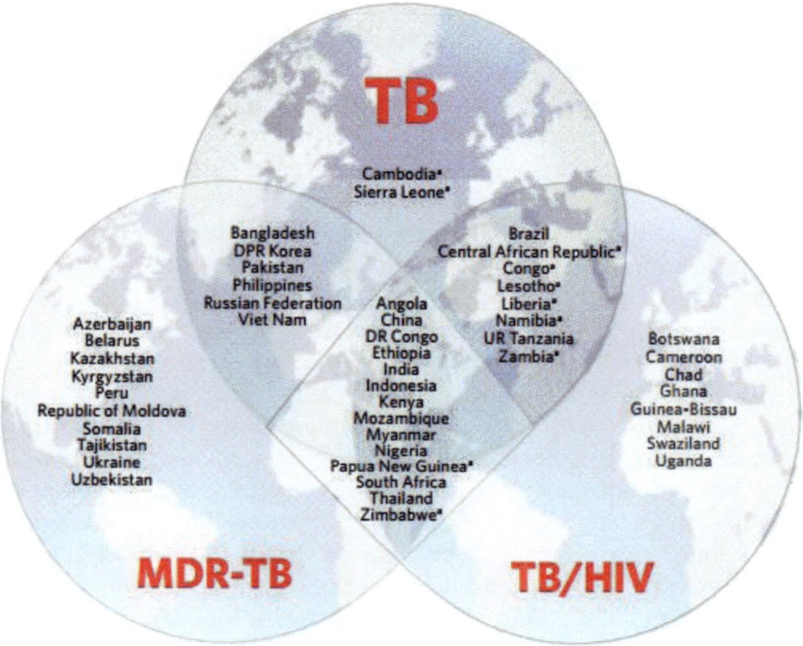

FIGURE 4-1 Countries with a high burden of TB, TB/HIV coinfection, and MDR-TB.
NOTES: Includes top 20 by absolute number of cases and an additional 10 countries that have the highest incidence rates per capita. HIV = human immunodeficiency virus; MDR-TB = multidrug-resistant tuberculosis; TB = tuberculosis; TB/HIV = tuberculosis/HIV coinfection.

[a] Indicates countries that are included in the list of 30 high-burden countries for TB on the basis of the severity of their TB burden (i.e., TB incidence per 100,000 population), as opposed to the top 20, which are included on the basis of their absolute number of incident cases per year.

SOURCE: Global Tuberculosis Report 2016
http://apps.who.int/iris/bitstream/10665/250441/1/9789241565394-eng.pdf?ua=1
ISBN 978 92 4 156539 4
Figure 2.2: Countries in the three TB high-burden country lists that will be used by WHO during the period 2016–2020, and their areas of overlap. Page 12.

bilateral programs face. The center diamond in Figure 4-1 highlights where TB, MDR-TB, and TB/HIV coinfection occur at high rates.

Clearly, the current strategies used to treat and combat TB have not kept pace with the burden it poses. The mainstay of TB treatment is the directly observed treatment, short-course (DOTS) strategy,[20] which

[20] Though DOTS contains five elements (sustained political and financial commitment, diagnosis by quality-ensured sputum smear microscopy, standardized short-course anti-TB

was adopted by WHO in the mid-1990s largely as a branding strategy for global TB control. The evidence for the effectiveness of short-course therapy, which served as the foundation of DOTS, was limited to Malawi, Mozambique, and Tanzania in a 1991 study (Ogden et al., 2003). By 2001, 127 countries had adopted the DOTS policy (WHO, 2001). The logic behind DOTS is that through direct observation treatment failure would occur less frequently. However, meta-analyses of the literature have shown that DOTS (the directly observed component) is no more effective than self-administration of treatment (Karumbi and Garner, 2015; Pasipanodya and Gumbo, 2013).

Given the resource intensiveness of directly observed treatment and its relative ineffectiveness compared to self-administration, policy makers need to reconsider TB control strategies and a redirection of resources toward other causes of poor treatment outcomes. As TB is a disease of poverty, one option could be targeting the social determinants of TB, which include social circumstances and material resources, misunderstandings of the etiology of TB, stigma, fear of punitive sanctions due to a positive TB diagnosis, and a lack of social support during treatment (Noyes and Popay, 2007). However, this option would not target the fundamental problems that LMICs face in diagnosing TB and its drug-resistant strains and managing the complexities of treatment. Addressing these issues would require a substantial investment in TB diagnostics and drugs.

Research and Development for Tuberculosis Diagnostics and Drugs

Development of new diagnostic tools for TB has seen some progress. The most notable example is the GeneXpert molecular test, which can detect monoresistant, specifically Rifampicin-resistant, TB strains within 2 hours (Lawn et al., 2013; Sharma et al., 2015). Although this tool is highly accurate and has the potential to improve the accuracy and speed of TB diagnosis, it is also costly, which poses a hurdle for its implementation. WHO endorsement of the GeneXpert tool has resulted in donor support, but sustaining its use will fall to national governments. Regardless, rapid diagnostic tests are urgently needed to combat TB (Lawn et al., 2013). Similar to diagnostics, the development of new TB drugs also is needed to improve the outcomes of TB therapy in terms of shortening the length and improving therapy for MDR-TB and XDR-TB. Unfortunately, the new TB drug pipeline is almost empty. Only two new TB drugs (bedaquiline and delamanid) have been approved to treat MDR-TB, which marks the first

---

treatment given under direct and supportive observation, a regular supply of high-quality anti-TB drugs, and standardized recording and reporting), it is mostly known for its direct observation of treatment.

time in more than 50 years that a new drug has been approved for this use (Zumla et al., 2015). Though 16 additional drugs are in preclinical and clinical development (Zumla et al., 2015), research and development for TB drugs is particularly complex due to the need to establish efficacy of a new agent in the context of combination therapy, which can make the clinical phase of development last up to two decades (Ginsberg and Spigelman, 2007). Streamlining the development of TB drugs will require novel research strategies, possibly including the use of biomarkers (discussed in Chapter 7).

U.S. Strategy for Tuberculosis

The U.S. government, through USAID, started its TB program in 1998. Global TB funding has increased since then, and the United States is now the largest international funder for TB, with its bilateral programs reaching more than 50 countries (KFF, 2017b). Since the initiation of its TB program, the U.S. government has contributed to the gains made against TB, saving 37 million lives between 2000 and 2013 (USAID, 2015). The current U.S. policy for global TB is guided by the Global Tuberculosis Strategy: 2015–2019, which assigns clear roles to U.S. government agencies for TB activities. USAID is designated as the lead agency in international TB control, including MDR-TB[21] and XDR-TB; PEPFAR is established as the lead actor for U.S. government response to TB/HIV coinfection; CDC is responsible for providing technical support (surveillance and laboratory networks) to ministries of health and U.S. agencies, in addition to conducting operational research; and the National Institute of Allergy and Infectious Diseases is responsible for U.S. international TB-related research (USAID, 2015). However, the current strategy failed to designate a single entity to direct and coordinate resources. This U.S. TB strategy mirrors WHO's End TB Strategy and has ambitious goals of achieving a 95 percent reduction in TB deaths and a 90 percent reduction in TB incidence by 2035 (USAID, 2015). The U.S. government has also created an MDR-TB–specific strategy, the National Action Plan for Combating Multidrug-Resistant Tuberculosis,[22] which emphasizes improving access to diagnostics and treatment internationally and accelerating research and development for MDR-TB (White House, 2015).

Unfortunately, U.S. funding for global TB has not been commensurate

---

[21] USAID has recently entered into a partnership with Janssen, the company that developed bedaquiline, to guarantee that the company's donations of the MDR-TB drug are implemented effectively into treatment programs in its partner countries (USAID, 2016).

[22] The National Action Plan was developed in response to President Obama's Executive Order 13676 and creates an interagency collaboration between USAID, PEPFAR, CDC, the National Institutes of Health, and the U.S. Department of Defense. It also includes specific goals to curb the burden of MDR-TB in the United States.

with its ambitious goals. Despite $4 billion being authorized under the 2008 Lantos-Hyde Act for FY2009–FY2013 for global TB programs, only 40 percent ever became appropriated (Nieburg and Jackson, 2016) in recent years, and the TB budget has hovered around $230–$240 million annually (KFF, 2017b). Furthermore, funding was contracted in the FY2017 budget request for TB, which was only $195 million, a 19 percent decrease from FY2016 (KFF, 2017a). Although this decrease in funding could be particularly detrimental for low-income countries that rely on international donors for 90 percent of their national TB program financing (WHO, 2016c), it is symptomatic of a broader issue: an underprioritization of TB. Underprioritization is not a sustainable course of action, as it will threaten gains made in key U.S. programs, particularly PEPFAR. Figure 4-1 displays those countries that have a high burden for TB, MDR-TB, and TB/HIV in the center diamond. Of the 14 countries listed, 11 are PEPFAR-supported countries. PEPFAR has allocated an average of $138 million toward integrated TB/HIV treatment programs, but this amounts to only 3 percent of its expenditures (Morrison and Neiburg, 2014). If additional resources and operational changes are not directed toward this need, PEPFAR could lose hard-won gains in the clinical management of HIV (IOM, 2013). To meet the goals set in the current U.S. strategy for TB, a fundamental rethinking is needed regarding the treatment programs deployed, the social interventions used, and the investment in research and development for diagnostics and drugs.

SUMMARY AND RECOMMENDATION

TB has historically been an underprioritized disease, and accordingly has not shown the same progress as HIV/AIDS. In fact, between 2000 and 2015, there was only a 1.4 percent reduction per year in the global incidence of TB and a 2.3 percent reduction per year in global mortality from the disease (WHO, 2016c). TB caused 1.4 million deaths in 2015, thus surpassing HIV/AIDS as the leading cause of death due to an infectious disease. Further complicating global efforts is a rise in drug resistance, with 3.9 percent of all new TB cases being drug-resistant. Treatment for TB, MDR-TB, and XDR-TB is lengthy and complex, and frequently fails. Furthermore, treatment for MDR-TB and XDR-TB can cost up to 100 times as much as treatment for nonresistant TB (Laurence et al., 2015; Nieburg et al., 2015; Pooran et al., 2013). With few drugs available to treat these resistant strains and little research and development on new treatment options, TB and its drug-resistant strains pose a growing threat to the health and health security of all countries, including the United States. Yet while TB has been a priority for the United States and was a focal point in a 2015 National Action Plan for Combating MDR-TB, it has been underprioritized financially.

Of the $4 billion authorized over 5 years under the 2008 Lantos-Hyde Act to implement the strategy, only 40 percent was ever appropriated, with the most recent budget request being reduced even further than previous years to just $195 million (KFF, 2017a; Nieburg and Jackson, 2016).

Conclusion: The threat of TB has been rising in recent decades, and levels of funding have been far short of the amounts needed to address this threat adequately. There are very few drugs or vaccines for TB in the development pipeline, and the growing number of resistant strains will make this threat even more alarming and complex to address if sufficient action is not taken. The U.S. government's underprioritization of TB undercuts its capability to reduce the burden of TB. Given that current strategies for combating the disease are not keeping pace with its burden and complexity, the U.S. government needs to significantly reevaluate its investment in and strategies for dealing with TB.

Recommendation 5: Confront the Threat of Tuberculosis

The U.S. Centers for Disease Control and Prevention, the National Institute of Allergy and Infectious Diseases, and the U.S. Agency for International Development should conduct a thorough global threat assessment of rising tuberculosis (TB) levels, including multidrug-resistant TB and extensively drug-resistant TB. They should then execute a plan of action, including governance structure and priority activities, for developing and investing in new diagnostics, drugs, vaccines, and delivery systems.

MALARIA

Malaria, one of the world's most widespread parasitic diseases, places approximately 3.2 billion people at risk of infection at all times (CDC, 2016c) and resulted in 212 million new cases and 429,000 deaths in 2015 (WHO, 2016d). The WHO African region faces the highest global burden, with 90 percent of cases and 92 percent of deaths. Furthermore, malaria disproportionately affects the poorest and most vulnerable populations (WHO, 2014), which includes pregnant women, infants, and children under 5 years old (WHO, 2017a). In fact, nearly 70 percent of malaria deaths worldwide in 2015 were children under the age of 5 (WHO, 2017a), with a child dying every 30 seconds. Malaria also poses an economic burden both to families and endemic countries. Families can lose more than one quarter of their income due to treatment costs and lost days of work, and malaria costs the African region upward of $12 billion each year in lost productivity (European Alliance against Malaria, 2007; UNICEF, 2004).

Global Commitment to Malaria

Although efforts to control malaria date back to the 19th century, true global commitment began in 1955 when WHO formed the Global Malaria Eradication Program (GMEP), which had ambitious goals to interrupt malaria transmission in all endemic areas, with the exception of sub-Saharan Africa. GMEP's expansive efforts resulted in 143 malaria-endemic countries becoming classified as malaria free in 1978 (Nájera, 2001; RBM, 2011). However, public support waned throughout the 1960s, which resulted in tightening of financial resources for global malaria control. Global support for GMEP became officially withdrawn at the 22nd World Health Assembly in 1969 (Nájera et al., 2011). The lack of public support and financial resources resulted in worldwide resurgence of malaria during the 1980s (RBM, 2011). The resurgence contributed to malaria climbing back up the global agenda, formalized with the launch of the Roll Back Malaria (RBM) partnership in 1998 and the adoption of the Millennium Development Goals (MDGs) in 2000. The political commitment and subsequent influx of funding have contributed to remarkable gains in malaria control. Between 2000 and 2015, 57 countries achieved the MDG of reducing the number of new malaria cases by at least 75 percent (WHO, 2015a). At the same time, the global incidence of malaria declined by 41 percent and global malaria mortality rates declined by 62 percent (WHO, 2016d).

Global Financing of Malaria Control and Elimination

The progress made toward malaria control and elimination since the turn of the century was possible in large part due to increases in financial support, which grew from under $100 million in 2000 (WHO, 2013) to $2.9 billion in 2015 (WHO, 2016d). Despite these increases, global funding for malaria still falls 46 percent short of the $6.4 billion needed to achieve the 2020 goals established by WHO's Global Technical Strategy. In 2015 the majority (68 percent) of funding for global malaria was provided by multilateral and bilateral programs, with the Global Fund accounting for nearly 45 percent of all international assistance. The United States continues to be the single largest international funder for malaria, accounting for approximately 35 percent of total malaria funding in 2015, including both the President's Malaria Initiative (PMI) and contributions to the Global Fund (WHO, 2016d). The remaining 32 percent of funding was provided by governments of endemic countries. Although investing in malaria may seem costly, the cost–benefit analysis modeling the effect of global malaria reduction and elimination found that the net gains in economic output would be worth $208.6 billion (Purdy et al., 2013). These gains would positively affect international travelers and endemic populations alike.

Malaria Elimination and Shrinking the Malaria Map

The success of global malaria programs has raised interest in the concept of malaria elimination, or the reduction of incidence of locally acquired malaria infection to zero as a result of deliberate efforts. This has become a focal point of WHO's Global Technical Strategy 2016–2030 and RBM's Action and Investment to Defeat Malaria 2016–2030. Both of these programs inform the current global malaria strategy, which uses 2015 as a baseline and has the goal of reducing malaria mortality and incidence by 40 percent and eliminating malaria from 10 countries by 2020. The final target of the global malaria agenda is to reduce malaria mortality and incidence by 90 percent and eliminate malaria from 35 countries by 2030 (RBM, 2015; WHO, 2015b). Elimination now is considered to be a realistic goal. In fact, between 2007 and 2013 alone, four countries have been declared malaria free (Newby et al., 2016). At the core of elimination is the idea of "shrinking the malaria map," which stipulates that as the incidence of malaria is reduced at its natural borders,[23] reducing incidence—and thereby achieving elimination—becomes easier in the endemic heartland (Feachem and MEG, 2009; Feachem and Sabot, 2008). That 35 countries have made political commitments toward malaria elimination serves as a testament to its feasibility (Newby et al., 2016).

Challenges

Malaria has suffered from the "out of sight, out of mind" perspective. Past investments in malaria led to reduced deaths, costs, and illness for millions, yet as discussed in Chapter 3, relaxation of mosquito control efforts in several countries resulted in a resurgence of the disease. A severe example occurred in Venezuela, which had eliminated malaria in 1961—one of the first countries to do so (WHO, 2012b)—but experienced a resurgence recently due to its collapsing economy and relaxation of spraying interventions. In addition to maintaining coverage of interventions, it is vital for the global community to maintain a vigilant eye on the growing challenge of drug resistance. As explained in the next paragraph, countries have begun to observe strains of malaria resistant to baseline therapy. If these strains are not contained, they threaten global successes in controlling and eliminating malaria.

[23] The endemic borders of malaria depend on a country's latitude, altitude, and climate. The edges of these borders have lower probability of reintroduction.

The epicenter of drug resistance is the Greater Mekong subregion in Southeast Asia,[24] but it could spread to India and Africa (where the largest burden lies) if governments, funders, and program implementers do not maintain vigilance (Hanboonkunupakarn and White, 2016). In addition to treatment resistance, insecticide resistance has also grown. Although insecticide control relies on four classes of compounds,[25] the pyrethroids are the most commonly used but unfortunately have the most widespread resistance—an issue that especially threatens sub-Saharan Africa (Hemingway et al., 2016; WHO, 2016d). The growing challenge of both types of resistance poses a significant obstacle toward the integrated management of malaria. Unless commitment is maintained and new tools and strategies are developed, further resistance is likely to spread.

Corporate Investments in Malaria

The private sector has played a particularly important role in malaria control and elimination, appreciating that malaria places a tremendous burden on the businesses and workforce in many LMICs. Corporate investments in malaria, which range from direct financing of interventions, to supply-chain strengthening, to workforce capacity support, occur through two approaches: (1) protecting employees and operational site communities and (2) forming broad partnerships with national programs (Brieger, 2013). The majority of direct financing and in-kind donations for malaria have been provided by the oil/gas and minerals industries. For example, ExxonMobil donated $500,000 to establish a malaria diagnostic laboratory in the HopeXchange Medical Center in Kumasi, Ghana (Menka, 2011), and it has also contributed to reducing malaria cases among workers through a chemoprophylaxis compliance testing program (Diara et al., 2012). AngloGold Ashanti developed its own malaria control program focused on indoor spraying in the Obuasi District in Ghana in 2005 that contributed to a 74 percent reduction in malaria cases (Brieger, 2013). Similarly, Kinross Gold Corporation launched a $3.2 million 4-year malaria program in the western region of Ghana to provide vector control interventions and treatment services that resulted in a 45 percent reduction of malaria incidence in the community (Stiles-Ocran, 2013).

---

[24] The Greater Mekong subregion, which comprises Cambodia, China (Yunnan Province), Lao PDR, and Myanmar (Burma), experiences multidrug resistance and insecticide resistance. Due to its geographical heterogeneity and the presence of multiple malaria parasites, the region is notoriously complex for malaria control and elimination. As a result, the Greater Mekong subregion is considered to be one of the most dangerous foci of malaria in Southeast Asia (Cui et al., 2012; WHO, 2016a).

[25] The four classes of insecticides are organochlorides, organophosphates, carbamates, and pyrethroids (WHO, 2016d).

Although multinational companies may have made such investments in isolation at first, now they often invest in coordination through involvement with the Global Business Coalition for Health, which has three key initiatives: leading the Corporate Alliance on Malaria in Africa, which has a membership of 15 companies (CAMA, 2016); serving as the focal point for the Global Fund's Private Sector Delegation (GBCHealth, 2014b); and the Private Sector Constituency of RBM (GBCHealth, 2014a). Because of their affiliation with the Global Business Coalition for Health, member organizations of the Corporate Alliance on Malaria in Africa have a unique interface with the global malaria space. Many of these corporate investments are examples of both social goals and corporate goals being achieved. For diseases such as malaria, which have commitment from multiple angles across the global landscape and can provide opportunity for private-sector involvement both to address the disease burden and help corporations' bottom line, the committee sees a continuing and important role for the private sector in this next stage of global health.

U.S. Commitment: President's Malaria Initiative

As noted, the United States is the single largest international funder for malaria, and in 2016 contributed $861 million for global malaria control, with the majority of the activities being conducted by PMI. Launched in 2005 to assist a set of 15 focus countries that had a high burden of malaria (PMI, 2017a), PMI is directed by the Global Malaria Coordinator within USAID. PMI now provides surveillance, prevention, treatment, research, and health system–strengthening services to 20 partner countries in Africa and Southeast Asia (PMI, 2017a). Through a focus on four key proven interventions,[26] PMI has been able to contribute to a global decline of malaria mortality by 48 percent, a decline of malaria cases by 37 percent, and an avoidance of 6.2 million deaths of children under five in sub-Saharan Africa (PMI, 2016b).

From many accounts, PMI is considered a successful program not only because of its coordination with global partners, but also because of its

---

[26] PMI focuses on four proven interventions: indoor residual spraying, artemisinin-based combination therapy, insecticide-treated mosquito nets and long-lasting insecticide-treated nets, and intermittent preventative treatment for pregnant women (PMI, 2016a). As PMI's approach is focused on achieving results, almost 50 percent of its funding is directed toward purchasing these commodities, including rapid diagnostic tests (Simon et al., 2011). In 2015 alone, PMI procured more than 42 million long-lasting insecticide-treated nets, conducted indoor residual spraying on more than 4 million houses (protecting more than 16 million people), conducted more than 21 million intermittent preventative treatments for pregnant women, and administered more than 57 million artemisinin-based combination therapies and 54 million rapid diagnostic tests (PMI, 2016a).

strong interagency coordination (Simon et al., 2011). Unlike PEPFAR, PMI was launched when the global community had already established a framework for global malaria control and strong institutions, such as RBM and the Global Fund, were already in existence. Thus, PMI was never meant to lead the global response to malaria but rather had donor coordination as a key priority at its inception (Simon et al., 2011). In fact, PMI's decision to partner with its initial 15 focus countries was made because the Global Fund had functioning grants in place (Simon et al., 2011).

PMI has also been successful in coordinating the interagency[27] programs involved in global malaria control. Although this success is partly due to the leadership of the Global Malaria Coordinator, which has been Admiral Timothy Ziemer since PMI's inception, it is also due to the mechanism by which funding is allocated to the agencies involved (Simon et al., 2011). PMI funding decisions start at the country level, where a detailed malaria operation plan is prepared for each year of funding that describes what inputs and activities a national malaria program needs to reach targets. Each malaria operation plan covers the four priority interventions, but the balance among them is determined by the local epidemiology of malaria. After a malaria operation plan is reviewed by the PMI leadership,[28] funds are moved to the implementation level. The process by which this occurs improves the interagency coordination, as allocations are made not only based on the needs of the country but also on the capability of each partner.[29]

Thus, just as with PEPFAR, much of PMI's successes can be linked to the influence of its "presidential" aspect, showing how effective U.S. government programs can be when there is political commitment at the highest level of government, clear targets are set, and agency responsibility and authority are clearly designated.

SUMMARY AND RECOMMENDATION

Remarkable progress has been made in reversing the tide of malaria. From 2000 to 2015, the global community was able to reduce the number

[27] PMI is housed within USAID and coordinates both USAID and CDC for implementing programs. However, it is overseen by an Interagency Advisory Group comprising representatives from USAID, CDC and the U.S. Department of Health and Human Services, the U.S. Department of State, the U.S. Department of Defense, the National Security Council, and the Office of Management and Budget (PMI, 2017a).

[28] The leadership involved with the malaria operation plan review is the PMI Interagency Technical Working Group, the PMI Coordinator, and the PMI Interagency Steering Group (Simon et al., 2011).

[29] Personal communication with Michael Miller, The Kyle House Group, November 11, 2016.

of deaths due to malaria by 62 percent and the incidence of the disease by 41 percent (WHO, 2016d). This progress has been possible in large part as a result of increases in global programmatic and financial support—from \$100 million in 2000 to \$2.9 billion in 2015 (WHO, 2013, 2016d). As a result, elimination of malaria has become a realistic goal, with many countries not only making commitments to elimination but also declaring themselves malaria-free. Much of this progress has been possible through U.S. support, notably through the PMI, which has been praised for its ability to coordinate the interagency response to global malaria; collaborate with global partners; and, most important, deliver results. However, malaria still imposes a major burden of disease, with 212 million cases occurring in 2015 and enormous financial costs for affected families and countries' economies (WHO, 2016d). Furthermore, the global community is witnessing a rise in malaria's resistance to drugs and insecticides, which threatens the hard-won gains that have been achieved.

> *Conclusion: As a result of the continuing threat of malaria, it is vital for the United States to remain engaged in the global fight against the disease. The President's Malaria Initiative (PMI) program has been highly successful within the U.S. Agency for International Development under the leadership of the PMI coordinator. The committee concludes that PMI is a well-designed interagency model that warrants continuous and sustainable funding.*

Recommendation 6: Sustain Progress Toward Malaria Elimination

> **Relevant agencies of the U.S. government should continue their commitment to the fight against malaria through the President's Malaria Initiative and collaborative work with all partners toward elimination of the disease.**

PUBLIC HEALTH COMPLACENCY AND RESISTANCE: A RATIONALE FOR CONTINUED INVESTMENT

There is no doubt that gains have been made against HIV/AIDS, TB, and malaria. Because of the investments by the United States and the global community, HIV is no longer necessarily a death sentence for the poorest in the world, millions of deaths due to TB have been averted, and malaria elimination has become a real possibility for many countries. Maintaining programmatic and financial commitment toward these diseases is vital if these gains are to be sustained. All too often, a reduction of the burden can result in complacency and cause prioritization to subside. Lapses in commitment occurred with both TB and malaria in the mid-1900s, followed by outbreaks and resurgence of both diseases worldwide in the 1980s. These disastrous results were incredibly expensive to reverse, especially for TB. New York City alone spent $1 billion to curb a TB epidemic in the 1990s (Frieden et al., 1993). The ability of these diseases to rebound should serve as a cautionary tale for public health vigilance and as a rationale for continued U.S. investments in PEPFAR, global TB control, and PMI.

HIV/AIDS has thus far not suffered from this cycle of neglect and panic. However, if interest wanes, it is likely that resurgence of HIV will also occur, a predictable but avoidable result. With 9.5 million people directly benefitting from PEPFAR-provided antiretroviral therapy in 2015, and many more secondarily benefitting through decreased rates of HIV transmission, a decrease in PEPFAR funding could be disastrous to the communities that PEPFAR serves. PEPFAR acknowledged this possibility in its 2016 *Annual Report to Congress*, noting that countries like Uganda demonstrate how easily progress can be reversed if continual focus and pandemic control efforts are not maintained (PEPFAR, 2016a).

In addition to the risk of resurgence, sustained involvement is important to contain the spread of antimicrobial resistance. As discussed in the previous sections, resistance has created a global emergency for TB and significantly threatens the progress of integrated malaria control. As national borders become more porous and globalization increases global travel, coordination among neighboring countries becomes vital to contain resistance. This need is most apparent for malaria, as indicated by the massive efforts by PMI and global partners to contain artemisinin and insecticide resistance in the Greater Mekong subregion in Southeast Asia (PMI, 2017b; WHO, 2016b). If resistance in this region were to spread to nearby countries, such as India, or the African continent, progress toward global malaria control efforts could be not only halted but also reversed (Cui et al., 2012). This concern goes beyond just neighboring countries as well, as four patients in the United Kingdom recently recorded failure of frontline drug treatment after returning home from visiting countries in Africa in 2015–2016 (UCLH, 2017).

To finish the work that began decades ago and build the capacity of so many countries, it is important to address the three unfinished agendas for HIV/AIDS, TB, and malaria. However, the rise in resistance for all three diseases threatens the completion of these agendas. Although recent advancements in research and development, such as bedaquiline for MDR-TB, are praiseworthy, a sustained, concerted effort to contain resistance is crucial to ensure that the global community's hard-won gains are not lost. Public health complacency has reversed progress in the past. If the United States and its partners do not want to see history repeat itself, then a continued investment in the agendas of HIV, TB, and malaria is imperative.

REFERENCES

AVERT (AVERTing HIV and AIDS). 2017. *Funding for HIV and AIDS*. http://www.avert.org/professionals/hiv-around-world/global-response/funding (accessed November 15, 2016).

Brieger, W. 2013. *The corporate challenge: Help defeat malaria*. Cambridge, UK: Africa Health.

CAMA (Corporate Alliance on Malaria in Africa). 2016. *Corporate Alliance on Malaria in Africa*. New York: GBCHealth.

CDC (U.S. Centers for Disease Control and Prevention). 2013. Chapter 4: Diagnosis of tuberculosis disease. In *Core Curriculum on Tuberculosis: What the Clinician Should Know*. Atlanta, GA: Centers for Disease Control and Prevention.

CDC. 2016a. *Reported tuberculosis in the United States, 2015*. Atlanta, GA: Centers for Disease Control and Prevention.

CDC. 2016b. *Multidrug-resistant tuberculosis (MDR-TB)*. https://www.cdc.gov/tb/publications/factsheets/drtb/mdrtb.htm (accessed March 3, 2017).

CDC. 2016c. *Impact of malaria*. https://www.cdc.gov/malaria/malaria_worldwide/impact.html (accessed March 7, 2017).

Cegielski, J. P. 2010. Extensively drug-resistant tuberculosis: "There must be some kind of way out of here." *Clinical Infectious Diseases* 50(Supplement_3):S195-S200.

Cohen, J. 2016. AIDS epidemic nears control in three African countries. *Science* 354(6317):1213.

Cui, L., G. Yan, J. Sattabongkot, Y. Cao, B. Chen, X. Chen, Q. Fan, Q. Fang, S. Jongwutiwes, D. Parker, J. Sirichaisinthop, M. P. Kyaw, X. Z. Su, H. Yang, Z. Yang, B. Wang, J. Xu, B. Zheng, D. Zhong, and G. Zhou. 2012. Malaria in the greater Mekong subregion: Heterogeneity and complexity. *Acta Tropica* 121(3):227-239.

Daschle, T., and B. Frist. 2015. *The case for strategic health diplomacy: A study of PEPFAR*. Washington, DC: Bipartisan Policy Center.

Desikan, P. 2013. Sputum smear microscopy in tuberculosis: Is it still relevant? *The Indian Journal of Medical Research* 137(3):442-444.

Diara, M., A. Nowosiwsky, S. Harmen, N. Burke, and M. Alilio. 2012. Enabling factors for improved malaria chemoprophylaxis compliance. *The American Journal of Tropical Medicine and Hygiene* 87(5):960-961.

European Alliance against Malaria. 2007. *Malaria and poverty*. http://www.malariaconsortium.org/userfiles/file/Past%20events/factsheet2%20-%20malaria%20and%20poverty.pdf (accessed March 7, 2017).

Feachem, R., and O. Sabot. 2008. A new global malaria eradication strategy. *The Lancet* 371(9624):1633-1635.

Feachem, R. G. A., and MEG (The Malaria Elimination Group). 2009. Shrinking the malaria map: A guide on malaria elimination for policy makers. San Francisco: The Global Health Group, Global Health Sciences, University of California, San Francisco.

Frieden, T. R., T. Sterling, A. Pablos-Mendez, J. O. Kilburn, G. M. Cauthen, and S. W. Dooley. 1993. The emergence of drug-resistant tuberculosis in New York City. *New England Journal of Medicine* 328(8):521-526.

Frieden, T. R., P. I. Fujiwara, R. M. Washko, and M. A. Hamburg. 1995. Tuberculosis in New York City—turning the tide. *New England Journal of Medicine* 333(4):229-233.

GBCHealth. 2014a. *Roll Back Malaria private sector constituency*. http://www.gbchealth.org/focal-point-roles/roll-back-malaria-private-sector-constituency (accessed February 15, 2017).

GBCHealth. 2014b. *Global Fund private sector delegation*. http://www.gbchealth.org/focal-point-roles/global-fund-private-sector-delegation (accessed February 13, 2017).

Getahun, H., C. Gunneberg, R. Granich, and P. Nunn. 2010. HIV infection–associated tuberculosis: The epidemiology and the response. *Clinical Infectious Diseases* 50(Supplement_3):S201-S207.

Ginsberg, A. M., and M. Spigelman. 2007. Challenges in tuberculosis drug research and development. *Nature Medicine* 13(3):290-294.

Global Fund (Global Fund to Fight AIDS, Tuberculosis and Malaria). 2016. *The Global Fund strategy 2017-2022: Investing to end epidemics.* Geneva, Switzerland: Global Fund to Fight AIDS, Tuberculosis and Malaria.

Global Fund. 2017. *Sourcing & management of health products.* https://www.theglobalfund.org/en/sourcing-management (accessed April 25, 2017).

Green, A. 2016. NIH project focuses on integration of HIV and NCD care. *Lancet* 388(10054):1869.

Hanboonkunupakarn, B., and N. J. White. 2016. The threat of antimalarial drug resistance. *Tropical Diseases, Travel Medicine and Vaccines* 2(1):10.

Harries, A. D., D. Maher, and P. Nunn. 1998. An approach to the problems of diagnosing and treating adult smear-negative pulmonary tuberculosis in high-HIV-prevalence settings in sub-Saharan Africa. *Bulletin of the World Health Organization* 76(6):651-662.

Hemingway, J., H. Ranson, A. Magill, J. Kolaczinski, C. Fornadel, J. Gimnig, M. Coetzee, F. Simard, D. K. Roch, C. K. Hinzoumbe, J. Pickett, D. Schellenberg, P. Gething, M. Hoppé, and N. Hamon. 2016. Averting a malaria disaster: Will insecticide resistance derail malaria control? *The Lancet* 387(10029):1785-1788.

HHS (U.S. Department of Health and Human Services). 2016. *Global statistics.* https://www.aids.gov/hiv-aids-basics/hiv-aids-101/global-statistics (accessed February 1, 2017).

IOM (Institute of Medicine). 2013. *Evaluation of PEPFAR.* Washington, DC: The National Academies Press.

Karumbi, J., and P. Garner. 2015. Directly observed therapy for treating tuberculosis. *The Cochrane Database of Systematic Reviews*(5):1-56.

Kates, J., A. Wexler, and E. Lief. 2016. *Financing the response to HIV in low- and middle-income countries.* Washington, DC: Henry J. Kaiser Family Foundation; UNAIDS.

Kemp, J. R., G. Mann, B. N. Simwaka, F. M. Salaniponi, and S. B. Squire. 2007. Can Malawi's poor afford free tuberculosis services? Patient and household costs associated with a tuberculosis diagnosis in Lilongwe. *Bulletin of the World Health Organization* 85(8):580-585.

Keshavjee, S., and P. E. Farmer. 2012. Tuberculosis, drug resistance, and the history of modern medicine. *New England Journal of Medicine* 367(10):931-936.

KFF (Kaiser Family Foundation). 2017a. *U.S. global health funding: Bilateral tuberculosis (TB), FY2001-FY2017 request.* http://kff.org/global-health-policy/slide/u-s-global-health-funding-global-tuberculosis-tb , July 20. http://www.kff.org/global-health-policy/fact-sheet/the-u-s-government-and-global-tuberculosis-efforts (accessed March 13, 2017).

KFF. 2017b. *The U.S. government and global tuberculosis efforts.* http://www.kff.org/global-health-policy/fact-sheet/the-u-s-government-and-global-tuberculosis-efforts (accessed March 13, 2017).

KFF. 2017c. *The U.S. President's Emergency Plan for AIDS Relief (PEPFAR).* http://kff.org/global-health-policy/fact-sheet/the-u-s-presidents-emergency-plan-for (accessed March 3, 2017).

Laurence, Y. V., U. K. Griffiths, and A. Vassall. 2015. Costs to health services and the patient of treating tuberculosis: A systematic literature review. *Pharmacoeconomics* 33(9):939-955.

Laurenzi, M., A. Ginsberg, and M. Spigelman. 2007. Challenges associated with current and future TB treatment. *Infectious Disorders–Drug Targets* 7(2):105-119.

Lawn, S. D., P. Mwaba, M. Bates, A. Piatek, H. Alexander, B. J. Marais, L. E. Cuevas, T. D. McHugh, L. Zijenah, N. Kapata, I. Abubakar, R. McNerney, M. Hoelscher, Z. A. Memish, G. B. Migliori, P. Kim, M. Maeurer, M. Schito, and A. Zumla. 2013. Advances in tuberculosis diagnostics: The Xpert MTB/RIF assay and future prospects for a point-of-care test. *Lancet Infectious Diseases* 13(4):349-361.

Lima, V. D., R. Granich, P. Phillips, B. Williams, and J. S. G. Montaner. 2013. Potential impact of The U.S. President's Emergency Plan for AIDS Relief on the tuberculosis/HIV coepidemic in selected sub-Saharan African countries. *The Journal of Infectious Diseases* 208(12):2075-2084.

Menka, E. 2011. ExxonMobil Foundation provides $500,000 for malaria diagnosis in Ghana. *Ghana Business News,* July 20. https://www.ghanabusinessnews.com/2011/07/20/exxonmobil-foundation-provides-500000-for-malaria-diagnosis-in-ghana (accessed March 13, 2017).

Morrison, J. S., and P. Neiburg. 2014. *Strategic U.S. leadership—essential to address the global tuberculosis pandemic.* Washington, DC: Center for Stratgic and International Studies.

Nachega, J. B., and R. E. Chaisson. 2003. Tuberculosis drug resistance: A global threat. *Clinical Infectious Diseases* 36(Supplement_1):S24-S30.

Nájera, J. A. 2001. Malaria control: Achievements, problems and strategies. *Parassitologia* 43(1-2):1-89.

Nájera, J. A., M. González-Silva, and P. L. Alonso. 2011. Some lessons for the future from the Global Malaria Eradication Programme (1955–1969). *PLOS Medicine* 8(1):e1000412.

Newby, G., A. Bennett, E. Larson, C. Cotter, R. Shretta, A. A. Phillips, and R. G. A. Feachem. 2016. The path to eradication: A progress report on the malaria-eliminating countries. *The Lancet* 387(10029):1775-1784.

Nieburg, P., and A. Jackson. 2016. *U.S. government roles in control of global tuberculosis: Opportunities for strengthening program effectiveness.* Washington, DC: Center for Strategic and International Studies.

Nieburg, P., T. Dubovi, and S. Angelo. 2015. *Tuberculosis: A complex health threat.* Washington, DC: Center for Strategic and International Studies.

NIH (National Institutes of Health) Fogarty International Center. 2016. *Partnership initiative for health professional education and research in selected PEPFAR countries.* https://www.fic.nih.gov/About/Advisory/Pages/funding-concepts.aspx#partnerhsip (accessed February 15, 2017).

Noyes, J., and J. Popay. 2007. Directly observed therapy and tuberculosis: How can a systematic review of qualitative research contribute to improving services? A qualitative meta-synthesis. *Journal of Advanced Nursing* 57(3):227-243.

OARAC (Office of AIDS Research Advisory Council). 2015. *OARAC meeting minutes.* https://www.oar.nih.gov/oarac/meetings/April_16_2015.asp (accessed December 10, 2016).

Ogden, J., G. Walt, and L. Lush. 2003. The politics of "branding" in policy transfer: The case of DOTS for tuberculosis control. *Social Science and Medicine* 57(1):179-188.

Oomman, N., M. Bernstein, and S. Rosenzweig. 2007. *Following the funding for HIV/AIDS: A comparative analysis of the funding practices of PEPFAR, the Global Fund and World Bank map in Mozambique, Uganda, and Zambia.* Washington, DC: Center for Global Development.

Pasipanodya, J. G., and T. Gumbo. 2013. A meta-analysis of self-administered vs. directly observed therapy effect on microbiologic failure, relapse, and acquired drug resistance in tuberculosis patients. *Clinical Infectious Diseases* 57(1):21-31.

Patel, K. B., R. Belmonte, and H. M. Crowe. 1995. Drug malabsorption and resistant tuberculosis in HIV-infected patients. *New England Journal of Medicine* 332(5):336-337.

Pawlowski, A., M. Jansson, M. Sköld, M. E. Rottenberg, and G. Källenius. 2012. Tuberculosis and HIV co-infection. *PLOS Pathogens* 8(2):e1002464.

PEPFAR (The U.S. President's Emergency Plan for AIDS Relief). 2009. *Guidance for PEPFAR partnership frameworks and partnership framework implementation plans.* Washington, DC: The U.S. President's Emergency Plan for AIDS Relief.

PEPFAR. 2012a. *PEPFAR 3.0—controlling the epidemic: Delivering on the promise of an AIDS-free generation.* Washington, DC: The U.S. President's Emergency Plan for AIDS Relief.

PEPFAR. 2012b. *Report on costs of treatment in the President's Emergency Plan for AIDS Relief (PEPFAR).* Washington, DC: The Office of the U.S. Global AIDS Coordinator and Health Diplomacy, U.S. Department of State.

PEPFAR. 2015. *PEPFAR 2015 annual report to Congress.* Washington, DC: The Office of the U.S. Global AIDS Coordinator and Health Diplomacy, U.S. Department of State.

PEPFAR. 2016a. *PEPFAR 2016 annual report to Congress.* Washington, DC: The Office of the U.S. Global AIDS Coordinator and Health Diplomacy, U.S. Department of State.

PEPFAR. 2016b. *PEPFAR dashboards.* https://data.pepfar.net/global (accessed March 16, 2017).

PEPFAR. 2016c. *PEPFAR funding: Fiscal year 2014-2017.* Washington, DC: The Office of the U.S. Global AIDS Coordinator and Health Diplomacy, U.S. Department of State.

PEPFAR. 2017a. *PEPFAR 2017 annual report to Congress.* Washington, DC: The Office of the U.S. Global AIDS Coordinator and Health Diplomacy, U.S. Department of State.

PEPFAR. 2017b. *Working together for an AIDS-free future for girls and women.* https://www.pepfar.gov/partnerships/ppp/dreams (accessed December 10, 2016).

Petrakos, C. 1993. Catching a killer: Before we were stalked by AIDS, we were menaced by TB. *The Chicago Tribune.* http://articles.chicagotribune.com/1993-08-29/entertainment/9308290161_1_tb-tuberculosis-forgotten-plague (accessed January 18, 2017).

Pietersen, E., E. Ignatius, E. M. Streicher, B. Mastrapa, X. Padanilam, A. Pooran, M. Badri, M. Lesosky, P. van Helden, F. A. Sirgel, R. Warren, and K. Dheda. 2014. Long-term outcomes of patients with extensively drug-resistant tuberculosis in South Africa: A cohort study. *The Lancet* 383(9924):1230-1239.

PMI (President's Malaria Initiative). 2016a. *A decade of progress: Tenth annual report to Congress.* Washington, DC: The President's Malaria Initiative.

PMI. 2016b. *PMI by the numbers.* https://www.pmi.gov/docs/default-source/default-document-library/pmi-reports/pmi-by-the-numbers.pdf (accessed March 15, 2017).

PMI. 2017a. *About.* https://www.pmi.gov/about (accessed March 8, 2017).

PMI. 2017b. *Greater Mekong subregion.* https://www.pmi.gov/where-we-work/mekong (accessed March 19, 2017).

Pooran, A., E. Pieterson, M. Davids, G. Theron, and K. Dheda. 2013. What is the cost of diagnosis and management of drug resistant tuberculosis in South Africa? *PLOS ONE* 8(1):e54587.

Purdy, M., M. Robinson, K. Wei, and D. Rublin. 2013. The economic case for combating malaria. *The American Journal of Tropical Medicine and Hygiene* 89(5):819-823.

RBM (Roll Back Malaria Partnership). 2011. *Eliminating malaria: Learning from the past, looking ahead: Progress and impact series.* Geneva, Switzerland: Roll Back Malaria Partnership.

RBM. 2015. *Action and investment to defeat malaria: 2016-2030.* Geneva, Swizerland: Roll Back Malaria Partnership Secretariat, World Health Organization.

Resch, S., T. Ryckman, and R. Hecht. 2015. Funding AIDS programmes in the era of shared responsibility: An analysis of domestic spending in 12 low-income and middle-income countries. *The Lancet Global Health* 3(1):e52-e61.

Richter, R. 2012. *740,000 lives saved: Study documents benefits of AIDS relief program.* https://med.stanford.edu/news/all-news/2012/05/740000-lives-saved-study-documents-benefits-of-aids-relief-program.html (accessed January 5, 2017).

Shah, N. S., S. C. Auld, J. C. M. Brust, B. Mathema, N. Ismail, P. Moodley, K. Mlisana, S. Allana, A. Campbell, T. Mthiyane, N. Morris, P. Mpangase, H. van der Meulen, S. V. Omar, T. S. Brown, A. Narechania, E. Shaskina, T. Kapwata, B. Kreiswirth, and N. R. Gandhi. 2017. Transmission of extensively drug-resistant tuberculosis in South Africa. *New England Journal of Medicine* 376(3):243-253.

Sharma, S. K., M. Kohli, R. N. Yadav, J. Chaubey, D. Bhasin, V. Sreenivas, R. Sharma, and B. K. Singh. 2015. Evaluating the diagnostic accuracy of Xpert MTB/RIF assay in pulmonary tuberculosis. *PLOS ONE* 10(10):e0141011.

Simon, J., K. Yeboah-Antwi, A. Schapita, M. K. Cham, R. Barber-Maddan, and M. I. Brooks. 2011. *External evaluation of the President's Malaria Initiative: Final report.* Washington, DC: The QED Group LLC, Camris International, Social & Scientific Systems Inc.

Singhal, R., and V. P. Myneedu. 2015. Microscopy as a diagnostic tool in pulmonary tuberculosis. *International Journal of Mycobacteriology* 4(1):1-6.

Stiles-Ocran, J. 2013. *The Chirano Gold Standard: A successful private sector initiative against malaria.* Accra: Chirano Malaria Control Programme.

Sturchio, J. L., and G. M. Cohen. 2012. How PEPFAR's public-private partnerships achieved ambitious goals, from improving labs to strengthening supply chains. *Health Affairs (Millwood)* 31(7):1450-1458.

Suchindran, S., E. S. Brouwer, and A. Van Rie. 2009. Is HIV infection a risk factor for multi-drug resistant tuberculosis? A systematic review. *PLOS ONE* 4(5):e5561.

Tarnoff, C., and M. L. Lawson. 2016. *Foreign aid: An introduction to U.S. programs and policy.* Washington, DC: Congressional Research Service.

UNAIDS (Joint United Nations Programme on HIV/AIDS). 2014a. *90-90-90: An ambitious treatment target to help end the AIDS epidemic.* Geneva, Switzerland: Joint United Nations Programme on HIV/AIDS.

UNAIDS. 2014b. *The gap report.* Geneva, Switzerland: Joint United Nations Programme on HIV/AIDS.

UNAIDS. 2015a. *AIDS by the numbers 2015.* Geneva, Switzerland: Joint United Nations Program on HIV/AIDS.

UNAIDS. 2015b. *How AIDS changed everything—MDG6: 15 years, 15 lessons of hope from the AIDS response.* Geneva, Switzerland: Joint United Nations Programme on HIV/AIDS.

UNAIDS. 2015c. *On the fast-track to end AIDS: UNAIDS strategy 2016-2021.* Geneva, Switzerland: Joint United Nations Programme on HIV/AIDS

UNAIDS. 2015d. *People living with HIV (all ages).* Geneva, Switzerland: Joint United Nations Programme on HIV/AIDS.

UNAIDS. 2016a. *AIDSinfo.* http://aidsinfo.unaids.org (accessed March 1, 2017).

UNAIDS. 2016b. *Fact sheet November 2016.* http://www.unaids.org/en/resources/fact-sheet (accessed December 12, 2016).

UNICEF (United Nations International Children's Emergency Fund). 2004. *Fact sheet: Malaria, a global crisis.* New York: United Nations International Children's Emergency Fund.

University College London Hospitals. 2017. First recorded cases of frontline malaria drug failing to treat UK patients. London, UK: University College London Hospitals.

USAID (U.S. Agency for International Development). 2015. *United States government Global Tuberculosis Strategy: 2015-2019.* Washington, DC: United States Agency for International Development.

USAID. 2016. *USAID's bedaquiline donation program in partnership with Johnson and Johnson.* https://www.usaid.gov/what-we-do/global-health/tuberculosis/technical-areas/bedaquiline-donation-program (accessed March 19, 2017).

Wagner, Z., J. Barofsky, and N. Sood. 2015. PEPFAR funding associated with an increase in employment among males in ten sub-Saharan African countries. *Health Affairs (Millwood)* 34(6):946-953.

Whalen, C., C. R. Horsburgh, D. Hom, C. Lahart, M. Simberkoff, and J. Ellner. 1995. Accelerated course of human immunodeficiency virus infection after tuberculosis. *American Journal of Respiratory and Critical Care Medicine* 151(1):129-135.

White House. 2015. *National Action Plan for Combatting Multidrug-Resistant Tuberculosis.* Washington, DC: The White House.

WHO (World Health Organization). 2001. *Global tuberculosis control report, 2001.* Geneva, Switzerland: World Health Organization.

WHO. 2012a. *"Totally drug-resistant TB": A WHO consultation on the diagnostic definition and treatment options.* Geneva, Switzerland: World Health Organization.

WHO. 2012b. *World malaria report 2012.* Geneva, Switzerland: World Health Organization.

WHO. 2013. *World malaria report 2013.* Geneva, Switzerland: World Health Organization.

WHO. 2014. *World malaria report 2014.* Geneva, Switzerland: World Health Organization.

WHO. 2015a. *World malaria report 2015.* Geneva, Switzerland: World Health Organization.

WHO. 2015b. *Global Technical Strategy for Malaria: 2016-2030.* Geneva, Switzerland: World Health Organization.

WHO. 2016a. *Consolidated guidelines on the use of antiretroviral drugs for treating and preventing HIV infection: Recommendations for a public health approach.* Geneva, Switzerland: World Health Organization.

WHO. 2016b. *Eliminating malaria in the greater Mekong subregion: United to end a deadly disease.* Geneva, Switzerland: World Health Organization.

WHO. 2016c. *Global tuberculosis report 2016.* Geneva, Switzerland: World Health Organization.

WHO. 2016d. *World malaria report 2016.* Geneva, Switzerland: World Health Organization.

WHO. 2017a. *High-risk groups.* http://www.who.int/malaria/areas/high_risk_groups/en (accessed February 10, 2017).

WHO. 2017b. *Tuberculosis and HIV.* http://www.who.int/hiv/topics/tb/en (accessed March 10, 2017).

Zumla, A., J. Chakaya, R. Centis, L. D'Ambrosio, P. Mwaba, M. Bates, N. Kapata, T. Nyirenda, D. Chanda, S. Mfinanga, M. Hoelscher, M. Maeurer, and G. B. Migliori. 2015. Tuberculosis treatment and management: An update on treatment regimens, trials, new drugs, and adjunct therapies. *The Lancet Respiratory Medicine* 3(3):220-234.

PART 2:

ENHANCING PRODUCTIVITY AND ECONOMIC GROWTH

5

Investing in Women's and Children's Health

Significant and long-lasting benefits accrue from investing in the health, quality of life, productivity, and economic growth of women and children. Despite these benefits, glaring gaps must still be filled to reduce the mortality rate, provide equitable access to quality health care among women and children, and improve outcomes for children who survive past the age of 5. Because healthy women and children are the linchpin for healthy and thriving societies (see Figure 5-1), investing in the health of women and children is indispensable to achieving the new Sustainable Development Goals (SDGs) agenda. In low- and middle-income countries (LMICs), providing more education for children, especially girls, can result in greater accumulation of human capital, increased productivity, and increased income and economic development (UNICEF, 2015). In an analysis of multiple countries, a clear correlation was noted between average years of education and poverty rates: For each additional year of education among young adults ages 25–34, national poverty rates were 9 percent lower (UNICEF, 2015). Similarly, a study in Botswana found that each additional year of secondary schooling reduced cumulative human immunodeficiency virus (HIV) infection risk by 8.1 percent (De Neve et al., 2015). Based on such evidence for the connection between education and health, the Global Fund to Fight AIDS, Tuberculosis and Malaria and other HIV and acquired immunodeficiency syndrome (AIDS) organizations have even shown an interest in developing incentives to keep girls in school. The U.S. President's Emergency Plan for AIDS Relief's (PEPFAR's) Determined, Resilient, Empowered, AIDS-free, Mentored, and Safe women (DREAMS) program,

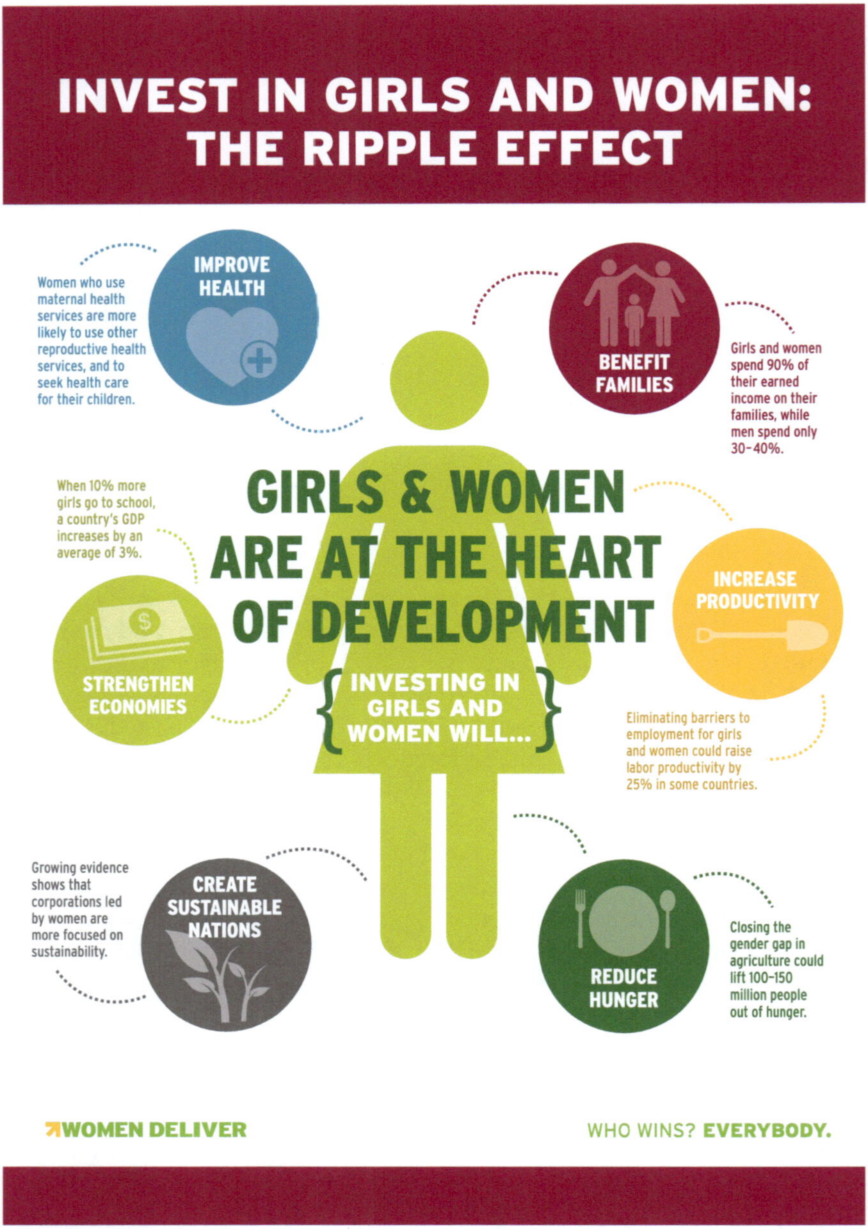
INVEST IN GIRLS AND WOMEN: THE RIPPLE EFFECT
IMPROVE HEALTH
Women who use maternal health services are more likely to use other reproductive health services, and to seek health care for their children.
BENEFIT FAMILIES
Girls and women spend 90% of their earned income on their families, while men spend only 30-40%.
When 10% more girls go to school, a country's GDP increases by an average of 3%.
GIRLS & WOMEN ARE AT THE HEART OF DEVELOPMENT
INCREASE PRODUCTIVITY
STRENGTHEN ECONOMIES
INVESTING IN GIRLS AND WOMEN WILL...
Eliminating barriers to employment for girls and women could raise labor productivity by 25% in some countries.
Growing evidence shows that corporations led by women are more focused on sustainability.
CREATE SUSTAINABLE NATIONS
REDUCE HUNGER
Closing the gender gap in agriculture could lift 100-150 million people out of hunger.
WOMEN DELIVER
WHO WINS? EVERYBODY.

FIGURE 5-1 Invest in girls and women: The ripple effect.
NOTE: GDP = gross domestic product.
SOURCE: Giberson and Taddoni, 2014.

explored in Chapter 4, highlights education key to reducing HIV infections in adolescent girls and young women.

In addition to the education benefits for young adults, children born to more educated mothers are better off financially and are more likely to receive vaccines and rehydration, sleep under insecticide-treated bed nets, and have other good health interventions available to them. Countries where women hold more than 30 percent of seats in political bodies are shown to be more inclusive, equitable, and democratic (USAID, 2015). The benefits of investment in women and children will extend beyond health and translate into increased economic prosperity, strengthened societal bonds, and improved community resilience. These benefits make it a wise investment opportunity for the United States.

This chapter begins by discussing the shift of the global development agenda related to women and children, from the unfinished Millennium Development Goals (MDGs) to the multidisciplinary SDGs, and the current state of their health with a focus on mortality rates. Next, it reviews the current efforts in this area, including those of the U.S. Agency for International Development (USAID), World Health Organization (WHO), and Global Financing Facility (GFF). The chapter then goes through the key themes of the WHO strategy, with a focus on "Survive, Thrive, and Transform," and highlights where gaps still remain in addressing health issues for women and children, and what can be done to accomplish the related targets of the SDGs over the next 15 years.

GLOBAL DEVELOPMENT AGENDA SHIFT: WOMEN AND CHILDREN

The MDGs adopted by world leaders in 2000 set forth the first global goals for women's and children's health, calling for a two-thirds reduction in the mortality rate for children under age 5, a three-quarter reduction in the maternal mortality ratio, and universal access to reproductive health by 2015 (UN, 2015c,d). Much progress has been made on all three fronts. Global mortality rates for children under 5 years were cut by more than half, dropping from 87 to 41 deaths per 1,000 live births between 1990 and 2015 (UN, 2015c). Global rates of maternal mortality were also reduced by nearly 50 percent between 1990 and 2015, from 385 to 216 deaths per 100,000 live births, with most of the reduction happening since 2000 (Kassebaum et al., 2016). Part of this reduction can be attributed to the rise in skilled birth attendants: In 2014, skilled personnel assisted in 71 percent of births globally, which is an increase from 59 percent in 1990 (UN, 2015d).

In spite of this progress, none of the maternal and child health-related goals were met by the time the MDGs expired in 2015, and now the objectives remain a critical unfinished agenda (UN, 2015c,d). The approach to global development has since evolved, shifting in focus to the more cross-sector SDGs. As discussed in Chapter 2, the SDGs were designed to cut across sectors to advance progress more quickly and achieve new global targets by 2030 by attacking issues comprehensively (UN, 2015a). SDG 3—ensure healthy lives and promote well-being for all at all ages—has three targets pertaining directly to women's and children's health:

1. Reduce the global maternal mortality ratio from the current rate, which is 216 maternal deaths for every 100,000 live births (UN, 2015a), to <70 maternal deaths per 100,000 live births.
2. End preventable deaths of newborns and children under 5 years of age in all countries (neonatal mortality: maximum 12/1,000 live births; under-5 mortality: maximum 25/1,000 live births) (UN, 2015a).
3. Ensure universal access to sexual and reproductive health care services, including family planning, information, and education, and the integration of reproductive health into national strategies and programs.

CURRENT STATE OF WOMEN'S AND CHILDREN'S HEALTH

Despite the tremendous strides made in reducing the deaths of women and children, 5.9 million children still die each year before their fifth birthday (WHO, 2016a), with 4.5 million of these dying in their first year of life (WHO, n.d.-a). The vast majority of these deaths are preventable as they are caused by preterm birth complications, pneumonia, and intrapartum-related events (e.g., birth asphyxia) (Liu et al., 2016). Infants and young children who live in LMICs experience a greater risk of death than their peers in wealthier countries and children living in poverty experience a greater risk of poor development. At least 250 million children (43 percent) under 5 years of age in LMICs suffer from suboptimal development, which has substantial short- and long-term negative consequences. These consequences include poorer health in childhood and later in life, lower educational attainment, poorer school performance, less social integration, and lower earning power (estimates suggest that 25 percent of average adult income is lost per year) (Black et al., 2017). These consequences contribute to the perpetuation of poverty and can result in a country's forfeiting up to twice its current gross domestic product (GDP) expenditure on health (Richter et al., 2017). In addition, more than 50 percent of the almost 60 million displaced people, or refugees, documented in 2014 were children—many under 5 years old (Edwards, 2016). The violent and austere environments in which these children live have grave effects on their developmental trajectories and stress response systems, which in turn influence their physical, social, and emotional health.

Almost all (99 percent) of the 303,000 women who die annually from causes related to pregnancy and childbirth die in LMICs (WHO, 2016d). Most of these deaths are preventable with access to appropriate health care, a skilled birth attendant, and the availability of emergency obstetric care (USAID, 2016). The maternal mortality rate in LMICs is 14 times higher than in high-income countries, in part because only half the women in LMICs receive adequate health care (GFF, 2016). However, high maternal mortality is not a problem isolated to LMICs or countries receiving financial assistance. The rate of maternal deaths in the United States jumped from 17.5 per 100,000 live births in 2000 to 26.4 per 100,000 live births in 2015 (Kassebaum et al., 2016). Texas recorded an even higher jump, from 18 maternal deaths per 100,000 live births in 2000 to more than 30 deaths per 100,000 live births in 2014 (MacDorman et al., 2016). These maternal mortality rates put the United States squarely in line with middle-income countries such as Chile, Mexico, and Turkey—clearly highlighting pregnancy- and childbirth-related maternal deaths as an area that would benefit from shared investment with other countries to achieve common solutions for improvement.

CURRENT EFFORTS TO PROMOTE WOMEN'S AND CHILDREN'S HEALTH

The concept of investing in the well-being of women and children is not new, and many organizations have already begun tailoring their programs to specifically address the health needs of women and children based on the evidence and successes of others. Below is a brief review of the women's and children's health activities of a few key organizations engaged in global efforts to promote women's and children's health.

U.S. Agency for International Development

In 2014, USAID's report *Acting on the Call: Ending Preventable Maternal and Child Deaths* operationalized the U.S. government strategy on maternal and child health (USAID, 2016). The aim of USAID's Ending Preventable Maternal and Child Deaths (EPMCD) program is to save the lives of 15 million children and 600,000 mothers by 2020 in 24 priority countries (USAID, 2016). To reach this goal, USAID's investments focus on the provision of routine immunizations; equity of care for childhood illnesses such as malaria, pneumonia, and diarrhea; family planning; maternal and newborn health; nutrition; and water, sanitation, and hygiene. Scaling up coverage of 11 of these innovations was projected to prevent up to

6 million maternal and child deaths (PATH, 2016). In 2016, total funding for the EPMCD program was $2.4 billion (USAID, 2016). Between 2012 and 2015, the average annual rate of reduction of under-5 deaths was 3.6 percent, which is short of the 4.1 percent required to meet the original MDG target. Furthermore, as of 2016, only 19 countries were on track to achieve the SDG's under-5 mortality target by 2030 (USAID, 2016). Given these findings, the committee sees an opportunity for USAID to accelerate implementation of the EPMCD program to achieve unfinished maternal and child health MDG targets by 2020 and under-5 targets by 2030. Strategies should focus on ensuring the highest impact through scaling innovative approaches, with rigorous monitoring and evaluation, with a focus on immunization; integrated management of child illness, nutrition, and prenatal care; and increasing access to contraceptives, including family planning.

World Health Organization

A new global agenda, WHO's Global Strategy for Women's, Children's, and Adolescents' Health (2016–2030), aims to support countries in finishing the unfinished MDG targets (WHO, 2016b). WHO's Global Strategy adopts a life-course perspective guided by a cross-cutting three-part framework: survive, thrive, and transform.[1] Several of the Global Strategy goals overlap with the SDGs' health-related targets (WHO, 2016b). In the survive domain, for example, targeted reductions in global rates of maternal, newborn, and under-5 mortality are aligned with SDG Goal 3. The thrive domain calls for ending all forms of malnutrition and addressing the nutritional needs of children, adolescent girls, and pregnant and lactating women (which is aligned with SDG Goal 2); ensuring universal access to sexual and reproductive health care services; substantially reducing pollution-related deaths and illnesses; and achieving universal health coverage. In the transform domain, the target of achieving universal and equitable access to safe drinking water, sanitation, and hygiene is aligned with SDG Goal 6.

Global Financing Facility

Achieving the SDG targets will require closing the $33.3 billion funding gap for reproductive, maternal, newborn, child, and adolescent health in high-burden LMICs (GFF, 2016). The GFF, the financing arm of Every

[1] The framework spans health-related domains as well as other areas such as promoting education for women, establishing legal identities, and eliminating gender-based discrimination and violence.

Woman Every Child,[2] was launched in 2015 and it seeks to address this funding gap in 63 target countries by supporting country-led efforts to build equitable and resilient health systems and promote long-term sustainable financing (Claeson, 2017). Furthermore, GFF establishes high-impact, evidence-based interventions unique to each country that have measurable results (Claeson, 2017). To help countries implement these interventions, GFF serves as an innovative financing pathfinder, shifting the focus from traditional development assistance toward four strategies: improving efficiency, increasing domestic resource mobilization, increasing and better aligning external financing, and leveraging private-sector resources (Claeson, 2017). Establishing GFF platforms in all high-burden countries by 2030 has the potential to prevent up to 3.8 million maternal deaths, 101 million child deaths, and 21 million stillbirths (GFF, 2016). This program has been met with optimism and excitement for the progress it can induce, but because it is so new, it is too difficult to assess yet, though the committee also remains hopeful for its success.

Opportunities for Investment and Intervention

Although gaps still exist in spite of widespread investments by various stakeholders, simple interventions without a large increase in cost can be implemented to address mother and child health issues. A strong evidence base supports the choice of interventions for the prevention of maternal and child deaths, with the current challenge found in the implementation and scaling up of these interventions. The programs described above largely continue to exclude adolescent girls, except when they are pregnant. A more effective strategy would be to focus on the life course, encouraging nutrition and health promotion for infants, children, adolescent girls, and women throughout adulthood, whether or not they are pregnant. In the sections below, the committee reviews the three key elements of WHO's Global Strategy's framework—survive, thrive, and transform—and offers potential investment and intervention strategies.

SURVIVE: CONTINUING TO DECREASE MORTALITY RATES

To continue the forward progress of the MDGs and address the weaknesses that prevent the elimination of preventable maternal and child

[2] Every Woman Every Child is a global movement that puts into action WHO's Global Strategy for Women's, Children's, and Adolescent's Health. Launched by the UN Secretary-General in 2010, Every Woman Every Child aims to mobilize national governments, international organizations, the private sector, and civil society to solve the health issues that women, children, and adolescents face around the world (Every Woman Every Child, 2016).

deaths, it is important to understand the remaining barriers in the current burden of disease in children and women. During the past 15 years, the most important successes in reducing child and maternal mortality have been through immunizations; improved sanitation; and social changes, such as improved access to voluntary family planning methods, that allow women to thrive and take charge of their own decision making (Bustreo and Mpanju-Shumusho, 2016).

Mortality Among Children Under 5 Years of Age

Immunizations alone are estimated to save 2 to 3 million lives per year (Bustreo and Mpanju-Shumusho, 2016). These advancements have, to a degree, shifted some of the causes of under-5 deaths globally since 1990, so that death rates caused by diseases such as measles have dropped by 65.5 percent (Wang et al., 2016). However, many of the causes of under-5 mortality remain the same. Preterm birth, neonatal encephalopathy, and lower respiratory infections remain in the top five causes of death in children globally, with preterm birth being the leading cause in 2015[3] (Wang et al., 2016). Additionally, environmental hazards such as air pollution, unsafe water, poor sanitation, and secondhand smoke are now found to be responsible for 26 percent of the nearly 6 million deaths each year of children under 5 years of age (WHO, 2017b). Undernutrition is linked to nearly half of all under-5 deaths (Black et al., 2017). Many of these deaths occur in regions nearly untouched by the lifesaving interventions and societal changes that have allowed such robust progress in other parts of the world. Children in rural areas are still 1.7 times more likely to die before their fifth birthday than children in urban areas, and children of mothers with no education are three times more likely to die than children with mothers who have a secondary or higher education (UN, 2015c).

Examining preterm birth as one of the top causes of death and disability in children highlights a need for an improvement in health care services for babies and their mothers, especially in LMICs, and also explains the important interplay between women's health and children's health. Preventing preterm birth requires both antenatal and postnatal care systems. Preterm birth complications can be prevented and addressed with cost-effective strategies provided by adequately trained midwives; these strategies can reduce prematurity by 24 percent (WHO, 2016e). Additionally, the healthy

[3] The top 20 causes of death for children under-5 are preterm birth, neonatal encephalopathy, lower respiratory infections, diarrheal diseases, congenital anomalies, malaria, neonatal sepsis, other neonatal disorders, protein-energy malnutrition, meningitis, sexually transmitted diseases, HIV/AIDS, hemoglobinopathies, measles, drowning, whooping cough, road injuries, neonatal hemolytic disease, encephalitis, and intestinal infections.

spacing of children plays an important role in the reduction of neonatal and under-5 deaths. Among the urban poor in LMICs, children born within 18 months of an older sibling are two times as likely to die, and children born between 18 and 23 months after an older sibling are 18 percent more likely to die as compared to children born 36 months after an older sibling (Fotso et al., 2013). Ensuring that mothers have access to modern contraceptives and birth spacing information will help to alleviate the burden of infant and under-5 deaths and increase the chance of childhood survival because the child does not have to compete for scarce resources, and also may reduce the likelihood of maternal depletion[4] (Fotso et al., 2013).

Maternal Mortality and Morbidity

Although unsafe abortion and hemorrhage remain among the most frequent causes of maternal mortality in low-income countries (Say et al., 2014), the underlying causes of maternal mortality worldwide have become more complex. Almost one-third of global maternal deaths now result from causes not directly related to pregnancy, including HIV/AIDS, malaria, cardiovascular disease, diabetes, and obesity. In the modern context of this disease burden, midwives and other deliverers of health care services face the additional task of addressing the health needs of pregnant women with chronic illnesses. In addition to causing greater risks for mothers, noncommunicable diseases (NCDs) or unhealthy lifestyles cause significant risks for the newborn. Mothers who smoke, for example, are likely to breastfeed for shorter periods of time, have less milk, and produce milk that is less nutritious; additionally, their secondhand tobacco smoke increases the risk of respiratory infections, sudden infant death syndrome, and asthma in their children (WHO, 2010). The goal of allowing more children to survive is contingent on having adequate health care systems for mothers that can provide care and support for routine pregnancies as well as high-risk ones.

Although the world has not yet reached the MDG 5—A goal of reducing maternal mortality by 75 percent (achieving fewer than 70 deaths per 100,000 live births), the gains that have been made allowed for women to have greater access to trained health care workers during pregnancy. As the world transitions to the SDGs, the improvement in access can provide an entry point for an integration of primary care services for reproductive-aged women. Just as many women in the United States ask their obstetricians questions relating to primary care, women in LMICs can likewise benefit from receiving primary care services during antenatal visits. This integra-

[4] Maternal depletion syndrome (MDS) is defined as poor maternal health and infant health in LMICs encompassing successive pregnancies, suggesting that short interbirth intervals create poor maternal health and pregnancy outcomes (Winkvist et al., 1992).

tion will be particularly important as the burden of disease in women shifts to NCDs, because women who are sick are more likely to give birth to babies who are sick: For example, babies born from diabetic mothers are more likely to develop respiratory problems than babies born from non-diabetic mothers (Lee, 2017). An integrated health care system that lowers the incidence of NCDs in reproductive-aged women will improve women's health overall and will allow women to give birth to healthier babies.

In addition to the management of physical health, ensuring the availability of mental health services is of utmost importance to ensure the health and safety of women and their babies; integrating these services in the primary care setting will increase the likelihood that women will take advantage of and benefit from them. It is known that prenatal depression in women is a major risk factor for postnatal depression, which has significant negative effects on the functioning of the mother and health of her baby. Prenatal and postnatal depression in mothers is linked to a higher risk of preterm birth, low birth weight, infant undernutrition, and increased disease incidence in their children (Shidhaye and Giri, 2014). Living in resource-poor areas and receiving poor family support exacerbates these risks (Shidhaye and Giri, 2014). Offering mental health services to women as they receive antenatal visits will help women avoid incurring extra costs to reach a specialized facility (Honikman et al., 2012). One study in South Africa revealed that among 5,407 women who received a mental health screening in a primary care setting during an antenatal visit, 32 percent were referred to an on-site counselor, and 62 percent of those who were referred agreed to receive services (Honikman et al., 2012). In a follow-up, 87.8 percent of women who received counseling services reported an improvement in their presenting problem, and 97.1 percent reported the experience as positive (Honikman et al., 2012). Treatment for maternal depression is feasible and provides significant benefits to the entire family. Offering these services at the primary-care level will decrease the barriers to receiving care and can promote healthier pregnancies in women.

Targeting Interventions to Maximize Survival

Although the scope of challenges across the entire sector of women's and children's health is extremely broad, many evidence-based practices and interventions can have a high level of impact in a cost-effective manner. The committee has selected five key areas (described in the sections below) in which it suggests investment and attention in order to maximize rates of survival for pregnant women and children: immunizations; integrated management of childhood illness; nutrition for pregnant women, newborns, infants, and children; keeping pregnant women safe; and access to contraceptives.

Immunizations

Immunizations are recognized as a "best buy" for global health, estimated to save 2 to 3 million lives each year. In one case—smallpox—vaccination led to disease eradication. Increased coverage of the measles vaccination alone is estimated to have saved 14 million lives since 2000 (Bustreo and Mpanju-Shumusho, 2016). However, infections leading to pneumonia and diarrhea—that could be prevented through immunization—are still some of the top contributors to mortality for children under 5. WHO estimates there are 1.5 million vaccine-preventable child deaths every year, 75 percent of which result from pneumococcus, *Haemophilus influenzae* serotype b (Hib), and rotavirus diarrhea (Gavi, 2015).

Global coverage for pneumococcal vaccine has reached only 35 percent of children under 5, and even that number is sometimes reduced because of supply issues (Gavi, 2015). Rotavirus coverage numbers are slightly lower with just 23 percent coverage (WHO, 2016c), also due to supply concerns and ill-equipped immunization systems in some countries. Although global coverage of three doses of Hib vaccine is estimated to be 64 percent, there is great variability across regions. In the Americas this number is as high as 90 percent, yet the Western Pacific only has 25 percent coverage (WHO, 2016c). To reach child mortality targets, it will be critical to scale up coverage for these three vaccines. Since its establishment in 2000, Gavi, the Vaccine Alliance (Gavi), has employed innovative mechanisms (discussed further in Chapter 8) to increase vaccination coverage and subsidize the costs of new vaccines that lack a commercial market. Additionally, it has established groups focused on pneumococcus, Hib, and rotavirus—the top three most frequent causes of pneumonia and diarrhea (Greenwood, 2014). As a result of these groups partnering with country governments, ministries of health and finance, and nongovernmental organizations (NGOs), there has been rapid introduction of the Hib and pneumococcal vaccines (Greenwood, 2014). As barriers to vaccination are better understood, strategies will be needed to address the inequities that contribute to disparities in access for vulnerable populations.

Integrated Management of Childhood Illness

Historically, treatment of the top causes of death among children (e.g., neonatal causes, diarrhea, pneumonia, AIDS, and malaria) occurred within vertical programs. In the 1990s, there was a push for integrated management of the sick child. Integrated Management of Childhood Illness (IMCI) was developed in 1995 by WHO and the United Nations Children's Fund to promote health and provide preventive and curative services for children under 5 in countries with high child mortality rates (WHO, 2016f). The approach focused on three key components of improving case management skills of health care staff, overall health systems, and family and community health practices. IMCI was expected to increase the probability that children would receive treatment for all major diseases and decrease the possibility that children would receive correct treatment for one disease and die from another unrecognized illness (Victora et al., 2006). In this integrated system, children are screened for risk factors, signs, and symptoms of the key diseases listed previously and treated based on needs. For proper management, children should be assessed for malnutrition, anemia, and vaccination status. Parents and caregivers of low-weight children receive nutrition counseling. Varying levels of classification are assigned based on needs, and children are discharged as those classifications designate. Evaluations of this approach have shown some reductions in child mortality and improved quality of care, but IMCI needs to be complemented with efforts to redesign and strengthen the health system, and significant reductions in mortality will not be realized until widespread intervention coverage is achieved (WHO, 2016f). Additionally, childhood mortality reductions were found to be limited when a country's approach lacked an emphasis on equity, community engagement, and linkages across sectors (e.g., water and sanitation or education).

Nutrition for Pregnant Women, Newborns, Infants, and Children

Children who survive undernutrition have diminished wellness and productivity trajectories, contributing up to a 12 percent reduction in a country's GDP (Soe-Lin et al., 2016). Because a child's nutrition starts in utero, maternal undernutrition has significant consequences for that child's future growth, health, and development (Black et al., 2013). The threat of stunting as a result of undernutrition is most serious in the 1,000 days from conception until the age of 2; this window is vital because the negative effects of undernutrition on the brain and on future development cannot be remediated (USAID, 2014). Consequently, the committee has identified nutritional interventions as possessing great potential not only for continuing to decrease the mortality rates of infants and young children, but for improving their developmental trajectories. Among many successful programs is USAID's Multi-Sectoral Nutrition Strategy, which targets its nutritional interventions to pregnant women and their children during the first 1,000 days (USAID, 2014). Through their interventions at several levels, the committee encourages the continuation of these cross-cutting efforts.

Ensuring babies are born at adequate birth weight starts with the mother's nutrition, even before she gets pregnant. Making certain that pregnant women have access to adequate food will ensure that the baby has nutrients to grow and develop in utero (USAID, 2014). The Multi-

Sectoral Nutrition Strategy addresses women's nutritional needs by increasing women's access to high-quality nutrition services to ensure they gain adequate weight during pregnancy, avoid anemia, and, for women with HIV, safely breastfeed after the baby is born (USAID, 2014).

One of the most widely supported interventions for nutrition after the baby is born is exclusive breastfeeding, including the provision of colostrum in the first few hours and days of a baby's life (Black et al., 2008; WHO, 2017a). In the 2016 *Lancet* series Breastfeeding, researchers found that the deaths of 823,000 children and 20,000 mothers each year could be averted through universal breastfeeding (Victora et al., 2016). Breastfeeding is essential to child survival in part because of its unique biological contribution to the child's immune response (Victora et al., 2016). Similar to the added benefits of sufficient nutrition for young children, breastfeeding can contribute to long-term positive effects such as reduction of the risk of diabetes and obesity later in life, as well as higher cognitive performance. A study in Brazil that followed participants for 30 years found a positive association with breastfeeding and adult earnings—roughly 20 percent of the average income level (Victora et al., 2015). The majority of this effect (72 percent) was explained by the direct benefits of breastfeeding on intelligence. The benefits of breastfeeding also extend to the mothers, and include a reduction in incidence of breast cancer, improvement in birth spacing, and possible reductions in women's risk of diabetes and ovarian cancer (Victora et al., 2016).

In addition to breastfeeding, micronutrient supplementation is a key intervention to improve maternal, infant, and child health. Ensuring mothers and children receive adequate nutrients will help them stay healthy, which has lasting effects on development. Iron and folate deficiencies, for example, which are two of the most common causes of anemia during pregnancy, can lead to pregnancy complications as well as poor development consequences for the baby (Darnton-Hill and Mkparu, 2015). Children need diversity as well as adequate amounts of nutrient-rich foods after the breastfeeding stage (USAID, 2014). Vitamin A, for example, is extremely important for the eyesight of mothers and children, as well as the immune system development of young children (WHO, n.d.-b). However, it is estimated that 250 million preschool children will be vitamin A deficient, leading to about 250,000 to 500,000 children losing their eyesight every year (WHO, n.d.-b). Supplementation with vitamin A keeps children healthy and is known to significantly reduce mortality for children under 5 years (USAID, 2014), and it keeps women healthy in the final trimester, when the demand for vitamin A is highest for the mother and unborn child (WHO, n.d.-b). USAID's Multi-Sectoral Nutrition Strategy seeks to improve intake of micronutrients, including vitamin A, by increasing the availability and quality of nutrient-rich foods for women, who in many contexts receive less food than other members of the family (USAID, 2014).

Nutrition interventions delivered via community health workers can be a key resource for reducing nutrition-related maternal, infant, and child mortality. For example, community health workers in rural Uganda decreased nutrition-related morbidity and mortality simply by offering health information to families with children under 5 years and encouraging families to attend health outreach activities (USAID, 2014). The community health worker, then, has the opportunity to build trust with mothers during pregnancy and immediately after birth to ensure a mother is empowered to make proper nutritional decisions for herself and her child, and can then follow the mother as the child grows and develops.

Keeping Pregnant Women Safe: Prenatal Care, Safe Delivery, and Access to Emergency Obstetrical Care

Although the number of women who die each year from pregnancy and childbirth complications has fallen by nearly half in the past 20 years, 303,000 women still die every year from these causes (WHO, 2016d). Almost all these deaths could be prevented if these women had access to skilled care, good hygiene, and available drugs to manage conditions (such as preeclampsia) caused by high-risk pregnancies (Bustreo and Mpanju-Shumusho, 2016). Various interventions during the prenatal period are relatively simple, such as the provision of supplements like iron and folic acid; exercising safely during pregnancy; and, more recently, a booster vaccine to protect against pertussis[5] to give protective benefits to the unborn child. With so many comorbidities contributing to more complex pregnancies, expanding the scope of training and skills for midwives and skilled birth attendants to include knowledge about hypertension, healthy nutrition, and other lifestyle factors can enhance the delivery of simple, life-saving interventions to women at risk of complex pregnancy and delivery.

Worldwide, at least 15 percent of pregnancies result in complications that require emergency obstetric care, including surgical management, and an estimated 951 million women are without access to this type of care (Meara et al., 2015). In 2010, the collective disability for all measured maternal disorders reached 16 million disability-adjusted life years, of which 3.3 million were attributed to maternal hemorrhage, 1.8 million to complications of obstructed labor, and 1.3 million to maternal sepsis (Murray et al., 2012). These numbers indicate the tremendous morbidity associated with surgically preventable obstetric complications that can be targeted worldwide.

Two interventions will have a major impact in reducing the toll of maternal death and disability: the presence of a trained attendant at every

[5] This vaccine (Tdap) provides protection against tetanus, diphtheria, and pertussis (CDC, 2016).

birth and access to urgent obstetric care at every birth. Increasing the number of women giving birth in a facility or with a skilled attendant has been challenging, but rates are on the rise. One study in Tanzania showed that using simplified ultrasound scanning at the lowest levels of care led to mothers' increased attendance for future antenatal care and increased chances of a facility delivery (Mbuyita et al., 2015). This finding was reinforced with the finding that paraprofessionals with minimal training can perform sonographic procedures on rural pregnant women in Tanzania with consequent beneficial effects (Bellagio Study Group on Child Survival, 2003). A report from the *Lancet* Commission on Global Surgery determined that all people should have timely access to emergency surgical services, which includes the ability to "access, within 2 [hours], a facility that can do caesarean delivery. . . . 2 [hours] is a threshold of death from complications of childbirth" (Meara et al., 2015, p. 608). Several studies have shown that with the exception of very few countries, devoting appropriate financial resources to cesarean delivery, for example, could combat the catastrophic health consequences to mothers in an economically favorable fashion (Meara et al., 2015).

A combined set of relatively simple interventions integrated with appropriate task shifting and work force training within a functioning health system may have a tremendous effect on the overall well-being of any LMIC. Interventions should be aimed at streamlining care so that women in need of an emergent cesarean delivery are aware of facilities available, are properly diagnosed, can be transported to a referral hospital within a reasonable amount of time, and undergo safe cesarean delivery in a capable facility.

Access to Contraceptives

Access to modern contraceptives is a critical foundation for maternal and child health, according to the *Lancet* series Maternal Health (Ceschia and Horton, 2016). Preventing unwanted pregnancy, family planning, and delaying of pregnancy through healthy birth spacing are critical actions to reduce both maternal and infant death, as well as provide other health benefits to women (Ahmed et al., 2012). An analysis of 172 countries showed that family planning prevents approximately 272,000 maternal deaths worldwide each year (Ahmed et al., 2012). Countries with the highest maternal mortality burden also have low contraceptive prevalence rates. In many of these countries, the unmet need for contraception is even higher than the prevalence of contraceptive use (Ahmed et al., 2012). The London Summit on Family Planning (the FP2020 initiative) in 2012 committed countries to providing access to contraceptives to an additional 120 million women by 2020, requiring 15 million to gain access each year (Ceschia and

Horton, 2016). As of October 2016, 8 million additional women are accessing modern contraceptive methods each year. Though they are off track for achieving the goal, the FP2020 initiative has increased contraceptive users by 30.2 million since 2012, putting the total at 300 million in the world's 69 poorest countries, a huge milestone. As a result of this increase in contraceptive use, between July 2015 and July 2016, the FP2020 initiative estimated that globally, 82 million unintended pregnancies were prevented, 25 million unsafe abortions were averted, and 124,000 maternal deaths were averted (FP2020, 2016).

At a more granular level, when contraceptive prevalence in Kazakhstan increased by 50 percent between 1990 and 2000, abortion rates decreased by 50 percent in the same time frame (Westoff, 2000). More recently, a study in Ghana found that lack of access to contraceptives likely caused the observed 12 percent increase in rural pregnancies, leading to 200,000 additional abortions and more than 500,000 additional unwanted births (Jones, 2011). The researchers also found the unwanted children were less likely to have proper nutrition and development (Jones, 2011). Moving forward, the challenge will be examining country-level inequities and issues and understanding why some countries have been quick to implement this commitment to contraception access, while others lag behind.

The United States has long supported international family planning and population issues, and it is the largest donor to global family planning and reproductive health efforts. The Senate Appropriations Committee, with bipartisan support, recently approved its version of a fiscal year (FY) 2017 U.S. Department of State foreign operations appropriations bill that funds the operations of the U.S. government's foreign assistance program, including international family planning and reproductive health (PAI, 2016). This continued support will be critical to achieve the maternal and child health-related SDG targets.

SUMMARY AND RECOMMENDATION

Despite the tremendous strides made in reducing mortality among women and children, nearly 6 million children still die annually before their fifth birthday, and an estimated 303,000 women die each year from preventable pregnancy- and childbirth-related causes (WHO 2016a,d). Maternal mortality stands at 216 per 100,000 births, while child deaths are at 41 per 1,000 live births (Kassebaum et al., 2016; UN, 2015c). Investing in women and children yields proven short- and long-term benefits for a country's economy. USAID has increased its investments in reducing maternal, newborn, and child deaths and recently launched the Ending Preventable Maternal and Child Death initiative, but gaps still exist with respect to subnational inequity in access to care. Many of the causes of death that still plague both women and children are preventable; for example, undernutrition is linked to nearly half of all deaths of children under 5 (Black et al., 2017). Extremely strong evidence supports the most effective interventions for preventing maternal and child deaths, yet the remaining challenge is to implement and scale up these interventions in locations that have the highest level of need.

> *Conclusion: Current mortality rates for both mothers and children under age 5 are still unacceptably high. Sustained investments in cost-effective, evidence-based interventions are needed to prevent the deaths of infants, children, adolescents, and pregnant and lactating women.*

Recommendation 7: Improve Survival in Women and Children

> **Congress should increase funding for the U.S. Agency for International Development to augment the agency's investments in ending preventable maternal and child mortality, defined as global maternal mortality rates of fewer than 70 deaths per 100,000 live births by 2020 and fewer than 25 child deaths per 1,000 live births by 2030. Investments should focus on the most effective interventions and be supported by rigorous monitoring and evaluation. These priority interventions include**
>
> - **immunizations;**
> - **integrated management of child illness;**
> - **nutrition (pregnant women, newborns, infants, children);**
> - **prenatal care and safe delivery, including early identification of at-risk pregnancies, safe delivery, and access to emergency obstetrical care; and**
> - **access to contraceptives and family planning.**

THRIVE: MEETING DEVELOPMENT POTENTIAL AND BUILDING COUNTRY FUTURES

In LMICs, 250 million children (43 percent of the population) younger than 5 years do not reach their developmental potential because of extreme poverty and stunting (Black et al., 2017). Saving lives is critical, but simply keeping children from dying around the world is not enough. As child mortality declines, the focus correctly shifts to thriving, or maximizing the cognitive, language, and emotional development of children. In addition to developmental interventions, efforts must also include nurturing care, that is, the supportive environment in which a child grows and develops.

Nurturing care is a core principle underlying the support for children to thrive (Britto et al., 2017). This concept is realized by having a stable home environment that is sensitive to children's health and nutritional needs, responsive, emotionally supportive, and developmentally stimulating and appropriate, with opportunities for play and exploration and protection from adversities (Britto et al., 2017). Such early child development practices translate into significant lifelong benefits in terms of labor market participation and earnings (Richter et al., 2017). Early and continued investments in children can help them grow and develop into healthy and productive adults, ultimately contributing to economic growth.

Links Between Adverse Childhood Experiences and Diminished Adult Outcomes

Children who live in poverty in LMICs and are exposed to negative stressors such as violence or abuse are subject to many repercussions into adulthood (Currie and Vogl, 2013). Research continues to emerge on the strong links between adverse childhood experiences and physical, emotional, and social outcomes in adulthood. When children are exposed to violence or abuse at a young age, their brains are physically altered by the stress, and their executive functioning is adversely affected (Hertzman and Boyce, 2010). Children with greater exposure to violence may grow up to become perpetrators of violence or revictimized in adulthood (Moylan et al., 2010; Widom et al., 2008). The documented associations between low socioeconomic status in early childhood and brain development (Noble et al., 2015) may explain the well-established associations between poverty and low cognitive, academic, and behavioral performance (Hair et al., 2015). These long-term effects of early life experiences make it critically important for service providers and stakeholders to change their thinking to accurately target interventions and services to prevent and mitigate those problems.

Scientific evidence supports the notion that the period from conception to age 3 years is a crucial time for interventions (Black et al., 2017). The early years in a child's life are critical for investments for physical growth and cognitive and socioemotional development. For example, the association of linear growth and cognitive development is stronger for children under 2 than for older children, although the association appears to persist beyond the first 2 years of a child's life (Sudfeld et al., 2015). Gearing assistance and evidence-based interventions for young children toward their physical, cognitive, and social-emotional development offers clear long-term returns on investment.

Fostering Positive Environments for Children and Families

The social, economic, political, climatic, and cultural context can provide broad support and guidance for the implementation of family-friendly systems that enable nurturing care to support children best (Britto et al., 2017). Positive and healthy environments for children and families should be prioritized. For example, social protection programs are designed to reduce poverty and provide opportunities to improve child development (Britto et al., 2017). Supportive environments are then likely to extend past the individual and immediate family and often create a ripple effect throughout the community. Previous attempts to create packages of effective interventions have focused either on grouping interventions because they should happen at the same time (e.g., packaging interventions that co-occur during the same age period of the child) or packaging interventions that are delivered through the same system (e.g., maternal health). The recent *Lancet* series Early Child Development proposed a set of packages that consider these factors while also incorporating nurturing care and protection and tailoring the packages to unique sets of risks and adversities that characterize complex environments (Britto et al., 2017). The packages proposed in the review are

- family support and strengthening (i.e., increasing access to quality care, building skills, and providing social-sector support);
- "caring for the caregiver" (i.e., caring for and protecting the parent's physical and mental health with a life-cycle approach); and
- early learning and protection package (i.e., supporting parents, teachers, and caregivers in learning programs) (Britto et al., 2017).

Promoting positive environments for children and families often does not require new services or programs, but instead demands the integration of existing programs, structures, and systems of service delivery under a more holistic lens. This integration should be considered across health care and social services, nurturing care and parenting support, violence prevention and mitigation, poverty assistance, and early childhood education.

Health Care and Social Services

Maternal and newborn health programs should be designed and conducted as an integrated whole, rather than separate programs for two types of patients, as is currently the case in many places. The *Lancet* series Maternal Mortality recently found that linking health care for a mother and her baby not only promotes greater efficiency and lowers costs, but also maximizes the effect on their health and survival (Lassi et al., 2013). Having a mother visit one clinic for her own maternal care and another clinic at a different time, and often in a separate location, for her newborn's care is duplicative and inefficient. Such an arrangement creates an added burden and may make women more likely to miss appointments. For example, until recently, HIV/AIDS services and maternal and newborn health services were not available at the same service delivery points, making it difficult for women and their newborns to receive both types of necessary care (SMGL, 2014). Many opportunities for this type of packaging and collaboration can take place without new infrastructure or funding of new programs. However, success will require both teamwork among global health actors and alignment of efforts to achieve specific, country-appropriate goals. With a recent study finding depression as the largest contributor to disability globally for the 20- to 24-year-old age group (Vos et al., 2016), this imperative is clear to ensure all medical appointments are attended and that with each interaction, a trained provider is available to check on the mother's well-being and mental health to ensure her safety and the safety of the baby.

Nurturing Care and Parenting Support

In addition to providing simple health-related services like immunizations and nutrition—both critical to encouraging a healthy life for a child—the health care delivery system is also an opportunity to integrate nonhealth services such as nurturing care and parenting support. Support for caregivers' nutrition and mental and physical health provides secondary benefits in children's growth and development and enhances caregiver receptiveness to parenting programs. Rahman and colleagues (2013) found the relationship between maternal mood and infant health and development is not unidirectional (Rahman et al., 2013). Interventions engaging mothers on how to improve infant development had positive impacts on maternal mood, and other interventions designed to improve maternal mood had positive effects on the infant's development (Rahman et al., 2013). Studies from across the globe, including Jamaica (Gertler et al., 2014; Grantham-McGregor et al., 1997; Walker et al., 2005), Pakistan (Yousafzai et al., 2014), and Turkey (Kagitcibasi et al., 2009), illustrated by the *Lancet* series Early Childhood Development, have shown that incorporating nurturing care components into interventions significantly improved childhood development and even later adult outcomes (see Box 5-1). Additionally, members of the *Lancet* Commission on Early Childhood Development found that programs providing parental support for child development within the context of larger social protection efforts in Latin America have shown substantial benefits for child development (Fernald et al., 2017).

BOX 5-1
Case Studies of Nurturing Care Components Across the Globe

Jamaica: Weekly visits over a 2-year period were conducted by community health workers who taught parenting skills and encouraged mothers and children to interact in ways that develop cognitive and socioemotional skills, including weekly 1-hour play sessions at home with community health aides. Nutritional supplementation was provided in the form of 1 kg of formula containing 66 percent of daily recommended calories, protein, and micronutrients. Study participants were resurveyed 20 years later, and it was found that the stimulation group earned 25 percent more than those in the control group. These findings show a simple psychosocial intervention in early childhood for disadvantaged children can have a substantial effect on labor market outcomes and compensate for developmental delays.

Pakistan: Using the Lady Health Worker program, the study investigated the feasibility and effectiveness of integrating interventions directed at children under 2 years of age to enhance child development and growth outcomes. All interventions were integrated within existing services through home visits and group meetings. The enhanced nutrition group received nutrition education and multiple-micronutrient powder. The responsive stimulation group encouraged activities between the child and caregiver, observed and coached by the lady health worker. Responsive stimulation had significant benefits on early child cognitive, language, and motor development outcomes.

Turkey: The Turkish Early Enrichment Project carried out two interventions with 4- to 6-year-old children from deprived backgrounds. One intervention was a training program for mothers that emphasized educational activities with the child at home plus support for the mother, and the other was an educational preschool environment. In a 19-year follow-up, the researchers found that participants who had been exposed to either type of early enrichment exhibited higher school attainment, began their working lives at a later age, and had higher occupational status than those who had not been exposed.

SOURCES: Gertler et al., 2014; Kagitcibasi et al., 2009; Yousafzai et al., 2014.

Prevention and Mitigation of Violence

The 2014 *Global Status Report on Violence Prevention* includes data from 133 countries on violence prevalence and prevention, including child abuse and neglect (WHO, 2014b). In spite of the (1) global acceptance of child rights, (2) recognition of the harmful effects of violence exposure and maltreatment on children, and (3) endorsement of home visiting and parent education as effective in reducing risk factors for child maltreatment (Mikton and Butchart, 2009), there have been few evaluations of programs to protect children from violence and maltreatment in LMICs (Black et al., 2017). Given the lack of knowledge around risks children face in conflict and as refugees and the effectiveness of interventions in fragile countries and failed states, program evaluation is an area where more research is needed. The United Nations International Children's Emergency Fund (UNICEF) recommends that efforts along six dimensions are needed as part of a global violence prevention strategy (UNICEF, 2014):

1. Support caregivers.
2. Help children manage risks.
3. Change attitudes and norms that encourage violence.
4. Provide support services for children.
5. Implement child protection laws.
6. Conduct data collection and research.

One intervention that can address some of these dimensions is registering births. In 2012, only 49 percent of births were registered in the first year of life worldwide. This percentage drops even lower for regions such as South Asia (37 percent) and sub-Saharan Africa (38 percent), although country rates within a region can vary greatly (Lawn et al., 2014). A birth certificate provides the child with an identity and nationality that will allow him or her to access fundamental social services, including medical care and education, as well as allowing the child to obtain a driver's license or marriage license later in life. Possession of a birth certificate is linked to higher rates of finishing primary school (Corbacho et al., 2012), countering early marriage before girls are legally eligible, protecting children who are trafficked, ensuring children are enrolled in school, and providing access to immunization and health care (UNICEF, n.d.-a,-b). The biggest hindrance to obtaining birth certificates for children is that parents often need to present documentation such as a marriage license and visit multiple government agencies to obtain the certificate (Mailman School of Public Health, 2016). Ensuring that all births are registered is of critical importance to countries as they evaluate national priorities and international aid. Birth certificates allow countries to make policies based on facts as opposed to ideologies (Mikkelsen et al., 2015), and they help to better evaluate international aid needs (Mailman School of Public Health, 2016). Because the absence of this crucial information negatively affects policy making and development, it is a strategic objective of WHO's Every Newborn Action Plan to End Preventable Deaths (WHO, 2014a).

Poverty Assistance and Cash Transfers

Social safety-net programs support vulnerable populations by distributing cash transfers to low-income households to prevent shocks, protect the chronically poor, promote capabilities and opportunities for vulnerable households, and transform systems of power that exclude certain marginalized groups (e.g., women, children, rural poor, indigenous). The economic rationale for cash transfer programs is that they can be an equitable and efficient way to address market failures and reach the most vulnerable populations (Fiszbein et al., 2009). Most LMICs spend 1–2 percent of their GDP on social transfer programs. Conditional cash transfer programs and microcredit usually target the transfer to mothers based on evidence that money controlled by mothers is spent on more child-centered goods and services than money controlled by fathers (Thomas, 1990). Social safety-net programs are hypothesized to improve outcomes via the family investment model (i.e., having more money to spend on inputs or more time to spend with children) and family stress model (i.e., decreased maternal depression due to increased household resources). A recent review shows mostly positive effects of cash transfer programs on some child outcomes, including birth weight; infant mortality; illness or morbidity; and cognitive, language, and behavioral development. Strong positive effects of cash transfers on promoting participation in prenatal care, giving birth in the presence of a skilled birth attendant, and growth monitoring have been reported (De Walque et al., 2017).

Early Childhood Education

For the post-2015 agenda, the SDGs call for all children by 2030 to "have access to quality early child development, care and preprimary education so that they are ready for primary education" (UN, 2015b). Achievement of this goal will require greater coordination of early child development programming within the broader education infrastructure, with attention to equity in both access and quality of services. Education and intellectual support of young children can take many forms. Low-cost activities such as storytelling, singing, and playing with household objects expose young children to a rich and varied social network that promotes early development (Black et al., 2017).

High-quality early child development programs and opportunities for early learning, such as day care, child care, and preschool, improve child outcomes during later schooling (Britto et al., 2017). The inclusion of early child development in the first of six Education for All goals recognizes early child development as an essential component of the broader education agenda.[6] Additionally, education has been found to have downstream health effects, especially when one considers female schooling. For example, a meta-analysis conducted by Schäferhoff and colleagues (2015) found that a 1-year increment in female schooling is associated with a 6.5 to 9.9 percent reduction in mortality for children under 5 in LMICs. Furthermore, 39.6 percent and 17.5 percent of child mortality reduction between 1990–2000 and 2000–2011, respectively, can be attributed to increases in female schooling (Schäferhoff et al., 2015). A challenge in most countries is the lack of a robust system for education for children before they enter primary school. In the United States, for example, there is little support for public-sector day care, and private day care is in short supply, high demand, and comes with extremely high out-of-pocket costs. Even for countries with early childhood programs, the variability of quality is such that it is difficult to measure effects and attribution across the board.

Despite the measured benefits of investment in early education for children, many reports still indicate that governments and private donors consider it a low priority (UNESCO, 2006, 2011). Another option for providing supportive early learning environments is through media. A meta-analysis representing more than 10,000 children from 15 countries[7] found significant benefits in literacy and numeracy, health and safety, and social reasoning and attitudes toward others—all from watching *Sesame Street* (Mares et al., 2015). Although shows like *Sesame Street* are a relatively easy way to bring learning opportunities to children who cannot join formal learning environments before age 5, gaps remain that need to be addressed for children to be mentally and socially prepared to enter school.

SUMMARY AND RECOMMENDATION

In LMICs, 250 million children younger than age 5 (43 percent) fail to reach their developmental potential because of extreme poverty and stunting (Black et al., 2017). With the decline of nutrition- and infection-related child mortality and the push for universal primary school, the support and promotion of child development is crucially important. The SDGs call for all children to "have access to quality early child development, care, and preprimary education so that they are ready for primary education" by 2030 (UN, 2015b). Recent evidence indicates that there are significant long-term effects of early investments in child cognitive and language de-

[6] Education for All is a global movement led by UNESCO (United Nation Educational, Scientific and Cultural Organization) that aims to meet the learning needs of all children, youth, and adults by 2015.

[7] Countries analyzed included Australia, Bangladesh, Canada, Egypt, India, Indonesia, Israel, Kosovo, Mexico, Nigeria, Northern Ireland, Palestine, South Africa, Tanzania, and Turkey (Mares and Pan, 2013).

velopment, which translate into lifelong benefits in terms of labor market participation, lifetime earnings, productivity, health, and economic growth (Gertler et al., 2014; Kagitcibasi et al., 2009; Yousafzai et al., 2014). Thus, a "thrive" agenda in addition to the existing "survival" agenda can be an important focal point for investment.

> *Conclusion: There is a need for greater investment in building enabling, nurturing, and cognitively enriching environments (which include responsive and emotionally supportive parenting, opportunities for play and learning, and support for early education) for vulnerable children under age 5 and their mothers. These programs can fit within the health, education, or social services sector.*

Recommendation 8: Ensure Healthy and Productive Lives for Women and Children

> **The U.S. Agency for International Development, The U.S. President's Emergency Plan for AIDS Relief, their implementing partners, and other funders should support and incorporate proven, cost-effective interventions into their existing programs for ensuring that all children reach their developmental potential and become healthy, productive adults. This integration should embrace principles of country ownership, domestic financing, and community engagement. These interventions should include the following:**
>
> - **Provide adequate nutrition for optimal infant and child cognitive development.**
> - **Reduce childhood exposure to domestic and other violence.**
> - **Detect and manage postpartum depression and other maternal mental health issues.**
> - **Support and promote early education and cognitive stimulation in young children.**

TRANSFORM: DEVELOPING WHOLE SYSTEMS OF CARE

Many of the strategies and opportunities for investments related to reducing maternal and child mortality described above do not necessarily require new and separate funding streams or a novel and dedicated workforce. Instead, a change of thinking is required that starts with an examination of all parts of the existing services delivery and support system to see what can be amended to maximize efficiency and effectiveness. The many opportunities for transformation are most easily and effectively pursued through broadening the delivery system to include social determinants (e.g., poverty and education), expanding the workforce skillsets, and bundling different types of services to optimize the interaction between patient and provider and improve adherence to treatments or behaviors.

Altering the Approach for Increased Survival

Shifting from a condition-based care and support model for a particular disease to a whole-person approach allows health care and social service workers to address risk and protective factors across the life span. For example, USAID's AIDS, Population, and Health Integrated Assistance Plus program, which integrates family planning into PEPFAR-platform HIV/AIDS services for women in Kenya (Fleischman and Peck, 2015), has been commended as a game changer. Such a program could be used as a model for other approaches to integrate essential maternal and child services, such as breast and cervical cancer screening.

Program administration that permits funding flexibility and connectivity of U.S.-supported efforts will go a long way to ensure that integrative models are successful. However, the successful scaling, adoption, and sustainability of integrative models requires investments in workforce development. Training community health workers to share the tasks of physicians and nurses serves as an effective means to increase awareness in low-resource settings about NCDs (e.g., high blood pressure), and they can help to disseminate information about particular diseases with the community's needs and culture in mind (Abrahams-Gessel et al., 2015). Skilled birth attendants and midwives can also be effectively used to increase their patients' awareness of breast or cervical cancer screening programs.

Expanding the Effort to Strengthen Health Systems

In many countries, early child development services are delivered through a disconnected set of organizations, primarily NGOs, often with few regulatory guidelines and little coordination with other services or sectors (Black et al., 2017). As the emphasis on early childhood has increased over the past decade and governments look to increase access to early child development programs, finding effective ways to leverage the nongovernmental sector to increase access and ensure quality is critically important (Black et al., 2017). Platforms for early child development services include home visits, clinical contacts, and community-based group sessions as well as newer approaches, such as media (Black et al., 2017). Overall, successful programs are not universal and need more research and contextual understanding. The factors that influence health and development often go well beyond the health sector and include the nutrition, education, and social sectors (Britto et al., 2017). Thus, to truly improve the health and well-being of populations, which is a desired outcome inherent in the design of the SDGs, policy and practice professionals need to go beyond the health sector to make the needed changes and integrate services across sectors. Integrated approaches should ideally include all sectors and share messages and opportunities for synergy. Several key improvements within the sector of women's and children's health would be relatively easy to implement and would result in multiple dividends, especially as such interventions often act synergistically with women and children. Consider the examples from Rahman and colleagues (2013) noted previously: Multiple studies show strong effects of improved maternal mood and infant health and development simply by having supervised, nonspecialist community health workers conduct culturally competent interventions (Rahman et al., 2013). Simple improvements to the health systems in countries could also include workforce development changes, mental health support for women and families, increased focus on nutrition to address remaining survival issues as well as enhanced thriving, and finally, increased cross-sector partnerships at the ground level to provide integrated services.

Within the category of workforce development, it is important to ensure that skilled birth attendants, community health workers, nurses, and primary care physicians have appropriate training in exclusive breastfeeding promotion and can ensure proper nutrition for newborns (WHO, 2017a). Refocusing the health system to include an emphasis on nutrition from pregnancy across the life cycle can ameliorate under-5 mortality and stunting and promote healthy growth as children grow into adolescents and adults. For women, this focus could translate to improved nutrition during pregnancy, ideally propagating the cycle of health and wellness (USAID, 2014). Moreover, because primary care health workers often do not possess the essential knowledge and skills to promote early child development, providing a basic training curriculum could assist in the identification of children who are at risk of delayed development at age-appropriate times. This approach would also enable providers to identify optimal opportunities to intervene to promote development.

Public–Private Partnerships with a Multisector Focus

Creating multisector partnerships with community organizations and the numerous NGOs throughout the global health community is another way to transform the system of care. As noted in Chapter 4, PEPFAR's DREAMS partnership is still nascent, but its goals to address poverty, gender inequality, lack of education, and sexual violence—even with a bottom-line focus of reducing HIV infection rates—demonstrate a promising cross-sector example of this type of partnership. Saving Mothers, Giving Life is another public–private partnership. Launched in 2012, it partners with donor and recipient governments, NGOs, the private sector, and representatives from provider associations to test an integrated approach to significantly reduce maternal deaths (SMGL, 2014). In its first year alone, the program upgraded 68 facilities in Zambia and 11 facilities in Uganda to provide basic emergency obstetric and newborn care (Kruk et al., 2014). Additionally, the program trained 1,010 health workers in Zambia and 4,004 in Uganda to promote delivery in facilities and in birth preparedness, and it trained 179 health workers in Zambia and 238 health workers in Uganda to provide emergency obstetric care, newborn resuscitation, or surgery (Kruk et al., 2014). Saving Mothers, Giving Life's latest report showed a 55 percent reduction in maternal mortality in target facilities in Zambia as a result of its interventions, and target districts in Uganda saw a 44 percent reduction in maternal mortality (SMGL, 2016), showing the partnership is helping women from all over the community, not just those who make it to the facility (see Figure 5-2).

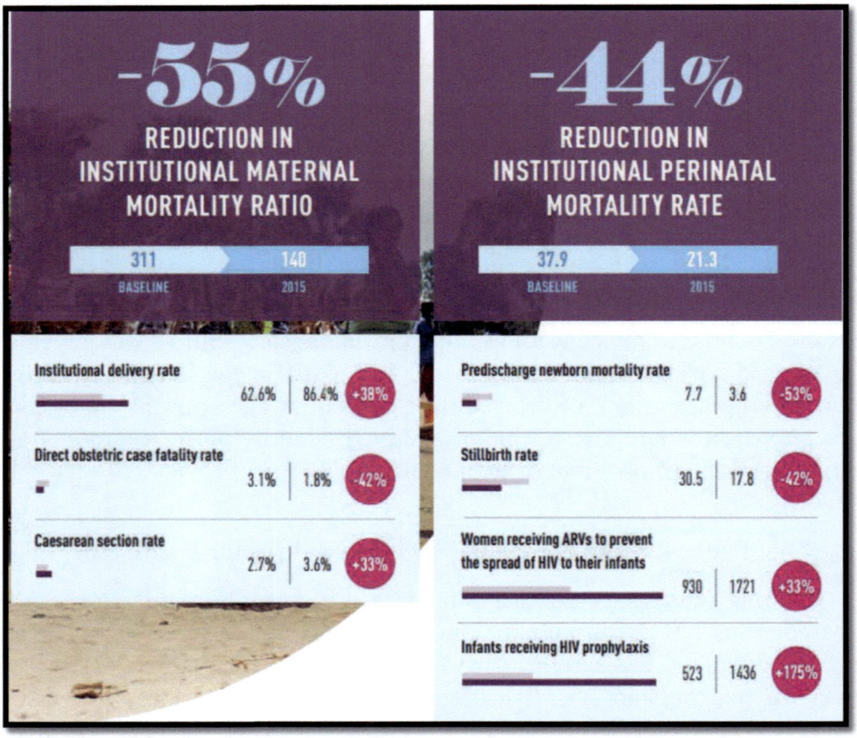

FIGURE 5-2 Results of the Saving Mothers, Giving Life program in Zambia after 4 years.
SOURCE: SMGL, 2016.

Among the successful private-sector partners in this partnership is Merck through its Merck for Mothers program. Merck for Mothers, part of the Saving Mothers, Giving Life initiative, supports on-the-ground program evaluation and program implementation (Merck for Mothers, 2013). More partnerships that pair the expertise of the public and private sectors are needed to take cross-sector intervention approaches, show results, and help to change the system.

REFERENCES

Abrahams-Gessel, S., C. A. Denman, C. M. Montano, T. A. Gaziano, N. Levitt, A. Rivera-Andrade, D. M. Carrasco, J. Zulu, M. A. Khanam, and T. Puoane. 2015. The training and fieldwork experiences of community health workers conducting population-based, noninvasive screening for CVD in LMIC. *Global Heart* 10(1):45-54.

Ahmed, S., Q. Li, L. Liu, and A. O. Tsui. 2012. Maternal deaths averted by contraceptive use: An analysis of 172 countries. *The Lancet* 380(9837):111-125.

Bellagio Study Group on Child Survival. 2003. Knowledge into action for child survival. *The Lancet* 362(9380):323-327.

Black, M. M., S. P. Walker, L. C. Fernald, C. T. Andersen, A. M. DiGirolamo, C. Lu, D. C. McCoy, G. Fink, Y. R. Shawar, J. Shiffman, A. E. Devercelli, Q. T. Wodon, E. Vargas-Baron, and S. Grantham-McGregor. 2017. Early childhood development coming of age: Science through the life course. *The Lancet* 389(10064):77-90.

Black, R. E., L. H. Allen, Z. A. Bhutta, L. E. Caulfield, M. de Onis, M. Ezzati, C. Mathers, and J. Rivera. 2008. Maternal and child undernutrition: Global and regional exposures and health consequences. *The Lancet* 371(9608):243-260.

Black, R. E., C. G. Victora, S. P. Walker, Z. A. Bhutta, P. Christian, M. De Onis, M. Ezzati, S. Grantham-Mcgregor, J. Katz, R. Martorell, and R. Uauy. 2013. Maternal and child undernutrition and overweight in low-income and middle-income countries. *The Lancet* 382(9890):427-451.

Britto, P. R., S. J. Lye, K. Proulx, A. K. Yousafzai, S. G. Matthews, T. Vaivada, R. Perez-Escamilla, N. Rao, P. Ip, L. C. H. Fernald, H. MacMillan, M. Hanson, T. D. Wachs, H. Yao, H. Yoshikawa, A. Cerezo, J. F. Leckman, and Z. A. Bhutta. 2017. Nurturing care: Promoting early childhood development. *The Lancet* 389(10064):91-102.

Bustreo, F., and W. Mpanju-Shumusho. 2016. Great progress in global health: Unfinished business remains. *Harvard International Review* 25 January.

CDC (U.S. Centers for Disease Control and Prevention). 2016. *Pregnant? Get Tdap in your third trimester*. https://www.cdc.gov/features/tdap-in-pregnancy (accessed February 28, 2017).

Ceschia, A., and R. Horton. 2016. Maternal health: Time for a radical reappraisal. *The Lancet* 388(10056):2064-2066.

Claeson, M. 2017. The Global Financing Facility: Towards a new way of financing for development. *The Lancet* 389(10079):1588-1592.

Corbacho, A., S. Brito, and R. Rivas. 2012. *Birth registration and the impact on educational attainment*. Washington, DC: Inter-American Development Bank.

Currie, J., and T. Vogl. 2013. Early-life health and adult circumstances in developing countries. *Annual Review of Economics* 5:1-36.

Darnton-Hill, I., and U. C. Mkparu. 2015. Micronutrients in pregnancy in low- and middle-income countries. *Nutrients* 7(3):1744-1768.

De Neve, J. W., G. Fink, S. V. Subramanian, S. Moyo, and J. Bor. 2015. Length of secondary schooling and risk of HIV infection in Botswana: Evidence from a natural experiment. *The Lancet Global Health* 3(8):e470-e477.

De Walque, D., L. Fernald, P. Gertler, and M. Hidrobo. 2017. *Cash transfers and child and adolescent development.* Disease Control Priorities, Third Edition: Volume 8. Child and Adolescent Health and Development. Part 4: Packages and Platforms to Promote Child and Adolescent Development. Washington, DC: World Bank.

Edwards, A. 2016. *Global forced displacement hits record high.* http://www.unhcr.org/afr/news/latest/2016/6/5763b65a4/global-forced-displacement-hits-record-high.html (accessed March 19, 2017).

Every Woman Every Child. 2016. *About.* https://www.everywomaneverychild.org/about (accessed April 15, 2017).

Fernald, L. C., R. M. Kagawa, H. A. Knauer, L. Schnaas, A. G. Guerra, and L. M. Neufeld. 2017. Promoting child development through group-based parent support within a cash transfer program: Experimental effects on children's outcomes. *Developmental Psychology* 53(2):222-236.

Fiszbein, A., N. Schady, F. Ferreira, M. Grosh, N. Keleher, P. Olinto, and E. Skoufias. 2009. *Conditional cash transfers: Reducing present and future poverty.* Washington, DC: World Bank.

Fleischman, J., and K. Peck. 2015. *Family planning and women's health in Kenya.* Washington, DC: Center for Strategic and International Studies.

Fotso, J. C., J. Cleland, B. Mberu, M. Mutua, and P. Elungata. 2013. Birth spacing and child mortality: An analysis of prospective data from the Nairobi Urban Health and Demographic Surveillance System. *Journal of Biosocial Science* 45(6):779-798.

FP2020 (Family Planning 2020). 2016. Report: More than 300 million women and girls in world's poorest countries using modern contraceptives at midpoint of FP2020 initiative. Washington, DC: Family Planning 2020.

Gavi (Gavi, the Vaccine Alliance). 2015. *Keeping children healthy: The Vaccine Alliance progress report 2015.* Washington, DC: Gavi, the Vaccine Alliance.

Gertler, P., J. Heckman, R. Pinto, A. Zanolini, C. Vermeersch, S. Walker, S. M. Chang, and S. Grantham-McGregor. 2014. Labor market returns to an early childhood stimulation intervention in Jamaica. *Science* 344(6187):998.

GFF (Global Financing Facility). 2016. *Global financing facility: Introduction.* https://www.globalfinancingfacility.org/introduction (accessed December 19, 2016).

Giberson, C., and V. Taddoni. 2014. Invest in girls and women: The ripple effect. Women Deliver. womendeliver.org/resources (accessed August 2, 2017).

Grantham-McGregor, S. M., S. P. Walker, S. M. Chang, and C. A. Powell. 1997. Effects of early childhood supplementation with and without stimulation on later development in stunted Jamaican children. *The American Journal of Clinical Nutrition* 66(2):247-253.

Greenwood, B. 2014. The contribution of vaccination to global health: Past, present and future. *Philosophical Transactions of the Royal Society of London. Series B, Biological Sciences* 369(1645):20130433.

Hair, N. L., J. L. Hanson, B. L. Wolfe, and S. D. Pollak. 2015. Association of child poverty, brain development, and academic achievement. *The Journal of the American Medical Association Pediatrics* 169(9):822-829.

Hertzman, C., and T. Boyce. 2010. How experience gets under the skin to create gradients in developmental health. *Annual Review of Public Health* 31:329-347.

Honikman, S., T. van Heyningen, S. Field, E. Baron, and M. Tomlinson. 2012. Stepped care for maternal mental health: A case study of the perinatal mental health project in South Africa. *PLOS Medicine* 9(5):e1001222.

Jones, K. M. 2011. *Evaluating the Mexico City policy: How U.S. foreign policy affects fertility outcomes and child health in Ghana.* Washington, DC: International Food Policy Research Institute.

Kagitcibasi, C., D. Sunar, S. Bekman, N. Baydar, and Z. Cemalcilar. 2009. Continuing effects of early enrichment in adult life: The Turkish early enrichment project 22 years later. *Journal of Applied Developmental Psychology* 30(6):764-779.

Kassebaum, N. J., R. M. Barber, Z. A. Bhutta, L. Dandona, P. W. Gething, S. I. Hay, Y. Kinfu, et al. 2016. Global, regional, and national levels of maternal mortality, 1990–2015: A systematic analysis for the Global Burden of Disease Study 2015. *The Lancet* 388(10053):1775-1812.

Kruk, M. E., M. Rabkin, K. A. Grepin, K. Austin-Evelyn, D. Greeson, T. B. Masvawure, E. R. Sacks, D. Vail, and S. Galea. 2014. "Big push" to reduce maternal mortality in Uganda and Zambia enhanced health systems but lacked a sustainability plan. *Health Affairs (Millwood)* 33(6):1058-1066.

Lassi, Z. S., A. Majeed, S. Rashid, M. Y. Yakoob, and Z. A. Bhutta. 2013. The interconnections between maternal and newborn health—evidence and implications for policy. *The Journal of Maternal-Fetal & Neonatal Medicine* 26 (Suppl 1):3-53.

Lawn, J. E., H. Blencowe, S. Oza, D. You, A. C. C. Lee, P. Waiswa, M. Lalli, Z. Bhutta, A. J. D. Barros, P. Christian, C. Mathers, and S. N. Cousens. 2014. Every newborn: Progress, priorities, and potential beyond survival. *The Lancet* 384(9938):189-205.

Lee, K. G. 2017. *Neonatal repiratory distress syndrome.* https://medlineplus.gov/ency/article/001563.htm (accessed February 14, 2017).

Liu, L., S. Oza, D. Hogan, Y. Chu, J. Perin, J. Zhu, J. E. Lawn, S. Cousens, C. Mathers, and R. E. Black. 2016. Global, regional, and national causes of under-5 mortality in 2000–15: An updated systematic analysis with implications for the Sustainable Development Goals. *The Lancet* 388(10063):3027-3035.

MacDorman, M. F., E. Declercq, H. Cabral, and C. Morton. 2016. Recent increases in the U.S. maternal mortality rate: Disentangling trends from measurement issues. *Obstetrics & Gynecology* 128(3).

Mailman School of Public Health. 2016. *Why birth certificates are so important.* https://www.mailman.columbia.edu/public-health-now/news/why-birth-certificates-are-so-important (accessed February 13, 2017).

Mares, M.-L., and Z. Pan. 2013. Effects of *Sesame Street*: A meta-analysis of children's learning in 15 countries. *Journal of Applied Developmental Psychology* 34(3):140-151.

Mares, M.-L., G. Sivakumar, and L. Stephenson. 2015. From meta to micro. *American Behavioral Scientist* 59(14):1822-1846.

Mbuyita, S., R. Tillya, R. Godfrey, I. Kinyonge, J. Shaban, and G. Mbaruku. 2015. Effects of introducing routinely ultrasound scanning during Ante Natal Care (ANC) clinics on number of visits of ANC and facility delivery: A cohort study. *Archives of Public Health* 73(1):36.

Meara, J. G., A. J. M. Leather, L. Hagander, B. C. Alkire, N. Alonso, E. A. Ameh, S. W. Bickler, L. Conteh, A. J. Dare, J. Davies, E. D. Mérisier, S. El-Halabi, P. E. Farmer, A. Gawande, R. Gillies, S. L. M. Greenberg, C. E. Grimes, R. L. Gruen, E. A. Ismail, T. B. Kamara, C. Lavy, G. Lundeg, N. C. Mkandawire, N. P. Raykar, J. N. Riesel, E. Rodas, J. Rose, N. Roy, M. G. Shrime, R. Sullivan, S. Verguet, D. Watters, T. G. Weiser, I. H. Wilson, G. Yamey, and W. Yip. 2015. Global surgery 2030: Evidence and solutions for achieving health, welfare, and economic development. *The Lancet* 386(9993):569-624.

Merck for Mothers. 2013. Saving Mothers, Giving Life interventions making an impact. Kenilworth, USA: Merck Sharp & Dohme Corp.

Mikkelsen, L., A. Lopez, and D. Phillips. 2015. *Why birth and death registration really are "vital" statistics for development*. http://hdr.undp.org/en/content/why-birth-and-death-registration-really-are-%E2%80%9Cvital%E2%80%9D-statistics-development (accessed February 13, 2017).

Mikton, C., and A. Butchart. 2009. Child maltreatment prevention: A systematic review of reviews. *Bulletin of the World Health Organization* 87:353-361.

Moylan, C. A., T. I. Herrenkohl, C. Sousa, E. A. Tajima, R. C. Herrenkohl, and M. J. Russo. 2010. The effects of child abuse and exposure to domestic violence on adolescent internalizing and externalizing behavior problems. *Journal of Family Violence* 25(1):53-63.

Murray et al. 2012. Disability-adjusted life years (DALYs) for 291 diseases and injuries in 21 regions, 1990-2010: A systematic analysis for the Global Burden of Disease study 2010. *The Lancet* 380(9859):2197-2223.

Noble, K. G., S. M. Houston, N. H. Brito, H. Bartsch, E. Kan, J. M. Kuperman, N. Akshoomoff, D. G. Amaral, C. S. Bloss, O. Libiger, N. J. Schork, S. S. Murray, B. J. Casey, L. Chang, T. M. Ernst, J. A. Frazier, J. R. Gruen, D. N. Kennedy, P. Van Zijl, S. Mostofsky, W. E. Kaufmann, T. Kenet, A. M. Dale, T. L. Jernigan, and E. R. Sowell. 2015. Family income, parental education and brain structure in children and adolescents. *Nature Neuroscience* 18(5):773-778.

PAI (Population Action Initiative). 2016. *Senate committee again approves bipartisan pro-family planning amendment*. https://pai.org/newsletters/senate-committee-approves-bipartisan-pro-family-planning-amendment-never-easy-looks (accessed April 8, 2017).

PATH. 2016. *Harnessing the power of innovation to save mothers and children: How 11 emerging innovations could save more than 6 million lives*. Seattle, WA: PATH.

Rahman, A., J. Fisher, P. Bower, S. Luchters, T. Tran, M. Yasamy, S. Saxena, and W. Waheed. 2013. Interventions for common perinatal mental disorders in women in low- and middle-income countries: A systematic review and meta-analysis. *Bulletin of the World Health Organization* 91:593-601.

Richter, L. M., B. Daelmans, J. Lombardi, J. Heymann, F. L. Boo, J. R. Behrman, C. Lu, J. E. Lucas, R. Perez-Escamilla, T. Dua, Z. A. Bhutta, K. Stenberg, P. Gertler, and G. L. Darmstadt. 2017. Investing in the foundation of sustainable development: Pathways to scale up for early childhood development. *The Lancet* 389(10064):103-118.

Say, L., D. Chou, A. Gemmill, Ö. Tunçalp, A.-B. Moller, J. Daniels, A. M. Gülmezoglu, M. Temmerman, and L. Alkema. 2014. Global causes of maternal death: A WHO systematic analysis. *The Lancet Global Health* 2(6):e323-e333.

Schäferhoff, M., D. Evans, N. Burnett, P. Komaromi, J. Kraus, C. D. Obure, E. Pradhan, C. S. Sutherland, E. Suzuki, and D. T. Jamison. 2015. *Estimating the costs and benefits of education from a health perspective*. Oslo: NORAD.

Shidhaye, P., and P. Giri. 2014. Maternal depression: A hidden burden in developing countries. *Annals of Medical and Health Sciences Research* 4(4):463-465.

SMGL (Saving Mothers, Giving Life). 2014. *Saving mothers, giving life: Primer.* Saving Mothers, Giving Life.

SMGL. 2016. *2016 annual report: Reducing maternal mortality in sub-Saharan Africa*. Saving Mothers, Giving Life.

Soe-Lin, S., A. Jaspers, and R. Hecht. 2016. *Renewing U.S. leadership to end stunting.* Washington, DC: Center for Strategic and International Studies Global Policy Center.

Sudfeld, C. R., D. C. McCoy, G. Danaei, G. Fink, M. Ezzati, K. G. Andrews, and W. W. Fawzi. 2015. Linear growth and child development in low- and middle-income countries: A meta-analysis. *Pediatrics* 135(5):e1266-e1275.

Thomas, D. 1990. Intra-household resource allocation: An inferential approach. *The Journal of Human Resources* 25(4):635-664.

UN (United Nations). 2015a. *Goal 3: Ensure healthy lives and promote well-being for all at all ages.* New York: United Nations.

UN. 2015b. *Goal 4: Ensure inclusive and quality education for all and promote lifelong learning.* New York: United Nations Sustainable Development Goals.

UN. 2015c. *Goal 4: Reduce child mortality.* New York: United Nations.

UN. 2015d. *Goal 5: Improve maternal health.* New York: United Nations.

UNESCO (United Nations Educational, Scientific and Cultural Organization). 2006. Strong foundations—Early childhood care and education: Education for All Global Monitoring Report 2007. Paris, France: United Nations Educational, Scientific and Cultural Organization.

UNESCO. 2011. The hidden crisis: Armed conflict and education. Paris, France: United Nations Educational, Scientific and Cultural Organization.

UNICEF (United Nations International Children's Emergency Fund). 2014. *Hidden in plain sight: A statistical analysis of violence against children.* New York: United Nations International Children's Emergency Fund.

UNICEF. 2015. *The investment case for education and equity.* New York: United Nations International Children's Emergency Fund.

UNICEF. n.d.-a. *Factsheet: Birth registration.* https://www.unicef.org/newsline/2003/03fsbirthregistration.htm (accessed February 14, 2017).

UNICEF. n.d.-b. *Why is birth registration important?* http://unicef.in/Story/365/Why-is-birth-registration-important (accessed February 14, 2017).

USAID (U.S. Agency for International Development). 2014. *Multi-Sectoral Nutrition Strategy 2014-2025.* Washington, DC: U.S. Agency for International Development.

USAID. 2015. *Why invest in women?* Washington, DC: U.S. Agency for International Development.

USAID. 2016. *Acting on the call: Ending preventable child and maternal deaths: A focus on equity.* Washington, DC: U.S. Agency for International Development.

Victora, C. G., T. Adam, and J. Bryce. 2006. Integrated management of the sick child. In *Disease control priorities in developing countries.* 2nd ed, edited by D. Jamison, J. Breman and A. Measham. New York: Oxford University Press.

Victora, C. G., B. L. Horta, C. L. de Mola, L. Quevedo, R. T. Pinheiro, D. P. Gigante, H. Gonçalves, and F. C. Barros. 2015. Association between breastfeeding and intelligence, educational attainment, and income at 30 years of age: A prospective birth cohort study from Brazil. *The Lancet Global Health* 3(4):e199-e205.

Victora, C. G., R. Bahl, A. J. D. Barros, G. V. A. França, S. Horton, J. Krasevec, S. Murch, M. J. Sankar, N. Walker, and N. C. Rollins. 2016. Breastfeeding in the 21st century: Epidemiology, mechanisms, and lifelong effect. *The Lancet* 387(10017):475-490.

Vos, T., C. Allen, M. Arora, R. M. Barber, Z. A. Bhutta, A. Brown, A. Carter, et al. 2016. Figure 3: Leading ten level 3 causes of global age-specific years lived with disability in 2015. *In Global, Regional, and National Incidence, Prevalence, and Years Lived with Disability for 310 Diseases and Injuries, 1990-2015: A Systematic Analysis for Global Burden of Disease Study 2015. The Lancet* 388(10053):8-14.

Walker, S. P., S. M. Chang, C. A. Powell, and S. M. Grantham-McGregor. 2005. Effects of early childhood psychosocial stimulation and nutritional supplementation on cognition and education in growth-stunted Jamaican children: Prospective cohort study. *The Lancet* 366(9499):1804-1807.

Wang, H., Z. A. Bhutta, M. M. Coates, M. Coggeshall, L. Dandona, K. Diallo, E. B. Franca, et al. 2016. Global, regional, national, and selected subnational levels of stillbirths, neonatal, infant, and under-5 mortality, 1980–2015: A systematic analysis for the Global Burden of Disease Study 2015. *The Lancet* 388(10053):1725-1774.

Westoff, C. 2000. *The substitution of contraception for abortion in Kazakhstan in the 1990s*. Calverton, Maryland: DHS Analytical Studies.

WHO (World Health Organization). 2010. *Global status report on noncommunicable diseases 2010*. Geneva, Switzerland: World Health Organization.

WHO. 2014a. *Every newborn: An action plan to end preventable deaths*. Geneva, Switzerland: World Health Organization

WHO. 2014b. *Global status report on violence prevention 2014*. Geneva, Switzerland: World Health Organization.

WHO. 2016a. *Children: Reducing mortality fact sheet*. Geneva, Switzerland: World Health Organization.

WHO. 2016b. *The Global Strategy for Women's, Children's, and Adolescents' Health (2016–2030)*. Geneva, Switzerland: World Health Organization.

WHO. 2016c. *Immunization coverage fact sheet*. http://www.who.int/mediacentre/factsheets/fs378/en (accessed February 14, 2017).

WHO. 2016d. *Maternal mortality fact sheet*. Geneva, Switzerland: World Health Organization.

WHO. 2016e. *Preterm birth fact sheet*. http://www.who.int/mediacentre/factsheets/fs363/en (accessed February 14, 2017).

WHO. 2016f. *Towards a grand convergence for child survival and health: A strategic review of options for the future building on lessons learnt from Integrated Management of Newborn and Childhood Illness (IMNCI)*. Geneva, Switzerland: World Health Organization.

WHO. 2017a. *Early initiation of breastfeeding to promote exclusive breastfeeding*. http://www.who.int/elena/titles/early_breastfeeding/en (accessed March 19, 2017).

WHO. 2017b. *Inheriting a sustainable world? Atlas on children's health and the environment*. Geneva, Switzerland: World Health Organization.

WHO. n.d.-a. *Infant mortality: Situation and trends*. Geneva, Switzerland: World Health Organization.

WHO. n.d.-b. *Micronutrient deficiencies: Vitamin A deficiency*. http://www.who.int/nutrition/topics/vad/en (accessed March 17, 2017).

Widom, C. S., S. J. Czaja, and M. A. Dutton. 2008. Childhood victimization and lifetime revictimization. *Child Abuse & Neglect* 32(8):785-796.

Winkvist, A., K. M. Rasmussen, and J. P. Habicht. 1992. A new definition of maternal depletion syndrome. *American Journal of Public Health* 82(5):691-694.

Yousafzai, A. K., M. A. Rasheed, A. Rizvi, R. Armstrong, and Z. A. Bhutta. 2014. Effect of integrated responsive stimulation and nutrition interventions in the lady health worker programme in Pakistan on child development, growth, and health outcomes: A cluster-randomised factorial effectiveness trial. *The Lancet* 384(9950):1282-1293.

6

Promoting Cardiovascular Health and Preventing Cancer

As a result of successes in infectious disease prevention and sanitation improvement, the burden of disease in low- and middle-income countries (LMICs) is rapidly shifting from communicable to noncommunicable diseases, demonstrating a paradox of success in global health. As a greater proportion of children survive into adulthood, and changes in diet and lifestyle occur, many countries now face a rise in chronic illnesses, such as cardiovascular disease (CVD), chronic obstructive pulmonary disease (COPD), cancer, and diabetes, all of which are often associated with behavioral factors such as tobacco use, physical inactivity, and diets high in calories, sugar, and salt (WHO, 2017b). Globally, these chronic or noncommunicable diseases (NCDs) kill 40 million people per year, almost three-quarters of whom reside in LMICs (WHO, 2017b). Though media attention often portrays NCDs as a western, high-income country health challenge, the burden of NCDs disproportionately affects the poor in middle-income countries—a trend that will continue to grow alongside rising urbanization and globalization.

In a global trade environment, U.S. interests are affected by the rise of NCDs in LMICs and their resultant human and economic effects. Countries with a high NCD burden tend to have lower national productivity and higher health and welfare expenditures (Bloom et al., 2011). The costs resulting from productivity losses associated with disability, unplanned absences from work, and increased rates of accidents are as much as 4 times the cost of treatment. Research also has shown that investors, including U.S. businesses, are less likely to enter markets where the labor force suffers a heavy disease burden.

The committee has chosen to focus this chapter on cardiovascular disease and cancer (specifically vaccine-preventable cancers, such as cervical cancer and liver cancer), not only because of their global burden but also because of the amount of research and knowledge that exists and the opportunity for intervention worldwide. This chapter begins by characterizing the economic and epidemiological burden of NCDs, and demonstrates how they are both projected to rise in the next 20 years if no action is taken to curb rising incidence. It then explores motivations for U.S. involvement, and highlights existing cost-effective, successful interventions found globally for prevention and early treatment of CVD and select cancers. Finally, this chapter emphasizes a need to transform health systems to be more capable of managing these chronic conditions, particularly highlighting the potential of public–private partnerships.

THE RISING ECONOMIC BURDEN OF NONCOMMUNICABLE DISEASES

A study conducted by the World Economic Forum and the Harvard School of Public Health estimated that the projected increase in the global economic burden of five NCDs (CVD, chronic respiratory disease, cancer, diabetes, and mental health) would result in cumulative output losses of $47 trillion by 2030, which is roughly 75 percent of the 2010 global gross domestic product (GDP) (Bloom et al., 2011).[1] CVDs were a primary contributor to lost output (33 percent), with 18 percent attributed to cancers (Bloom et al., 2011). As of 2015, the estimated annual global cost of CVD is expected to increase by 16 percent from $906 billion to more than $1 trillion by 2030 (see Figure 6-1). Furthermore, total output losses are projected to increase sharply over time (see Figure 6-2).

Researchers from the Netherlands conducted a series of systematic reviews to examine the global impact of NCDs at the macroeconomic level, including productivity, health care spending, and national income (Muka et al., 2015). CVD accounts for the highest health care expenditure in most countries, ranging from 12 to 16.5 percent of the overall health care budget (other NCDs ranged between 0.7 and 7.4 percent) (Muka et

[1] These estimates were generated using EPIC, a tool developed by the World Health Organization to simulate the economic impact of diseases on aggregate economic output. EPIC links the value of economic output to quantities of labor and capital inputs, as well as to technology. The EPIC model adjusts labor and capital inputs according to population health. Namely, labor is diminished by disability and death caused by NCDs. Capital is also reduced because costs of screening, treatment, and care claim resources that would otherwise be available for public and private investment. The EPIC model predicts losses caused by different health conditions in terms of their effect on the value of economic output (WEF and WHO, 2011).

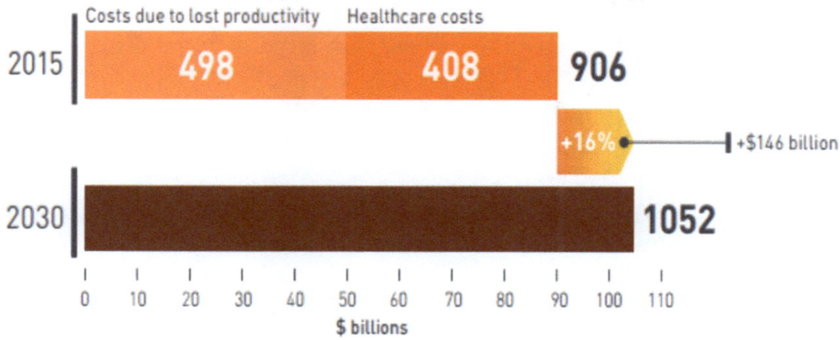

FIGURE 6-1 Global costs of cardiovascular disease.
SOURCE: Reddy et al., 2016.

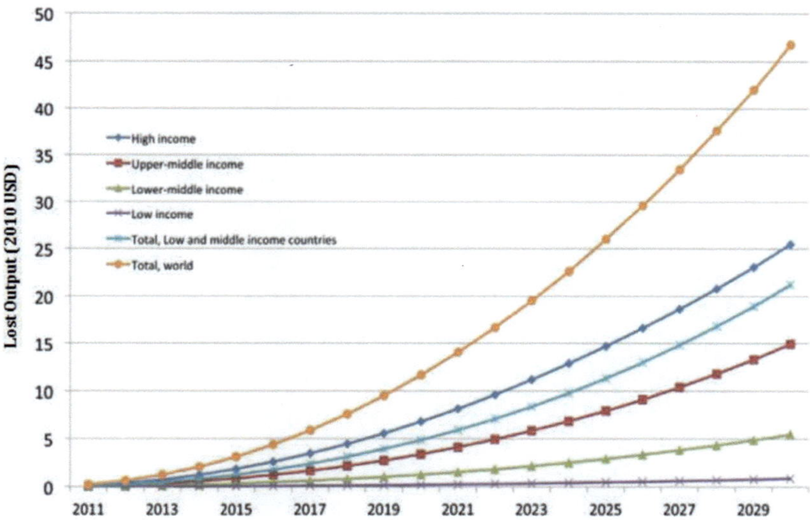

FIGURE 6-2 Output losses over time by income status.
SOURCES: Bloom et al., 2011; World Economic Forum.

al., 2015). Additional analyses found a large economic impact of NCDs on productivity across WHO regions, albeit with large regional differences in disability-adjusted life years (DALYs)[2] (Chaker et al., 2015).

Similarly, annual cancer costs worldwide were estimated at approximately \$1.16 trillion[3] in 2010, the equivalent of more than 2 percent of the global GDP (Stewart and Wild, 2014), with projections reaching \$8.3 trillion in annual costs by 2030 (Bloom et al., 2011). Yet, investing in cancer care and control could result in millions of avoidable deaths, achieving between \$100 and \$200 billion in global economic savings (Stewart and Wild, 2014). These costs are astronomical for many countries, even those with high-income status, and demonstrate the imperative behind addressing these two major health burdens.

Finding: CVDs and cancers comprise more than 51 percent of the projected \$47 trillion in cumulative lost output resulting from the increase in the global economic burden of five NCDs.

THE RISING EPIDEMIOLOGICAL BURDEN OF NONCOMMUNICABLE DISEASES

Of the 40 million deaths per year caused by NCDs, 17 million are considered to be "premature" (below the age of 70), and 87 percent of these occur in LMICs (WHO, 2017b). Tables 6-1 and 6-2 depict the heterogeneity of conditions that contribute to morbidity and mortality in 14 LMIC regions, and demonstrate the increasing burden of NCDs relative to communicable diseases in many parts of the world. Importantly, the health burden resulting from communicable and noncommunicable diseases is not always distinct. Recent studies have linked infections with the onset of chronic non-communicable diseases later in life. Following the 2009 H1N1 outbreak, multiple studies found an association between type 1 diabetes onset later in life and those who were diagnosed with H1N1 (Nenna et al., 2011; Piccini et al., 2012). This demonstrates a need for comprehensive preparedness and prevention efforts within a strong public health system to effectively combat NCDs as well as infectious disease threats—and their downstream consequences.

[2] The burden of disability associated with a disease or disorder can be measured in units called disability-adjusted life years (DALYs). DALYs represent the total number of years lost to illness, disability, or premature death within a given population. See more at https://www.nimh.nih.gov/health/statistics/global/index.shtml (accessed April 1, 2017).

[3] This figure is the sum of the costs of prevention and treatment, plus the annual economic value of DALYs lost as a result of cancer. It does not include the longer-term costs to families or the value that patients and families place on human suffering.

Cardiovascular Disease

Mortality due to CVDs has been growing around the world, with an increase of 12.5 percent between 2000 and 2015 (Wang et al., 2016). Though many incorrectly think that CVD and relevant risk factors are unique to high-income countries, the increase in global mortality is actually attributed to an increasing incidence of CVD in LMICs. In fact, 80 percent of all CVD related deaths occur in LMICs (Lozano et al., 2012; Pena and Bloomfield, 2015). CVD is now recognized as the leading cause of death globally, and in 2015 was responsible for nearly 18 million global deaths. The global burden of CVD is expected to continue to rise; premature deaths will increase from 5.9 million to 7.8 million between 2013 and 2025 if current risk factors for CVD do not change (O'Rourke, 2017).

Cancer

Cancer is the second largest cause of death worldwide, responsible for 8.8 million deaths (15.7 percent) globally in 2015 (Wang et al., 2016). The majority of the 14 million people diagnosed with cancer each year live in LMICs, where more deaths are caused by cancer than by human immunodeficiency virus/acquired immunodeficiency syndrome (HIV/AIDS), malaria, and tuberculosis (TB) combined (Ferlay et al., 2013; WHO, 2014). Around two-thirds of the 8.8 million global cancer deaths each year occur in LMICs because of late detection and poor access to treatment (WHO, 2017c), and this number is expected to triple by 2030 (Nyambura, 2017). Experts estimate that between 30 and 50 percent of cancers can currently be prevented, through evidence-based prevention strategies and reducing risk factors, meaning that up to 3.7 million lives can be saved each year, 80 percent of whom reside in LMICs (Stewart and Wild, 2014). Early detection and management can also contribute to the reduction of the cancer burden (WHO, 2017a). Nearly 70,000 women are diagnosed annually with cervical cancer in Africa alone, contributing to 22 percent of all cancers in women (Nyambura, 2017). As discussed later in this chapter, this and other types of cancer have been shown to be vaccine preventable; thus, there is a potential to substantially reduce cancer deaths by increasing vaccine coverage. In addition to mortality, cancer can also affect an individual's ability to work, which extends negative effects to the broader productivity of a country. For cervical cancer in particular, the percentage of attributable absolute DALYs varied across countries, for example from 1.6 percent in New Zealand to 13.4 percent in Brazil (Chaker et al, 2015).

TABLE 6-1 Morbidity (DALY) Ranking of Top NCDs and Communicable Diseases

	DALY Ranking					
Diseases	United States	Southern Latin America	Central Asia	Central Latin America	Andean Latin America	Caribbean
Cardiovascular Diseases	1	1	1	1	1	1
Cerebrovascular Diseases	11	4	3	11	10	3
Chronic Respiratory Diseases	3	3	9	7	7	8
Diabetes	4	7	13	3	9	4
Chronic Kidney Disease	18	15	22	5	11	16
HIV/AIDS	63	48	70	32	50	5
Tuberculosis	192	112	28	85	38	66
Malaria	256	244	247	226	220	196
Lower Respiratory Infection	25	5	4	9	2	6
Upper Respiratory Infection	113	128	158	111	119	142
Hepatitis	171	176	112	164	174	164
Chronic Liver Disease	21	17	6	10	13	26
Road Traffic Injury	12	8	12	6	4	10
Cancer	[redacted]					
Cervical	100	46	73	60	45	51
Liver	52	69	47	70	59	65
Breast	24	26	41	49	55	37
Tracheal, Bronchus, and Lung Cancer	5	14	25	44	47	24

NOTE: DALY = disability-adjusted life year; HIV/AIDS = human immunodeficiency virus/acquired immunodeficiency syndrome; NCD = noncommunicable disease.
SOURCE: *Global Burden of Disease Study 2015*. Institute for Health Metrics and Evaluation 2016. http://ghdx.healthdata.org/gbd-results-tool (accessed March 10, 2017). See Annex 6-1 for details on reconstructing the tables.

Tropical Latin America	East Asia	Southeast Asia	South Asia	N. Africa/ Middle East	Southern Africa	West Africa	East Africa	Central Africa
1	1	1	1	1	4	8	5	3
3	2	2	9	6	12	13	13	14
6	5	5	4	9	11	16	17	13
7	13	6	12	8	8	29	24	26
17	22	14	18	20	27	39	57	56
22	52	25	26	91	1	4	1	5
76	54	9	10	55	6	17	11	12
219	245	63	40	70	54	1	6	1
11	20	7	6	7	5	3	3	2
126	118	143	156	131	144	160	152	141
149	129	112	58	129	169	86	101	118
18	23	11	20	19	40	19	31	32
4	7	8	13	5	9	24	18	16
[redacted]								
59	80	67	101	141	43	81	67	66
69	10	33	107	65	62	44	70	63
39	45	36	63	47	48	98	79	79
30	8	27	54	38	36	105	129	104

TABLE 6-2 Mortality Ranking of Top NCDs and Communicable Diseases

	Mortality Rankings					
Diseases	United States	Southern Latin America	Central Asia	Central Latin America	Andean Latin America	Caribbean
Cardiovascular Diseases	1	1	1	1	1	1
Cerebrovascular Diseases	11	4	3	11	10	3
Chronic Respiratory Diseases	3	3	9	7	7	9
Diabetes	4	7	13	3	9	7
Chronic Kidney Disease	18	15	22	5	11	12
HIV/AIDS	63	48	70	32	50	10
Tuberculosis	192	112	28	85	38	46
Malaria	256	244	247	226	220	157
Lower Respiratory Infection	25	5	4	9	2	4
Upper Respiratory Infection	113	128	158	111	119	172
Hepatitis	171	176	112	164	174	131
Chronic Liver Disease	21	17	6	10	13	18
Road Traffic Injury	12	8	12	6	4	17
Cancer	[redacted]					
Cervical	100	46	73	60	45	32
Liver	52	69	47	70	59	33
Breast	24	26	41	49	55	21
Tracheal, Bronchus, and Lung Cancer	5	14	25	44	47	13

NOTE: HIV/AIDS = human immunodeficiency virus/acquired immunodeficiency syndrome; NCD = noncommunicable disease.
SOURCE: *Global Burden of Disease Study 2015*. Institute for Health Metrics and Evaluation 2016. http://ghdx.healthdata.org/gbd-results-tool (accessed March 10, 2017). See Annex 6-1 for details on reconstructing the tables.

Tropical Latin America	East Asia	Southeast Asia	South Asia	N. Africa/ Middle East	Southern Africa	West Africa	East Africa	Central Africa
1	1	1	1	1	3	2	1	1
3	2	2	5	3	7	8	6	5
5	5	5	3	10	10	18	14	12
8	21	8	11	9	8	19	22	22
13	19	12	14	13	18	29	50	46
22	40	20	24	68	1	5	2	4
53	36	9	9	38	9	15	8	9
172	184	69	38	70	56	1	9	3
6	14	6	6	8	6	3	3	2
179	173	177	179	182	180	171	172	166
109	90	81	50	82	135	76	82	101
14	18	11	16	12	28	14	20	19
10	11	13	15	7	11	20	18	16
[redacted]								
39	48	43	61	78	29	49	38	41
38	9	18	59	33	42	22	45	35
27	30	27	40	29	34	61	58	53
15	8	14	25	19	21	51	68	55

Barriers to Adequate Care

Whereas the populations of high-income countries benefit from quality health care centers, well trained health care providers, and regulations on harmful substances, such as tobacco, those in LMICs often lack adequate health care infrastructure (Wirtz et al., 2011) and policy safeguards. Compounding the challenge, health systems in LMICs are typically designed to handle infectious disease, not to provide the continuity of care needed for NCDs. The *Lancet* report on Prevention and Management of Chronic Disease explains:

> Chronic illness demands a complex health-systems response that needs to be sustained across a continuum of care. Evidence-based interventions should be delivered by health professionals with diverse skills. . . . Such interventions are possible only with a functioning health system, which can deliver disease prevention and education services alongside integrated care and intersectoral collaboration that extends beyond the health sector. (Samb et al., 2010, pp. 1785–1786)

In addition to ill-fitted health systems, traditional health care systems in LMICs often lack the fiscal infrastructure to meet patients' long-term health needs. In many LMICs, out-of-pocket expenses account for approximately 50 percent of total health expenditures, which may only be lowered by increased central government investment in health (Zhang and Liu, 2014). However, increased decentralization of health care spending suggests that local governments in low-income countries will lack the capital to provide for their citizens' health care needs, making this government investment more difficult. For many patients, high out-of-pocket expenditures lead them to opt out of seeking medical care and leave the hospital before it is recommended by their physicians (Babiarz et al., 2012). Increasing the number of patients who seek treatment and maintain their therapy regimen continues to be a challenge and hinders the efforts of global health actors and national governments in achieving CVD and cancer prevention targets.

Many countries experience difficulties effecting change in national policy and spending in part because NCDs like CVD are not prioritized in political agendas, despite their significant health and economic burden. In addition, the slow epidemic of NCDs does not create the type of panic or rapid response that infectious diseases like Ebola, multidrug-resistant tuberculosis (MDR-TB), or HIV/AIDS can generate (Reddy et al., 2016). The World Innovation Summit for Health 2016 Behavioral Insights report explains that it can be difficult for policy makers, politicians, and health care professionals to emphasize preventative care because of a tendency to "focus on the immediate problem in front of us, rather than the potential future problems that seem distant and abstract" (Hallsworth et al., 2016).

Finding: Although the mortality and morbidity burdens of CVD and cancers are high, there is evidence that investing in comprehensive health systems and prevention strategies can save millions of lives. Political challenges remain in mobilizing resources and support for NCDs that may not be seen as immediate priorities.

MOTIVATION FOR U.S. INVOLVEMENT

The growing global burden of mortality due to CVD and cancer poses a significant strategic problem that the United States cannot ignore. A 2014 Council on Foreign Relations Task Force report confirms this stance, stating that U.S. interests will be affected by the rise of NCDs in LMICs because of their human and economic impacts (Daniels et al., 2014). The majority of U.S. spending on global health is directed toward HIV/AIDS, TB, malaria, and other infectious diseases, in addition to maternal and child health, nutrition, and family planning. While some funding is directed toward strengthening health systems, there are no dedicated funding streams specifically for NCDs and no presidential initiatives established to reduce their burden. Even global dialogue about strengthening health systems neglects most chronic diseases (Samb et al., 2010). The 2014 Council on Foreign Relations Task Force report outlines steps the United States can take now to address the critical issues of NCDs, including promotion of cardiovascular health, and vaccination and screening programs to prevent cancer (Daniels et al., 2014). Many of these services can often be integrated into existing U.S. global health programs and platforms, motivated by three key benefits, which are discussed further in the sections below:

1. universal purpose
2. economic prosperity and trade benefits
3. safeguarding U.S. global health investments

Universal Purpose

Because NCDs are a leading cause of morbidity and mortality in high-, middle-, and low-income countries, there is a tremendous opportunity for a shared innovation approach to developing solutions to common problems. By investing in CVD and cancer prevention programs abroad, the United States can identify cost-effective strategies to target these diseases domestically. The potential of this approach has already been demonstrated through a program in King County, Washington, that implemented a mobile health solution for NCD management based on interventions used in Bangladesh, China, and India (Global to Local, n.d.). Additionally, research conducted in other countries, such as that done on Cuba's CIMAvax vaccine, may help to accelerate the discovery of cures and more effective treatments for cancers (Keck, 2016). For rare diseases in particular, expanding research efforts outside the United States could generate more opportunities for testing and information sharing.

Economic Prosperity and Trade Benefits

In today's global travel and trade environment, when other countries have a healthy population and workforce, the United States benefits. According to the 2013 report by the *Lancet* Commission on Investing in Health, approximately 11 percent of economic growth in LMICs is attributable to reductions in mortality (Jamison et al., 2013). Healthy populations lead to more stable economies, and this increased stability can encourage business expansion and additional consumption of U.S. goods. When multinational businesses open in a new country, it is in their interest to ensure their workforce is healthy and productive.

Safeguarding U.S. Global Health Investments

Many patients suffering from chronic conditions have already been recipients of U.S. global health aid for communicable diseases such as tuberculosis, malaria, and HIV/AIDS. If those patients are unable to work or die prematurely because of CVD or cancer, then the return on investment is lost. This holds especially true in the case of The U.S. President's Emergency Plan for AIDS Relief (PEPFAR) investments. In 2015, the PEPFAR program provided antiretroviral therapy for 9.5 million people (PEPFAR, 2017); it is critical to ensure these significant investments are not lost to morbidity and mortality attributable to NCDs. If these patients die prematurely from chronic illness, much of the progress gained from healthier societies and restabilized economies in PEPFAR partner countries could be at risk.

COST-EFFECTIVE AND HIGH-IMPACT GLOBAL INTERVENTIONS

A 2011 World Economic Forum report identified a set of highly cost-effective population- and individual-based "best buy" interventions for NCDs that can feasibly be implemented in resource-constrained LMIC health systems (WEF and WHO, 2011) (see Table 6-3). The cost of implementing the full suite of interventions across all LMICs between 2011 and 2025 would total $170 billion, representing less than 5 percent of overall health spending in those countries (WEF and WHO, 2011). Scaling up only the best buy interventions for CVD during that same time period, at a cumulative cost of $120 billion, would drive a 10 percent decrease in CVD-

TABLE 6-3 Cost-Effective Interventions for NCDs in Resource-Constrained Environments

Risk Factor/Disease	Interventions
Tobacco use	• Tax Increases • Smoke-free indoor workplaces and public places • Health information and warnings • Bans on tobacco advertising, promotion, and sponsorship
Harmful alcohol use	• Tax increases • Restricted access to retailed alcohol • Bans on alcohol advertising
Unhealthy diet and physical inactivity	• Reduced salt intake in food • Replacement of trans fat with polyunsaturated fat • Public awareness through mass media on diet and physical inactivity
Cardiovascular disease (CVD) and diabetes	• Counseling and multidrug therapy for people with a high risk of developing heart attacks and strokes (including those with established CVD) • Treatment of heart attacks with aspirin
Cancer	• Hepatitis B immunization to prevent liver cancer (already scaled up) • Screening and treatment of precancerous lesions to prevent cervical cancer

NOTE: NCD = noncommunicable disease.
SOURCE: WEF and WHO, 2011.

attributable mortality and a $377 billion projected cumulative economic benefit (WEF and WHO, 2011).

Similarly, a 2015 working paper for the Disease Control Priorities project found that substantially increasing the coverage of four prevention and treatment interventions, gradually over 15 years, would reduce projected NCD mortality by 25 percent in LMICs (Nugent, 2015). The analysis demonstrated an average benefit-cost ratio of 8:1, with annual benefits of $63.3 billion at a global cost of only $8.5 billion per year (see Table 6-4).

In examining these "best buy" interventions at a more granular level, the suggested practices can either be classified as policies targeted at the population level, or at the point of service delivery. A growing body of research demonstrates that interventions, such as fiscal and regulatory policies, that target behavioral and environmental risk factors that contribute to NCDs have a positive impact on health outcomes and can be cost effec-

TABLE 6-4 Cost–Benefit Analysis of Increasing Coverage of Interventions

Target	Annual Benefits (in $ millions)	Annual Costs (in $ millions)	Benefit for Every Dollar Spent
Aspirin therapy at the onset of AMI (75% coverage)	$836	$27.40	$31
Reduce salt content in manufactured foods by at least 30%	$12,121	$638	$19
Increase tobacco price by 125% through taxation	$37,194	$3,548	$10
Secondary prevention of CVD with polydrug (70% coverage)	$13,116	$3,850	$3
Total	$63,267	$8,063.40	$8

NOTE: AMI = acute myocardial infarction, CVD = cardiovascular disease.
SOURCE: Nugent, 2015.

tive (Cecchini et al., 2010; WEF and WHO, 2011). Of note, 7 of the top 10 risk factors contributing to global DALYs affect cardiovascular health (Forouzanfar et al., 2016).[4] Given that risk behaviors associated with the onset of CVD later in life often form during childhood and adolescence, a life course approach is critical to the prevention of NCDs (Lobstein et al., 2015). It is therefore important to target interventions in a comprehensive manner and develop approaches and interventions that change the nature of the consumer environment across the life course (e.g., changing availability, price, marketing practices that influence food choices and preferences) (Hawkes et al., 2015).

In addition to targeting risk factors through policy and regulatory means, communities and institutions can reduce CVD and cancer risk and thereby improve the health and well-being of their population by targeting service delivery. A critical component of this approach includes vaccination campaigns and screening programs, which can prevent the disease or catch it in its early stages before it devolves into a life-threatening illness or adverse event. The reach of policies and programs can be expanded by targeting points where the population already interfaces with the health care delivery system. Examples include integrating additional services into health care visits and conducting screening programs in high-traffic locations.

[4] These include blood pressure, smoking, fasting plasma glucose, body mass index, total cholesterol, alcohol use, and sodium intake. For more, see http://www.thelancet.com/journals/lancet/article/PIIS0140-6736(16)31679-8/abstract, Figure 7 (accessed April 20, 2017).

Across these various types of policy or health services interventions, the committee chose to prioritize prevention and early diagnosis. The committee urges U.S. global health programs to hone in on prevention and screening efforts to reduce disease incidence, contain disease progression in early stages, and decrease the economic burden in countries with high rates of CVD and cancer. Solutions for prevention of these diseases may also have a parallel impact on many other health outcomes as well, as many NCDs share risk factors. Moreover, solutions developed in other countries have the potential for application in the United States, as Americans also suffer from high burdens of CVD and cancer.

Fiscal and Regulatory Policies to Reduce Risk Factors for NCDs

Changes in individual behavior are difficult to achieve and maintain and the effects of behavior changes manifest over a long period of time. Fiscal and regulatory population-based approaches, which have been successful in reducing NCD risk factors such as smoking and alcohol consumption, are among the most effective means to curb the burden of CVD and cancer. Examples of such policies are discussed in the sections below.

Fiscal Policies

Fiscal approaches, often considered as part of a philosophy of "nudging," are an attempt to change behaviors through taxation or subsidization (Hector, 2012). In a study comparing interventions to address obesity (e.g., food labeling, fiscal measures, worksite interventions, mass media) in Brazil, China, India, Mexico, Russia, and South Africa, fiscal measures were consistently found to be cost saving and generated the largest or second largest health effects in 20- and 50-year projections, in comparison to the other interventions (Cecchini et al., 2010). Another recent review and meta-analysis showed that a 10 percent price reduction or subsidy increases consumption of healthful foods and beverages by 14 percent, whereas the same price increase or tax reduces consumption of unhealthy foods or beverages by 7 percent (Afshin et al., 2015). For example, a sugar tax employed in Mexico, where a one peso per liter tax was levied on sugar-sweetened beverages, resulted in an overall 7.6 percent reduction in sugar-sweetened beverage purchases 2 years after the tax was levied (Colchero et al., 2017). The decrease in purchase rate was even greater among low-socioeconomic status households (11.6 percent) (Colchero et al., 2017), demonstrating how these fiscal and regulatory policies often benefit a country's poorest the most. The health effects of this tax from 2013 to 2022 are likely to include substantially lower incidence of type 2 diabetes cases, strokes, and myocardial infarctions, and fewer deaths. As a result, the tax is projected to save Mexico $983 million (Sánchez-Romero et al., 2016).

Fiscal approaches have also been proven as an effective means to curb tobacco use. Over 100 studies, including those done in LMICs, have shown that taxation has a major effect on rates of smoking (Summers and Jamison, 2013). The *Lancet* Commission on Investing in Health found that adding a 50 percent price increase in cigarettes through tax in China would avert 20 million deaths and generate an extra $20 billion in revenue over the next 50 years (Summers and Jamison, 2013). Additionally, a study in China that analyzed the impact of a tax of 50 percent on tobacco products revealed that the tax would most benefit the poor: Of the 231 million years of life gained as a result of the tax over 50 years, one-third of those are expected to be gained by the lowest socioeconomic quintile, and of the $24 billion of decreased expenditures on tobacco-related disease, 28 percent would benefit the lowest quintile (Verguet et al., 2015).

Regulatory Policies

In addition to fiscal measures, policy makers have used regulatory means to influence behavioral and environmental factors contributing to NCD burden. For tobacco use, for example, a widely used approach is the requirement of warning labels, which has proven be to effective in raising awareness of the dangers of tobacco and reducing consumption (Mallikarjun et al., 2014). For example, a study set in India revealed that for those who noticed the labels on tobacco products, 71.5 percent reported that the labels made them think about quitting smoking, and those individuals had much greater knowledge about the relationship between tobacco use and lung cancer (Mallikarjun et al., 2014). Given that tobacco-related illnesses are projected to kill 8 million people per year by 2030 (ASH, 2015), a dual pronged prevention strategy using taxation and regulation can assist in decreasing the burden of cigarette smoking.

Another key risk factor for many NCDs, often related to cigarette smoking, is air quality. In fact, approximately 2 billion children live in areas where pollution levels exceed the minimum air quality standards set by the World Health Organization (WHO) (UNICEF, 2016). Every year, nearly 600,000 children under the age of 5 die from diseases either caused or exacerbated by indoor or outdoor air pollution. With the growing trends of globalization and urbanization, many experts expect this number to climb unless conditions are improved. Improving air quality through reductions in pollution will not only help the children exposed, but will also realize benefits for the whole society—through increased productivity and more sustainable development (UNICEF, 2016). Given that deaths from air pollution cost the global economy $225 billion in lost labor income and more than $5 trillion in welfare losses in 2013 (World Bank and IHME, 2016), a concerted effort toward improving air quality is needed. Opportunities for regulation exist to address air pollution from several angles, including limiting the open burning of waste or developing regulations for the detection of environmental diseases. For example, Israel's Clean Air Law of 2008 set limits for emissions on major industrial polluters, in addition to spot checks and penalties for violation, and the Pollution Control Department in Thailand adopted new vehicle emissions standards and low sulphur fuel, decreasing Bangkok's air pollution (UNEP, 2014). When done in cooperation with the private sector, air quality can be improved in a sustainable and cost-effective manner—leading to reduced mortality rates and economic burden.

Screening Programs for Early Detection and Treatment of Cardiovascular Disease

Blood pressure screening is a relatively inexpensive and simple health service that could easily be integrated with the existing health services offered through established U.S. global health programs. By offering blood pressure screening at the same location and using the same staff (after a period of training, as discussed below), U.S. global health programs could cost-effectively initiate CVD care in partner countries. Early screening alerts individuals that they are at risk for developing CVD, which can prompt behavior change and regular health care visits for improved management of the condition. Given the burden of CVD in LMICs, where 80 percent of deaths from CVD occur (Lozano et al., 2012; Pena and Bloomfield, 2015), and the knowledge that hypertension is a major risk factor for CVD screening will be a vital tool for reducing the burden of NCDs.

However, due to the additional social, political, and economic concerns in LMICs, it is important to contextualize the screening programs being implemented, as they will be contingent on the care services available, the supply chain of treatment regimens, the abilities of the medical providers in different locations, and the physical infrastructure of the health facilities. Vedanthan et al. (2015) examined CVD programs in western Kenya, noting that screening programs are just the first step of many required to ensure successful CVD prevention, and argued that the entire care cascade must be used effectively in order for the programs to be successful (see Box 6-1).

Immunization Strategies for Vaccine-Preventable Cancers

In recent years, cancer prevention has moved beyond screenings and early detection into the realm of primary prevention—or the prevention of disease before it even occurs. The two most common cancers in Africa—

BOX 6-1
Blood Pressure Screening Programs

As an implementing partner of AstraZeneca's Healthy Heart Africa program, the Academic Model Providing Access to Healthcare (AMPATH) is able to provide integrated, high-quality cardiovascular disease care in Western Kenya. AMPATH's foundational principles to find, link, treat, and retain patients guide the organization to respond to the challenges of identification of patients, poor laboratory and diagnostic equipment, and mistrust of public-sector services among Kenya's people. AMPATH has responded to these challenges by providing door-to-door, home-based screening services; providing diagnostic materials to rural health centers; and improving the relationships with the community and tribal elders. Through their efforts, AMPATH has created an integrated chronic disease prevention and treatment system that maximizes the work of community health workers at the village level, ensures that referrals are made efficiently through open referral networks, and guarantees that patients have the medicines they need through revolving fund pharmacies to support government pharmacies.

SOURCE: Vedanthan et al., 2015.

cervical cancer and liver cancer—have been linked to infections with human papillomavirus (HPV) and hepatitis B, respectively. Consequently, the risk of developing these cancers can be substantially reduced through vaccination. Of the 250 million people chronically infected with hepatitis B worldwide, 600,000 die each year as a result of liver cancer or liver failure due to viral infection (Gavi, 2012). Similarly, HPV is estimated to cause 275,000 deaths annually through progression to cervical cancer, the majority of which occur in LMICs. Without changes in prevention and control measures, this number is projected to rise to more than 400,000 deaths by 2035 (Gavi, 2015). Vaccines against HPV and hepatitis B have the potential to prevent many of these deaths caused by cervical and liver cancers.

Mother-to-child transmission is the most common route of hepatitis B infection (Franco et al., 2012), although sexual contact is also an important mode. WHO's Sector Strategy to Prevent Viral Hepatitis calls attention to a timely hepatitis B virus birth-dose vaccination as a key method to prevent mother-to-child transmission, an approach that could be enhanced through antenatal testing and the use of antiviral drugs (WHO, 2016b). The WHO strategy sets targets for 50 percent coverage by 2020 and 90 percent coverage by 2030 (WHO, 2016b). By the end of 2014, all low-income countries had introduced the hepatitis B vaccine into routine immunization programs, and global childhood hepatitis B virus vaccination coverage had increased to more than 82 percent (WHO, 2016b). However, coverage of hepatitis B virus birth-dose lagged behind at just 38 percent (WHO, 2016b). Improving this birth-dose coverage could reduce the number of deaths related to hepatitis B.

Since 2006, HPV vaccination has contributed to a decrease in HPV incidence in young women in the United States by two-thirds (Hoffman, 2016), and a decline in cervical cancer rates are expected as vaccinated women age. With the help of Gavi, the Vaccine Alliance (Gavi), 1 million girls have been immunized against HPV in 19 countries since 2013 (Gavi, n.d.). This has been achieved through lowering the vaccine price, using schools and community centers to reach school-aged girls, integrating the vaccine with other routine vaccinations and adolescent health programs, and improving communication at the community level to raise awareness about HPV (Gavi, n.d.). However, a strategy beyond reliance on Gavi will be necessary, as many countries with a high HPV burden may not be Gavi eligible or may have recently graduated from its assistance, as is the case in southeast Asia (amfAR, 2016). In order to reach the largest number of girls and women at risk for developing cervical cancer, more comprehensive operations are needed. This may prove challenging, as barriers to increased vaccination rates in LMICs include mistrust of government health care programs and association of the vaccine with sexual activity (Agosti and Goldie, 2007), which plagues vaccine implementation in many high-income countries as well. Regardless, a concerted effort to increase HPV vaccination rates, thereby reducing the risk for cervical cancer, is a worthy endeavor, as cervical cancer now ranks as the fourth leading type of cancer for women across the world (WHO, 2016a). In response to this need, global support for HPV vaccination programs has grown in recent years. By building on the valuable efforts of Gavi and working to fill the gaps in HPV vaccine coverage, the United States can capitalize on this momentum and significantly contribute to the progress being made to reduce the burden of cervical cancer.

Although routine vaccines for cervical and liver cancers are effective low-cost preventive tools, early-stage detection is also critical for effective, less costly treatment for those not covered by preventive interventions or who have disease etiology that is not vaccine preventable. For example, a 4-year pilot project on early diagnosis achieved a 34 percent decrease in presentation of late-stage cervical cancer by enabling women to receive early stage treatment (Devi et al., 2007). Additional success has been shown in detection and treatment of early cervical cancer in Zambia, where simple interventions can be conducted without the need for costly infrastructure or highly trained specialists (see Box 6-2).

Finding: Evidence-based strategies and interventions exist to address CVD and cancers both at the population level (such as fiscal and regulatory policies) and at the health care delivery level (such as early screening and immunization campaigns).

TRANSFORMING HEALTH SYSTEMS FOR NONCOMMUNICABLE DISEASES

Instead of creating a new "vertical" or singular disease program for CVD or cancers, U.S. global health programs can leverage existing stakeholders and programs to address risk factors and care delivery more holistically. A great example of this is the newly launched Global Hearts initiative, a collaboration among WHO, the U.S. Centers for Disease Control and Prevention (CDC), the World Heart Federation, the World Stroke Organization, the International Society of Hypertension, and the World Hypertension League (WHO, 2016c). The initiative will provide governments with technical support needed to implement and scale up interventions—such as those highlighted in this chapter—to reduce blood pressure and prevent heart attacks and strokes. Beyond leveraging existing programs, changing the approach of health system design to be more integrated and holistic in nature, and decentralizing services at the community level can be beneficial for ensuring cost-effectiveness of programs and contextual sustainability.

Additionally, there is clear interest from the private sector for many reasons (Hancock et al., 2011; Sturchio and Goel, 2012). For multinational companies, keeping their workforce healthy and productive will improve their bottom line. For those companies in the health sector, there is an opportunity to create a market for themselves in LMICs that have a high burden of NCDs. Creating health systems that enable robust and sustainable care delivery will also improve the sustainability and growth of their company's business. For these reasons, the committee feels that optimizing available resources and stakeholders through changes in health system design will be highly effective for improving cardiovascular health and preventing cancer, as explored in sections below.

Integration of Services at the Community Level

The dual burden of NCDs and infectious diseases in LMICs is exacerbated by well-documented interactions between communicable and noncommunicable diseases. For example, TB has been linked to an increased risk for stroke (Sheu et al., 2010) and lung cancer (Simonsen et al., 2014; Yu et al., 2011). Similarly, HIV/AIDS has been linked to an increased risk of cardiovascular disease (Hsue et al., 2012), in part due to the transition of HIV/AIDS as a chronic condition and AIDS patients now often living to old age (Rabkin et al., 2012), and side effects of antiretroviral therapy (Subbaraman et al., 2007). HIV/AIDS also has been linked to a specific set of cancers (Grulich et al., 2007). Cervical cancer, for example, is four to five times more common in women who are HIV positive (PEPFAR, n.d.).

With these examples in mind, the traditional siloed, disease-specific care system will be hard pressed to address both communicable diseases and NCDs if done in isolation. Given that patients often suffer from both kinds of diseases, the effectiveness of health programs can be increased by integrating services—an approach that would seek to share locations, staff, systems, tools, and strategies (Rabkin et al., 2012). Such integration has been found to be successful in varying locations and approaches, with examples described in Box 6-2.

PEPFAR—a well-known successful investment—offers a unique opportunity for such integration. Along with the George W. Bush Institute, the Susan G. Komen Foundation, UNAIDS, and other partners, PEPFAR initiated the Pink Ribbon Red Ribbon (PRRR) campaign in 2011 (PRRR, n.d.). Since then, PRRR has screened thousands of women for cervical and breast cancer and provided HPV vaccinations (see Box 6-3). Continuing this vision of cross-sector services, PEPFAR entered into a public–private partnership with AstraZeneca in 2016 called Healthy Heart Africa, which integrates HIV infection reduction programs with hypertension screening targeting older men, a cohort often missed by standard HIV efforts (AstraZeneca, 2016). These types of focused partnerships featuring complementary goals and overlapping patient populations offer great opportunity to expand the reach and effectiveness of existing U.S. global health programs.

Decentralizing Services at the Community Level

Complementing the shift toward integration, the infrastructure and systems of LMICs must be transformed to meet the changing national health profiles in the long-term. While this will take time and sustained effort, there are short-term methods that can increase the capacity of countries to better address the burden of NCDs, including a broader use of the existing workforce. A 2015 assessment of community health workers in Bangladesh, Guatemala, Mexico, and South Africa found that health workers without formal professional training can be adequately trained to effectively screen for and identify people with a high risk of cardiovascular disease (Gaziano et al., 2015). Training existing staff to perform new tasks could free up the higher-level trained professionals to focus on those tasks requiring greater expertise. The concept of task shifting more generally has been found to be feasible in the management of hypertension and reducing cardiovascular risk (Poulter et al., 2015). This concept has also been successfully applied in cancer screening; the cervical cancer screening program in Zambia dis-

BOX 6-2
Case Studies on Integration of Services for Communicable and Noncommunicable Diseases

Integrating Cardiovascular Disease Care into Existing Tuberculosis and Human Immunodeficiency Virus (HIV) Programs in South Africa

Developed by the University of Cape Town Lung Institute, the Practical Approach to Care Kit (PACK) aims to empower front-line nurses where resources are scarce. Though originally designed to improve access to diagnoses and treatment for people with tuberculosis and human immunodeficiency virus (HIV), PACK was expanded to include a number of chronic conditions—including CVD. Since its inception, PACK has contributed to consistent improvements in health outcomes for patients—for both communicable and noncommunicable conditions. As a result of its success, PACK is being adapted and implemented in Malawi, The Gambia, Brazil, Mexico, and Botswana.

HIV/Acquired Immunodeficiency Syndrome (HIV/AIDS)–Hypertension Integrated Care in Cambodia

Cambodia struggles with an increasing burden of chronic diseases, with 12 to15 percent of the population being hypertensive. To address this issue, the Cambodian Ministry of Health and Médecins Sans Frontières established clinics to integrate chronic care (for hypertension and diabetes) with HIV/AIDS care in Takeo and Siem Reap. This not only resulted in an increased inflow of patients—indicating a desire for integrated services—but it also improved the health of patients. Through the combined services, hypertensive patients were able to reach healthy blood pressure targets of 160/90 mm Hg. This success signified the feasibility of providing integrated services and the adaptability of medical staff to assume a multidisciplinary role.

Integrating HIV/AIDS Care and Cervical Cancer Prevention in Zambia

Zambia has seen positive dividends from concerted efforts to train middle-level health practitioners in screening methods for early signs of cervical cancer. The World Health Organization's endorsement in 2013 of the screening method known as VIA (visual inspection with acetic acid) and cryotherapy-based "screen and treat" programs prompted questions on how to scale these services without a correlating vertical disease program. An evaluation of approaches to scale up the Cervical Cancer Prevention Program in Zambia found that successful expansion could be achieved by leveraging HIV/AIDS program investments to address the high burden of cervical disease at a population level. Researchers also found that focusing on the provision of services for high-risk HIV-infected women initially gave the program firm support within the HIV platform, but it did not preclude progression or expansion of the program to HIV-uninfected women in the community. Researchers noted that using existing infrastructure for screening implementation will have a positive effect on costs, expertise, and sustainability.

SOURCES: Janssens et al., 2007; Parham et al., 2015; and Reddy et al., 2016.

BOX 6-3
Impacts of the Pink Ribbon Red Ribbon Initiative

Partnership countries for the Pink Ribbon Red Ribbon initiative include Botswana, Ethiopia, Tanzania, and Zambia. As of 2016, 119,192 girls have received all doses of human papillomavirus vaccine, 341,863 women have received basic screening for cervical cancer, 24,478 women have been treated with cryotherapy or LEEP for cervical cancer, and 17,944 women have been screened for breast cancer.

NOTE: LEEP = loop electrosurgical excision procedure.
SOURCE: PRRR, 2016.

cussed in Box 6-2 promoted task shifting from doctors to nurses and used mobile technology to fill in any gaps and improve decision making (Parham et al., 2015). Box 6-4 provides an example of a community-based approach, including task-shifting to address CVD management.

Leveraging Private-Sector Involvement

Multinational companies understand the value of a healthier workforce in terms of increased productivity. In addition to being able to work for a greater number of years before retirement (and thus, spending more time contributing to society and less time deriving benefits from social welfare systems), healthier people are able to achieve higher-quality results in a shorter time period (Bloom et al., 2011).

Decades of work through existing platforms, such as those established by the U.S. Agency for International Development (USAID), the National Institutes of Health (NIH), PEPFAR, and others, have enabled U.S. global health programs to build strong international, national, and community-level networks. Leveraging this U.S. knowledge base and infrastructure, and creating an environment conducive to catalytic, innovative support and partnerships, can lead to more sustainable programs and improved outcomes. However, according to an insights report from the World Economic Forum's Future of Health project, the willingness of the private and public sectors to coinvest depends on the right investment mechanisms being in place, on there being proof that those returns will materialize, and on the existence of a business model that makes it possible to share the benefits (WEF, 2015). This willingness has been growing in recent years and at the

BOX 6-4
Case Study: The Need for Innovative Community-Based Approaches to Cardiovascular Disease Management and Control

The prevalence of hypertension in Ghana was recently estimated at 27 percent of the population, but only 4 percent of patients control their condition. An international public–private partnership is leading the evaluation and cost-effectiveness analysis of a community-based hypertension program (ComHIP) in a district in Ghana as an important contribution to the development of evidence-based innovative approaches to the management of noncommunicable diseases in low- and middle-income countries (LMICs). Individuals from the Novartis Foundation, the Ghana Health Service, FHI 360, the London School of Hygiene & Tropical Medicine, and the School of Public Health of the University of Ghana comprise the research team. Other local collaborators include the Ministry of Health, Ghana National Health Insurance Scheme, Ghana College of Physicians & Surgeons, Ghana Medical and Dental Council, the Pharmacy Council, Licensed Chemical Sellers Association, and Ghana Nursing Board. This innovative, community-based and technologically driven approach has the potential to enhance the delivery of affordable and effective approaches to hypertension management and control in LMIC.

Project Aims: Enhance the capacity of the Ghana Health Service through task shifting and innovative technology solutions to improve access to quality and affordable services for hypertension and other CVDs. The project also aims to improve the capacity of patients in managing their own conditions and risk factors.

World Economic Forum Annual Meeting in 2017, a collaborative initiative among more than 20 companies—Access Accelerated—was launched. Fifty million dollars was initially committed to improve access to NCD prevention, care, and treatment, in partnership with the Union of International Cancer Control and the World Bank (Access Accelerated, n.d.; IP Watch, 2017). There is potential to capitalize on this willingness and interest from the private sector to augment the current knowledge base and infrastructure to advance NCD efforts globally.

The committee believes the United States should build on such shared commitments and is poised to assist other companies and multilateral groups in contributing to the advancement of progress against NCDs. Although the existing U.S. vertical platforms can be leveraged for integrating services and expanding the scope of the current workforce, there will likely be difficulty and opposition to using existing funds to purchase commodities for treating international patients with conditions such as hypertension,

Program Components:

- *Health services strengthening:* Strengthening private- and public-sector capacity and collaboration to manage hypertension, including the establishment of a direct referral linkage between the public health system and private drug outlets.
- *Task shifting:*
    1. Shifting screening and monitoring of blood pressure from health facilities to community health officers and private drug outlets.
    2. Shifting management of moderate and noncomplicated hypertension from doctors to community-based nurses.
    3. Shifting dispensing of blood pressure medication from pharmacists to private drug outlets.
- *Self-management:* Empowering patients to self-manage hypertension and control other CVD risk factors.
- *Technological innovation:* Using information and communication technologies to improve communication, patient education, clinical management, adherence to therapy, and health information management.
- *Reduce out-of-pocket costs:* Minimizing out-of-pocket costs of hypertension by ensuring the provision of health coverage by the Ghana National Health Insurance Scheme.

SOURCES: FHI 360, 2014; Novartis Foundation, 2016; Peter Lamptey, personal communication, February 2, 2017.

which is often a manifestation of behavior choices. However, public–private partnerships present unique opportunities and have already demonstrated successful results in many areas. Consider the previous example of PEPFAR and AstraZeneca's partnership, as well as PEPFAR's Determined, Resilient, Empowered, AIDS-free, Mentored, and Safe women (DREAMS) initiative, where a pharmaceutical company is purchasing medication for treatment in young women who are not eligible for coverage under PEPFAR. Additionally, the practice of matching resources to incentivize private involvement has also proven useful for PEPFAR programs in the past, by leveraging established supply chains and developing reference laboratories (Sturchio and Cohen, 2012). This method has been recommended for maternal and child health issues, and could easily be applied to NCD-focused partnerships.

Health companies have a vested interest in reaching the populations throughout LMICs that suffer from CVDs and cancers. Because these

TABLE 6-5 Private Companies Investing Their Own Resources in NCDs in Developing Countries

Company	Disease Target	Impact
AstraZeneca	Hypertension	Through Healthy Heart Africa, AstraZeneca aimed to reach 10 million people with treatment for hypertension by 2025. By 2015, it had screened over 1 million people (AstraZeneca, 2015).
Novartis Access Program	CVD, diabetes, breast cancer, and respiratory illnesses	Novartis Access portfolio includes 15 on and off-patent medicines addressing CVD, type 2 diabetes, breast cancer, and respiratory illnesses. It is offered as a basket to countries for $1/treatment/month. Its goal is to provide access to 20 million patients annually by 2020 (Novartis, n.d.).
Pfizer	Healthy aging	Pfizer joined with HelpAge International in 2012 to reduce the NCD impact among the elderly in Tanzania. The partnership has led to the development of a tool that measures healthy aging in the elderly (Pfizer, 2016).
Medtronic Foundation "Health Rise" Program	CVD and diabetes	Health Rise is a 5-year, $17 million global effort funded by the Medtronic Foundation to expand access to care for CVD and diabetes among underserved populations in targeted areas in Brazil, India, South Africa, and the United States. It also works to strengthen health care delivery in the community and home-based settings (HealthRise, 2015).

NOTE: CVD = cardiovascular disease; NCD = noncommunicable disease.

populations may not have access to the right medications because of either systemic or financial barriers, there is a gap that can draw mutual interest. If companies can create opportunities for larger numbers of people to purchase and depend on their medications, vaccines, and devices, they can eventually translate that increase to larger profits and sustainable business growth. Many companies have already invested their own resources in curbing the human and cost burden of NCDs in many countries (explored in more detail in Chapter 8). As an overview of the breadth of this private-sector interest, Table 6-5 gives examples of companies already investing in reducing the burden of CVDs and cancers, among other NCDs, around the world, through their own motivation.[5]

[5] For a comprehensive listing of health development programs involving the research-based pharmaceutical industry, see the International Federation of Pharmaceutical Manufacturers and Associations Health Partnerships Directory at http://ncds.ifpma.org/partnerships-and-prevention/index.html (accessed March 19, 2017).

Finding: Integration, decentralization of services at the community level, and public–private partnerships are promising methods for transforming health systems in LMICs to provide better care for patients suffering from NCDs.

SUMMARY AND RECOMMENDATION

NCDs, such as CVD, COPD, and lung cancer, kill 40 million people annually, almost three-quarters of whom are in LMICs (WHO, 2017b). CVD is the leading cause of death worldwide, killing 18 million people in 2015. In addition, 14 million people are diagnosed with cancer each year, leading to 8.8 million deaths in 2015 (Stewart and Wild, 2014). In LMICs, more people die from cancer than from AIDS, TB, and malaria combined (Ferlay et al., 2013; WHO, 2014).

NCDs are projected to cause cumulative global economic output losses of $47 trillion by 2030, approximately 75 percent of the 2010 global GDP. The global cost of CVD alone was estimated at $906 billion in 2015, and it is projected to rise to more than $1 trillion annually in 2030 (Reddy et al., 2016). Global cancer costs are expected to reach $8.3 trillion annually by 2030, yet investing in cancer care and control could result in millions of avoidable deaths and up to $200 billion in global savings (Stewart and Wild, 2014).

With similar rising human and economic burdens in the United States, U.S. global health programs have a clear opportunity to address these conditions that contribute to an enormous global disease burden. However, NCDs often are incorporated into other programs as an afterthought, and an overall coordination mechanism or strategy for these diverse diseases is lacking. U.S. global health programs have established strong networks and knowledge bases in countries as a result of decades of effort by various agencies through infectious disease and maternal and child health platforms. There is an opportunity to integrate NCD prevention and care into these established platforms. Private, multinational companies also are becoming more invested in addressing chronic diseases, and there is an opportunity to leverage these established networks and this private-sector interest to develop coordinated public–private partnerships focused on high-impact, evidence-based interventions.

Conclusion: Without intervention, the burden of NCDs will grow in both epidemiological and economic terms. This burden of disease will have massive adverse effects on societies of all income levels, including high rates of premature death and lost productivity that will reverse trends of improved economic growth and stability in many countries.

Conclusion: Global health programs are not devoting adequate attention to the promotion of cardiovascular health and prevention of cancer. National governments, donor governments, and NGOs need to address these priorities through policy changes, vaccination against vaccine-preventable cancers, and programs that are community based and integrated into existing health services.

Conclusion: The private sector has strong interest in addressing NCDs globally owing to their clear effects on workforce productivity, but such private-sector efforts are not synergized across countries or health systems. To be effective, private-sector efforts need to be better coordinated with those of other stakeholders and networks.

Recommendation 9: Promote Cardiovascular Health and Prevent Cancer

The U.S. Agency for International Development, the U.S. Department of State, and the U.S. Centers for Disease Control and Prevention, through their country offices, should provide seed funding to facilitate the mobilization and involvement of the private sector in addressing cardiovascular disease and cancer at the country level. These efforts should be closely aligned and coordinated with the efforts of national governments and should strive to integrate services at the community level. The priority strategies to ensure highest impact are

- **target and manage risk factors (e.g., smoking, alcohol use, obesity) for the major noncommunicable diseases, particularly through the adoption of fiscal policies and regulations that facilitate tobacco control and healthy diets;**
- **detect and treat hypertension early;**
- **detect and treat early cervical cancer; and**
- **immunize for vaccine-preventable cancers (specifically human papilloma virus and hepatitis B vaccines).**

ANNEX 6-1

Steps to Reconstruct Tables 6-1 and 6-2

The data used to construct the tables were extracted from http://ghdx.healthdata.org/gbd-results-tool, and the same steps were used for both mortality and morbidity rankings. Once at the site, the following parameters were chosen:

- Context: Cause
- Age: All
- Sex: Both
- Measure: "Deaths" for mortality and "DALY" for morbidity
- Metric: Number
- Year: 2015
- Cause: All nonbolded causes from the list of causes, with the exception of hepatitis, liver cancer, cardiovascular diseases, cerebrovascular diseases, cirrhosis and other chronic liver diseases, chronic kidney disease, and road injuries.
- Location: United States, Southern Latin America, Central Latin America, Caribbean, Tropical Latin America, East Asia, N. Africa/Middle East, Southern Africa, West Africa, East Africa, and Central Africa

The nonbolded categories for "Cause" were included as the committee was interested in learning about their ranking as a whole when compared to the infectious diseases being targeted in the report. Furthermore, as the diseases of interest (cardiovascular diseases and cancers) have common determinants and interventions, the committee felt it would be beneficial to consider their ranking as a whole.

To obtain the rankings, all the parameters except location were selected for each region at a time. Then, once downloaded into Excel, the data was sorted by "Measure" and then ranked.

REFERENCES

Access Accelerated. n.d. *What is access accelerated.* http://www.accessaccelerated.org/about (accessed February 14, 2017).

Afshin, A., J. Penalvo, L. Del Gobbo, M. Kashaf, R. Micha, K. Morrish, J. Pearson-Stuttard, C. Rehm, S. Shangguan, J. D. Smith, and D. Mozaffarian. 2015. CVD prevention through policy: A review of mass media, food/menu labeling, taxation/subsidies, built environment, school procurement, worksite wellness, and marketing standards to improve diet. *Currrent Cardiology Reports* 17(11):98.

Agosti, J. M., and S. J. Goldie. 2007. Introducing HPV vaccine in developing countries—key challenges and issues. *New England Journal of Medicine* 356(19):1908-1910.

amfAR (American Foundation for AIDS Research). 2016. *Cervical cancer, human papillomavirus (HPV), and HPV vaccines in Southeast Asia: Key considerations for expanding vaccine coverage and improving population health.* New York: The American Foundation for AIDS Research.

ASH (Action on Smoking and Health). 2015. *Tobacco and the developing world fact sheet.* Washington, DC: Action on Smoking and Health.

AstraZeneca. 2015. *Access to healthcare sustainability update 2015.* https://www.astrazeneca.com/content/dam/az/our-company/Sustainability/accesstohealthcare/Access%20to%20healthcare%20update%202015.pdf (accessed February 10, 2017).

AstraZeneca. 2016. PEPFAR and AstraZeneca launch partnership across HIV and hypertension services in Africa. Washington, DC: AstraZeneca.

Babiarz, K. S., G. Miller, H. Yi, L. Zhang, and S. Rozelle. 2012. China's new cooperative medical scheme improved finances of township health centers but not the number of patients served. *Health Affairs (Millwood)* 31(5):1065-1074.

Bloom, D. E., E. T. Cafiero, E. Jané-Llopis, S. Abrahams-Gessel, L. R. Bloom, S. Fathima, A. B. Feigl, T. Gaziano, M. Mowafi, A. Pandya, K. Prettner, L. Rosenberg, B. Seligman, A. Z. Stein, and C. Weinstein. 2011. *The global economic burden of noncommunicable diseases.* Geneva, Switzerland: World Economic Forum.

Cecchini, M., F. Sassi, J. A. Lauer, Y. Y. Lee, V. Guajardo-Barron, and D. Chisholm. 2010. Tackling of unhealthy diets, physical inactivity, and obesity: Health effects and cost-effectiveness. *The Lancet* 376(9754):1775-1784.

Chaker, L., A. Falla, S. J. van der Lee, T. Muka, D. Imo, L. Jaspers, V. Colpani, S. Mendis, R. Chowdhury, W. M. Bramer, R. Pazoki, and O. H. Franco. 2015. The global impact of non-communicable diseases on macro-economic productivity: A systematic review. *European Journal of Epidemiology* 30(5):357-395.

Colchero, M. A., J. Rivera-Dommarco, B. M. Popkin, and S. W. Ng. 2017. In Mexico, evidence of sustained consumer response two years after implementing a sugar-sweetened beverage tax. *Health Affairs (Millwood)* 36(3):564-571.

Daniels, Jr., M. E., T. E. Donilon, and T. Bollyky. 2014. *The emerging global health crisis: Noncommunicable diseases in low- and middle-income countries.* Washington, DC: Council on Foreign Relations.

Devi, B. C., T. S. Tang, and M. Corbex. 2007. Reducing by half the percentage of late-stage presentation for breast and cervix cancer over 4 years: A pilot study of clinical downstaging in Sarawak, Malaysia. *Annals of Oncology* 18(7):1172-1176.

Ferlay, J., I. Soerjomataram, M. Ervik, R. Dikshit, S. Eser, C. Mathers, M. Rebelo, D. Parkin, D. Forman, and F. Bray. 2013. *GLOBOCAN 2012 v1.0: Cancer incidence and mortality worldwide.* Lyon, France: IARC CancerBase.

FHI 360 (Family Health International 360). 2014. *Community-based hypertension improvement project (comHIP).* https://www.fhi360.org/projects/community-based-hypertension-improvement-project-comhip (accessed March 24, 2017).

Forouzanfar, M. H., A. Afshin, L. T. Alexander, H. R. Anderson, Z. A. Bhutta, S. Biryukov, M. Brauer, et al. 2016. Global, regional, and national comparative risk assessment of 79 behavioural, environmental and occupational, and metabolic risks or clusters of risks, 1990–2015: A systematic analysis for the Global Burden of Disease Study 2015. *The Lancet* 388(10053):1659-1724.

Franco, E., B. Bagnato, M. G. Marino, C. Meleleo, L. Serino, and L. Zaratti. 2012. Hepatitis B: Epidemiology and prevention in developing countries. *World Journal of Hepatology* 4(3):74-80.

Gavi (Gavi, the Vaccine Alliance). 2012. *Vaccines and cancer control: From hepatitis B to HPV*. http://www.gavi.org/partnersforum2012/session-summaries/22-%E2%80%93-vaccines-and-cancer-control--from-hepatitis-b-to-hpv (accessed February 14, 2017).

Gavi. 2015. *Keeping children healthy: The Vaccine Alliance progress report 2015*. Washington, DC: Gavi, the Vaccine Alliance.

Gavi. n.d. *Human papillomavirus vaccine support*. http://www.gavi.org/support/nvs/human-papillomavirus (accessed February 14, 2017).

Gaziano, T. A., S. Abrahams-Gessel, C. A. Denman, C. M. Montano, M. Khanam, T. Puoane, and N. S. Levitt. 2015. An assessment of community health workers' ability to screen for cardiovascular disease risk with a simple, non-invasive risk assessment instrument in Bangladesh, Guatemala, Mexico, and South Africa: An observational study. *Lancet Global Health* 3(9):e556-e563.

Global to Local. n.d. *Global to Local: Mobile health program*. http://www.globaltolocal.org/programs/2016/4/5/mobile-health-program (accessed February 14, 2017).

Grulich, A. E., M. T. van Leeuwen, M. O. Falster, and C. M. Vajdic. 2007. Incidence of cancers in people with HIV/AIDS compared with immunosuppressed transplant recipients: A meta-analysis. *The Lancet* 370(9581):59-67.

Hallsworth, M. S., V. Snijders, H. Burd, J. Prestt, G. Judah, S. Huf, and D. Halpern. 2016. *Applying behavioral insights: Simple ways to improve health outcomes*. Doha, Qatar: World Innovation Summit for Health.

Hancock, C., L. Kingo, and O. Raynaud. 2011. The private sector, international development and NCDS. *Globalization and Health* 7(1):23.

Hawkes, C., T. G. Smith, J. Jewell, J. Wardle, R. A. Hammond, S. Friel, A. M. Thow, and J. Kain. 2015. Smart food policies for obesity prevention. *The Lancet* 385(9985):2410-2421.

HealthRise. 2015. *What is HealthRise?* https://www.health-rise.org/about-healthrise/what-is-healthrise (accessed February 14, 2017).

Hector, C. 2012. Nudging towards nutrition? Soft paternalism and obesity-related reform. *Food and Drug Law Journal* 67(1):iii-iv, 103-122,.

Hoffman, J. 2016. HPV sharply reduced in teenage girls following vaccine, study says. *The New York Times*, February 22.

Hsue, P. Y., S. G. Deeks, and P. W. Hunt. 2012. Immunologic basis of cardiovascular disease in HIV-infected adults. *Journal of Infectious Diseases* 205 (Suppl 3):S375-S382.

IP (Intellectual Property) Watch. 2017. Brief: Industry initiative against non-communicable diseases launched at WEF. *Intellectual Property Watch*, January 19.

Jamison, D., L. Summers, G. Alleyne, K. Arrow, S. Berkeley, A. Binagwaho, F. Bustreo, D. Evans, R. Feachern, J. Frenk, G. Ghosh, S. Goldie, Y. Guo, S. Gupta, R. Horton, M. Kruk, A. Mahmoud, L. Mohohlo, M. Ncube, A. Pablos-Mendez, S. Reddy, H. Saxenian, A. Soucat, K. Ulltveit-Moe, and G. Yamey. 2013. Global Health 2035: A world converging within a generation. *The Lancet* 382:1898-1955.

Janssens, B., W. Van Damme, B. Raleigh, J. Gupta, S. Khem, K. Soy Ty, M. Vun, N. Ford, and R. Zachariah. 2007. Offering integrated care for HIV/AIDS, diabetes and hypertension within chronic disease clinics in Cambodia. *Bulletin of the World Health Organization* 85(11):880-885.

Keck, C. W. 2016. The United States and Cuba—turning enemies into partners for health. *New England Journal of Medicine* 375(16):1507-1509.

Lobstein, T., R. Jackson-Leach, M. L. Moodie, K. D. Hall, S. L. Gortmaker, B. A. Swinburn, W. P. T. James, Y. Wang, and K. McPherson. 2015. Child and adolescent obesity: Part of a bigger picture. *The Lancet* 385(9986):2510-2520.

Lozano, R., M. Naghavi, K. Foreman, S. Lim, K. Shibuya, V. Aboyans, J. Abraham, et al. 2012. Global and regional mortality from 235 causes of death for 20 age groups in 1990 and 2010: A systematic analysis for the Global Burden of Disease Study 2010. *The Lancet* 380(9859):2095-2128.

Mallikarjun, S., A. Rao, G. Rajesh, R. Shenoy, and M. P. Bh. 2014. Role of tobacco warning labels in informing smokers about risks of smoking among bus drivers in Mangalore, India. *Asian Pac Journal of Cancer Prevention* 15(19):8265-8270.

Muka, T., D. Imo, L. Jaspers, V. Colpani, L. Chaker, S. J. van der Lee, S. Mendis, R. Chowdhury, W. M. Bramer, A. Falla, R. Pazoki, and O. H. Franco. 2015. The global impact of non-communicable diseases on healthcare spending and national income: A systematic review. *European Journal of Epidemiology* 30(4):251-277.

Nenna, R., P. Papoff, C. Moretti, A. Pierangeli, G. Sabatino, F. Costantino, F. Soscia, G. Cangiano, V. Ferro, M. Mennini, S. Salvadei, C. Scagnolari, G. Antonelli, and F. Midulla. 2011. Detection of respiratory viruses in the 2009 winter season in Rome: 2009 influenza A (H1N1) complications in children and concomitant type 1 diabetes onset. *International Journal of Immunopathology and Pharmacology* 24(3):651-659.

Novartis. n.d. *Novartis Access*. https://www.novartis.com/about-us/corporate-responsibility/expanding-access-healthcare/novartis-access (accessed February 14, 2017).

Novartis Foundation. 2016. *ComHIP*. http://www.novartisfoundation.org/_file/607/comhip-factsheet.pdf (accessed March 8, 2017).

Nugent, R. 2015. *Benefits and costs of the noncommunicable disease targets for the post-2015 development agenda*. Tewksbury, MA: Copenhagen Consensus Center.

Nyambura, Z. 2017. Cancer: Africa's new health burden. *Deutsche Welle*, February 4.

O'Rourke, K. 2017. *Projecting, reducing the burden of cardiovascular disease by 2025*. http://www.healthdata.org/acting-data/projecting-reducing-burden-cardiovascular-disease-2025 (accessed March 29, 2017).

Parham, G. P., M. H. Mwanahamuntu, S. Kapambwe, R. Muwonge, A. C. Bateman, M. Blevins, C. J. Chibwesha, K. S. Pfaendler, V. Mudenda, A. L. Shibemba, S. Chisele, G. Mkumba, B. Vwalika, M. L. Hicks, S. H. Vermund, B. H. Chi, J. S. A. Stringer, R. Sankaranarayanan, and V. V. Sahasrabuddhe. 2015. Population-level scale-up of cervical cancer prevention services in a low-resource setting: Development, implementation, and evaluation of the cervical cancer prevention program in Zambia. *PLOS ONE* 10(4):e0122169.

Pena, M. S. B., and G. S. Bloomfield. 2015. Cardiovascular disease research and the development agenda in low- and middle-income countries. *Global Heart* 10(1):71-73.

PEPFAR (The U.S. President's Emergency Plan for AIDS Relief). 2017. *Congressional budget justification supplement: President's Emergency Plan for AIDS Relief (PEPFAR)*. Washington, DC: U.S. Department of State.

PEPFAR. n.d. *Pink Ribbon Red Ribbon: A global partnership fighting women's cancers*. https://www.pepfar.gov/partnerships/ppp/prrr/index.htm (accessed February 14, 2017).

Pfizer. 2016. *Healthy aging*. https://www.pfizer.com/files/investors/financial_reports/annual_reports/2015/healthy-aging.htm (accessed February 14, 2017).

Piccini, B., S. Toni, L. Lenzi, M. Guasti, F. Barni, and M. De Martino. 2012. Type 1 diabetes onset and pandemic influenza A (H1N1). *International Journal of Immunopathology and Pharmacology* 25(2):547-549.

Poulter, N. R., D. Prabhakaran, and M. Caulfield. 2015. Hypertension. *Lancet* 386(9995): 801-812.

PRRR (Pink Ribbon Red Ribbon). 2016. *Our impact.* http://pinkribbonredribbon.org/our-impact (accessed February 14, 2017).

PRRR. n.d. *Pink ribbon red ribbon: Our story.* http://pinkribbonredribbon.org/our-story (accessed February 14, 2017).

Rabkin, M., M. E. Kruk, and W. M. El-Sadr. 2012. HIV, aging and continuity care: Strengthening health systems to support services for noncommunicable diseases in low-income countries. *AIDS* 26(Suppl 1):S77-S83.

Reddy, S., F. Riahi, G. Dorling, R. Callahan, and H. Patel. 2016. *Innovative approaches to prevention: Tackling the global burden of cardiovascular disease.* Doha, Qatar: World Innovation Summit for Health.

Samb, B., N. Desai, S. Nishtar, S. Mendis, H. Bekedam, A. Wright, J. Hsu, A. Martiniuk, F. Celletti, K. Patel, F. Adshead, M. McKee, T. Evans, A. Alwan, and C. Etienne. 2010. Prevention and management of chronic disease: A litmus test for health-systems strengthening in low-income and middle-income countries. *The Lancet* 376(9754):1785-1797.

Sánchez-Romero, L. M., J. Penko, P. G. Coxson, A. Fernández, A. Mason, A. E. Moran, L. Ávila-Burgos, M. Odden, S. Barquera, and K. Bibbins-Domingo. 2016. Projected impact of Mexico's sugar-sweetened beverage tax policy on diabetes and cardiovascular disease: A modeling study. *PLOS Medicine* 13(11):e1002158.

Sheu, J. J., H. Y. Chiou, J. H. Kang, Y. H. Chen, and H. C. Lin. 2010. Tuberculosis and the risk of ischemic stroke: A 3-year follow-up study. *Stroke* 41(2):244-249.

Simonsen, D. F., D. K. Farkas, M. Sogaard, C. R. Horsburgh, H. T. Sorensen, and R. W. Thomsen. 2014. Tuberculosis and risk of cancer: A Danish nationwide cohort study. *International Journal of Tuberculosis and Lung Disease* 18(10):1211-1219.

Stewart, B. W., and C. P. Wild. 2014. *World cancer report 2014.* Lyon, France: International Agency for Research on Cancer, World Health Organization.

Sturchio, J. L., and G. M. Cohen. 2012. How PEPFAR's public-private partnerships achieved ambitious goals, from improving labs to strengthening supply chains. *Health Affairs (Millwood)* 31(7):1450-1458.

Sturchio, J. L., and A. Goel. 2012. *The private-sector role in public health: Reflections on the new global architecture in health.* Washington, DC: Center for Strategic and International Studies.

Subbaraman, R., S. K. Chaguturu, K. H. Mayer, T. P. Flanigan, and N. Kumarasamy. 2007. Adverse effects of highly active antiretroviral therapy in developing countries. *Clinical Infectious Diseases* 45(8):1093-1101.

Summers, L., and D. Jamison. 2013. *Policy brief #3: Curbing non-communicable diseases and injuries.* New York: *The Lancet.*

UNEP (United Nations Environment Programme). 2014. *Actions on air quality: Policies & programmes for improving air quality around the world.* Washington, DC: United Nations Environment Programme.

UNICEF (United Nations International Children's Emergency Fund). 2016. *Clear the air for children: The impact of pollution on children.* New York: United Nations International Children's Emergency Fund.

Vedanthan, R., J. H. Kamano, G. S. Bloomfield, I. Manji, S. Pastakia, and S. N. Kimaiyo. 2015. Engaging the entire care cascade in western Kenya: A model to achieve the cardiovascular disease secondary prevention roadmap goals. *Global Heart* 10(4):313-317.

Verguet, S., C. L. Gauvreau, S. Mishra, M. MacLennan, S. M. Murphy, E. D. Brouwer, R. A. Nugent, K. Zhao, P. Jha, and D. T. Jamison. 2015. The consequences of tobacco tax on household health and finances in rich and poor smokers in China: An extended cost-effectiveness analysis. *The Lancet Global Health* 3(4):e206-e216.

Wang, H., M. Naghavi, C. Allen, R. M. Barber, Z. A. Bhutta, A. Carter, D. C. Casey, et al. 2016. Global, regional, and national life expectancy, all-cause mortality, and cause-specific mortality for 249 causes of death, 1980–2015: A systematic analysis for the Global Burden of Disease Study 2015. *The Lancet* 388(10053):1459-1544.

WEF (World Economic Forum). 2015. *Maximizing healthy life years: Investments that pay off.* Geneva, Switzerland: World Economic Forum.

WEF and WHO (World Health Organization). 2011. *From burden to "best buys": Reducing the economic impact of non-communicable diseases in low- and middle-income countries.* Geneva, Switzerland: World Economic Forum and World Health Organization.

WHO (World Health Organization). 2014. *Global health observatory: The data repository.* http://www.who.int/gho/database/en (accessed April 5, 2017).

WHO. 2016a. *Fact sheet: Human papillomavirus (HPV) and cervical cancer.* http://www.who.int/mediacentre/factsheets/fs380/en (accessed March 30, 2017).

WHO. 2016b. *Global health sector strategy on viral hepatitis 2016-2021: Towards ending viral hepatitis.* Geneva, Switzerland: World Health Organization.

WHO. 2016c. *New initiative launched to tackle cardiovascular disease, the world's number one killer.* Geneva, Switzerland: World Health Organization.

WHO. 2017a. *Cancer fact sheet.* http://www.who.int/mediacentre/factsheets/fs297/en (accessed April 4, 2017).

WHO. 2017b. *Noncommunicable diseases fact sheet.* http://www.who.int/mediacentre/factsheets/fs355/en (accessed March 20, 2017).

WHO. 2017c. *Yearly, 8.8 million people die from cancer.* Dhaka, Bangladesh: World Health Organization.

Wirtz, V. J., W. A. Kaplan, Y. S.-A. Téllez, and R. L. Ridaura. 2011. *Affordable, quality, long-term care and pharmacotherapy of chronic diseases: A framework for low and middle income countries.* Geneva, Switzerland: World Health Organization.

World Bank and IHME (Institute of Health Metrics and Evaluation). 2016. *The cost of air pollution: Strengthening the economic case for action.* Washington, DC: World Bank and Institute for Health Metrics Evaluation.

Yu, Y. H., C. C. Liao, W. H. Hsu, H. J. Chen, W. C. Liao, C. H. Muo, F. C. Sung, and C. Y. Chen. 2011. Increased lung cancer risk among patients with pulmonary tuberculosis: A population cohort study. *Journal of Thoracic Oncology* 6(1):32-37.

Zhang, L., and N. Liu. 2014. Health reform and out-of-pocket payments: Lessons from China. *Health Policy Plan* 29(2):217-226.

PART 3:

MAXIMIZING RETURNS

7

Catalyzing Innovation

There must be a willingness to change the way global health business is conducted to better enable innovation and truly achieve sustainable and resilient health systems in every country, fostering prosperity and development. Given the multisectoral nature of health, simply addressing individual challenges in a singular, siloed manner will never solve the overall problem. Challenges in the drug development process for infectious and neglected diseases have plagued researchers and developers since before human immunodeficiency virus/acquired immunodeficiency syndrome (HIV/AIDS) captivated the world's attention in the 1980s. But since then, the challenges have only expanded—many infectious diseases still plague the world without an effective cure or vaccine, and many chronic conditions or noncommunicable diseases (NCDs) in low- and middle-income countries (LMICs) face limited treatment options. The committee believes that, through innovations and the development of partnerships, critical medical product development can be accelerated and public health services can be provided in a more sustainable manner. Furthermore, the extraordinary advances in information technology have the potential to revolutionize global health and bypass the necessity of costly brick-and-mortar health services.

This chapter provides examples and strategies to catalyze these innovations to improve health outcomes, by first discussing the various ways to accelerate the development of medical products. This includes addressing multiple steps along the value chain, such as enabling innovative trial designs, streamlining regulation, ensuring both the supply and demand through manufacturing capacity and market incentives, and finally building research and development (R&D) capacity in LMICs. The chapter then proceeds to review progress in digital health tools and uses worldwide, highlights remaining gaps, and charts a path forward for the United States to better support global health investments through technology.

ENABLING INNOVATION: ACCELERATING THE DEVELOPMENT OF MEDICAL PRODUCTS

The market for global health products suffers numerous failures—including lack of manufacturing capacity, a costly approval process, uncertain commercial potential, and poor workforce and laboratory capacities in LMICs. From 1975 to 1999, only 1.1 percent of new drugs were developed for neglected diseases. Given the international support and political attention resulting from the Millennium Development Goals[1] in 2000 it would be expected that this percentage would climb. However, between 2000 and 2011, only 4 percent of new products were indicated for neglected diseases[2] (Pedrique et al., 2013). This dearth of available medical products results in patients suffering from diseases, such as tuberculosis, malaria, and other potential pandemic diseases, without access to essential medicines. Though there are many promising process innovations, the entire value chain for global health products needs re-tooling. The committee considered a variety of means to streamline the R&D pipeline for global health products and offers strategies that government agencies, industry, and global health players can explore. These include enabling innovative trial design approaches; streamlining regulation; ensuring supply; creating market incentives; and building capacity for medical products manufacturing in partner countries to foster global health security and better support local needs.

Enabling Innovative Trial Design Approaches

Traditional clinical trials, though the mainstay of clinical research, often have shortcomings because of their rigidity or poor adaptability of results in real-life circumstances. For example, randomized clinical trials (RCTs) may require a large sample size and lengthy study duration (Bhatt and Mehta, 2016). In part because of these requirements, the costs of drug

---

[1] The Millennium Development Goals are "The world's time-bound and quantified targets for addressing extreme poverty in its many dimensions—income poverty, hunger, disease, lack of adequate shelter, and exclusion—while promoting gender equality, education, and environmental sustainability. They are also basic human rights—the rights of each person on the planet to health, education, shelter, and security" (Millennium Project, 2006).

[2] For this analysis, the term neglected diseases includes 49 different diseases in five categories: malaria, tuberculosis, diarrheal diseases, the WHO list of 17 neglected tropical diseases, or other neglected diseases (19 of which did not fit into another category). See supplementary appendix of Pedrique et al. (2013) for a detailed listing.

development have increased nearly 100-fold between 1950 and 2010, when adjusting for inflation, despite fewer new drugs being approved by the U.S. Food and Drug Administration (FDA). The core problem of clinical trials seems to be that processes that support them have not been improved (Pammolli et al., 2011; Woodcock and Woosley, 2008). The committee believes that the costly drug development process could be improved to reduce costs and attract pharmaceutical companies to develop more products needed for neglected global health diseases. One way of accomplishing this goal is through the encouragement of manufacturers to use more innovative product development approaches that improve the effectiveness and efficiency of the clinical trial process. Three approaches emerged in recent years and include adaptive clinical trials, pragmatic clinical trials, and surrogate endpoints (or biomarkers).

Adaptive Trial Designs

Clinical trials are often hindered by the rigidity of the protocols. A traditional RCT may not offer the flexibility necessary to modify its study design based on interim data that emerges as a trial progresses (Mahajan and Gupta, 2010). The adaptive clinical trials method, an alternative approach to a traditional RCT, embraces more flexibility and efficiency. This provides manufacturers the opportunity to modify the study design and hypothesis based on the analysis of interim data (FDA, 2010), as well as possibility shortening the development time to speed up the process (Chow and Corey, 2011). Among other benefits, adaptive trials design allow a more rapid divestment from unsuccessful compounds without wasting as much time or resources. Importantly, though adaptive trials seek to make clinical research more efficient, they still involve randomization[3] (Mahajan and Gupta, 2010). An additional adaptive method, the use of platform trials, are appealing because of their potential improved efficiency in creating superior evidence compared to single-sponsor, single-drug trials (Trusheim et al, 2016). A platform trial is a clinical trial with a single master protocol that can evaluate multiple treatments simultaneously, and can result in fewer patient failures and a shorter timeline—improving overall financial sustainability (Saville and Berry, 2016). While there are many benefits to be realized, conducting these types of trials effectively will require overcoming

[3] Randomization in clinical trials means the random assignment of participants to treatment groups, which contributes to the efficacy and internal validity of a trial. Forms of randomization include simple randomization, in addition to block, stratified, and covariate adaptive randomization. Specific types of randomization used in adaptive trials are described by (Mahajan and Gupta, 2010). As each type has its advantages and disadvantages clinical trial teams will need to assess the context surrounding the trial before determining which type of randomization to use.

many operational and statistical challenges, such as coordinating multiple sponsoring companies in collaborative governance and ensuring standardized protocols are followed supported by adequate data sharing (Trusheim et al., 2016).

While FDA has issued draft guidance on the use of adaptive clinical trials (FDA, 2010), there is still lack of clarity on how they would be evaluated. However, with the passing of the 21st Century Cures Act in 2016,[4] FDA has been directed to host a public meeting to discuss the incorporation of complex adaptive and other novel trial designs into clinical protocols and new drug applications as well as to issue additional guidance regarding their use (Brennan, 2016b). This could potentially set up a more efficient, yet safe environment conducive to accelerating development for certain diseases. Despite the promise of adaptive trials though, there can be several operational challenges such as pre-planning protocol deviations, complicated mathematical modeling, and the risk of false effectiveness conclusions (Chow and Corey, 2011; FDA, 2016a). These challenges will require continued evaluation when designing trials within this adaptive and accelerated environment.

Pragmatic Trials

In addition to the rigidity of their protocols, traditional RCTs, through strict control for biases, produce results that are statistically credible but not always applicable to real life circumstances such as demographics of the trial population, proximity to a study site, or patient adherence (Zwarenstein and Oxman, 2006). However, the use of "real-world evidence," such as electronic health records, medical claims data, disease registries, and data gathered through personal devices, can complement the knowledge gained from clinical trials. As a result, researchers and medical product manufacturers have expressed interest in integrating such real world settings into clinical research (Sherman et al., 2016). As a result, pragmatic trials have emerged as a mechanism to incorporate such data into clinical trials so interventions are tested in the full range of clinical settings and the findings are more generalizable (Patsopoulos, 2011) to close the gap between research and care. Requirements for pragmatism are described by the PRECIS-2 tool,[5] but overall pragmatic trials involve heterogeneity of participants and study settings in addition to numerous interacting com-

---

[4] See https://www.congress.gov/bill/114th-congress/house-bill/34 (accessed April 6, 2017).

[5] The PRECIS-2 tool includes dimensions of investigator and participant eligibility, recruitment, and setting; the organization of the intervention; the flexibility in delivery and adherence of the intervention; the nature of the follow-up; and the determination and analysis of the primary outcome (Ford and Norrie, 2016).

ponents, such as other medications or health conditions participants may have (Ford and Norrie, 2016; Patsopoulos, 2011). Though pragmatic trials seek to relax the control aspect of a clinical trial,[6] they also still use randomization (Ford and Norrie, 2016) and often require a larger sample size as a result of the increased heterogeneity (Patsopoulos, 2011). Researchers should adopt features of pragmatic trials where feasible, but refrain if there are questions of trial quality compromise (Ford and Norrie, 2016).

Pragmatic trials and the use of real world data have been encouraged by the U.S. government, and future expanded use of this trial type looks promising. The American Recovery and Reinvestment Act included $1.1 billion for comparative effectiveness research (Patsopoulos, 2011). And with the passing of the 21st Century Cures Act, FDA is now required to develop a framework on evaluating real world evidence for drug regulation to guide its use in clinical trials (Hills and Zegarelli, 2017). However, pragmatic trials may present new challenges, such as participant recruitment and consent, practice variation, or risk determination (Anderson et al., 2015; Ford and Norrie, 2016; Sugarman and Califf, 2014), all of which will demand continued dialogue among multiple stakeholders to adequately address the scientific, ethical, and regulatory challenges.

Biomarkers as Surrogate Endpoints

The primary outcome of a clinical trial is known as a clinical endpoint, and it characterizes whether or not a participant develops a symptom, disease, laboratory anomaly, or even death in response to the disease course or treatment under study. While these are clear metrics for the success or failure of a treatment, some may occur years after the end of a trial. The use of biomarkers[7] that can provide interim evidence about safety and effectiveness is an advancement in clinical research that addresses this issue, and therefore speeds up the drug development process. Establishing a biomarker as a surrogate endpoint,[8] however, is difficult and requires strong evidence to validate its use.[9] As a result, FDA approves the use of

---

[6] A controlled trial is a type of clinical trial in which observations made during the trial are compared to a standard, called the control. The control may be observations of a group of participants in the same trial or observations from outside the trial—for example, from an earlier trial, which is called a historical control (NLM, 2017).

[7] Biomarker: A substance, structure, or process that can be measured and influence or predict a clinical outcome or disease (WHO, 2001).

[8] Surrogate endpoint: A well-characterized biomarker that can act as a substitute for a clinical endpoint (Strimbu and Tavel, 2010).

[9] Strong scientific evidence must show that a biomarker be objectively measured, strongly correlates with the clinical endpoint, has predictive power in other related studies, and that it can be relied on to serve as a surrogate in other related clinical endpoints (Strimbu and Tavel, 2010).

biomarkers as surrogate endpoints on a provisional basis, requiring phase IV[10] studies to prove correlation. It is important to note that even defined biomarkers may not always be an indicator of a clinical endpoint, and are likely to draw erroneous conclusions (Strimbu and Tavel, 2010). Thus, while biomarkers may improve the efficiency of clinical trials and their use has been encouraged by FDA (FDA, 2004), they must be further developed to improve their reliability. Encouraging researchers to identify biomarkers for use could be an integral step in this process, as this method will be difficult for FDA to review and assist without active participation through proposed biomarkers in relevant research. The committee hopes that, in compliance with the 21st Century Cures Act, FDA provides guidance on a review pathway (Brennan, 2016b) and collaborates with scientific partners to develop qualification plans. This would ensure a safe path forward for more rapid product development.

Communicating in Crisis

A trial design may use a combination of these approaches depending on the disease in question. As a result, early communication among researchers and regulators around the globe is vital to clarify the best approach and ensure study success. In fact, a 2017 National Academies of Sciences, Engineering, and Medicine report, *Integrating Clinical Research into Epidemic Response: The Ebola Experience*, noted that international researchers missed the opportunity to quickly and collaboratively come to an agreement on trial design, which stalled efforts (NASEM, 2017a). Furthermore, Peter Marx, director of the Center for Biologics Evaluation and Research at FDA, discussed early conversations of regulators with trial sponsors and suggested it could be beneficial to bring the scientific community and international regulators together during an international health emergency to review the results available from differing trial designs. Overall, all of these trial designs present alternative options to be explored, but continued investment and dedication from all parties, including regulators, industry, and academic researchers, will be needed to continue to shape the trials to produce safe and efficacious medical products and as efficiently as possible.

[10] Phase IV studies are done after the drug or treatment has been marketed to gather information on the drug's effect in various populations and any associated side-effects following long-term use. For more on clinical trial phases, see https://www.nlm.nih.gov/services/ctphases.html (accessed April 13, 2017).

Streamlining Regulation

As the oldest consumer protection agency in the United States, FDA requires drug manufacturers to prove the safety and efficacy of products before they enter the market, and continues these safety evaluations through post-market surveillance (Danzis, 2003; Merrill, 1996). Although the process of drug approval protects consumers, it is complex and costly, and it can take 12 to 15 years for a new drug to be developed and enter the market (see Figure 7-1). Furthermore, this process is a risky investment: The average cost of developing a drug is over $2.5 billion (DiMasi et al., 2016), and only 9.6 percent of all new drugs successfully progress from Phase 1 clinical trials to FDA approval (Thomas et al., 2015). Of all new drugs intended for infectious diseases, 19.1 percent are approved (Thomas et al., 2015). Private companies decide which products they will invest in based on a risk assessment to their business and potential for financial return. If a company believes the costs and risks for development are too high, or the market for the product is too uncertain and small, investment in this product is unlikely to occur.

To partially alleviate the gap in development for global health priorities, the Center for Drug Evaluation and Research (CDER), the division of FDA tasked with overseeing the approval process, offers a variety of alternative review mechanisms that can reduce costs and risks by speeding up the timeline. Typically, CDER is expected to review and act on 90 percent of new drug applications within 10 months. However, CDER employs four different regulatory mechanisms for expedited review: fast-track, breakthrough therapy, accelerated approval, and priority review, as described in Box 7-1. The expedited review mechanisms are an example of how the U.S. government can reduce or share the burden of development costs and risks with industry, effectively "pushing" a product through the pipeline.

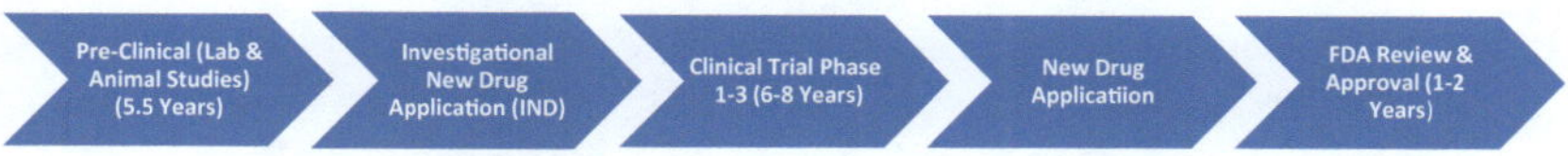

FIGURE 7-1 Timeline for drug or vaccine development.
SOURCES: Adapted from Ciociola et al., 2014; Thaul, 2012.

BOX 7-1
Mechanisms for Expedited Review

Fast-Track

Drugs that are meant to treat serious medical conditions and fill an unmet need are eligible for fast-track designation. The U.S. Food and Drug Administration (FDA) maintains more frequent communication with these manufacturers and uses mechanisms to expedite development and review. Drugs may be eligible for accelerated approval and priority review (discussed below), if criteria for those mechanisms are also met. This designation was used during the West Africa Ebola outbreak and it is the only FDA expedited review mechanism that is applicable to investigational products with only preclinical data.

Breakthrough Therapy

The breakthrough therapy mechanism expedites the development and review of new drugs that target serious conditions and suggest, based on clinical evidence, an improvement over available therapy. A manufacturer can request designation for a product no later than phase 2 clinical trials. Manufacturers with this designation receive all fast-track designation features and intensive guidance and commitment on behalf of FDA.

Accelerated Approval

The accelerated approval mechanism allows for a faster FDA approval process for drugs that are proven to treat a serious condition, provide meaningful advantage over currently available therapies, and demonstrate an effect based on a surrogate endpoint (a biomarker intended to substitute for a clinical endpoint). While this allows manufacturers to receive FDA approval faster, they need to confirm the initial results or risk losing approval.

Priority Review

To receive priority review, a manufacturer must show that their product represents an improvement in the safety or effectiveness of a treatment or has been designated as a qualified infectious disease product. Though not required by law, FDA by practice assigns priority review status to drugs that address an unmet need. Priority review shortens the length of FDA review from 10 to 6 months.

SOURCES: Aronson, 2005; FDA, 2014a,b,c; Thaul, 2012; Williams, 2016.

In addition to expedited review, Congress has implemented mechanisms related to regulation to incentivize industry partners to develop needed global health products that may not have a clear commercial market. Examples include the Orphan Drug Act, the Priority Review Voucher (PRV), and the Generating Antibiotic Incentives Now (GAIN) Act, which are described in the section below. While each mechanism has elements designed to attract manufacturers, they have not been used as widely as needed to have a clear effect on the dearth of critical products. The committee believes that this is partially because these incentives do not compensate enough for the costs of regulatory approval, and sees an opportunity for reassessment and expansion of these mechanisms to further streamline the approval process for critical global health products.

Orphan Drug Act

The Orphan Drug Act of 1983 was introduced to incentivize drug development for rare diseases[11] by providing pharmaceutical companies a 7-year market exclusivity, a tax credit that covers 50 percent of clinical trial costs, R&D grants, fast-track approval, and a waiver of the user fee associated with the application (Franco, 2013). As of November 2013, FDA has granted 2,923 diseases orphan status (relying on sponsors to request designation) (FDA, 2016b) but only granted market approval to 447 drugs (FDA, 2017).

The diseases receiving orphan designation have mostly been cancers with relatively few of them being neglected diseases. Those neglected diseases that have been given orphan status, such as malaria, tuberculosis, and leishmaniasis (Sachs-Barrable et al., 2014), are mostly prevalent among the U.S. military and travelers (Villa et al., 2009). Because the Orphan Drug Act was developed to address diseases in domestic markets (Villa et al., 2009) and neglected infectious diseases typically affect the world's poorest, most pharmaceutical companies do not frequently pursue drug development for these diseases through this act (Warshaw, 2015). Leveraging the Orphan Drug Act to spur development for neglected diseases has been suggested, with one solution proposed in a past bill (HR 3156) submitted to the 111th Congress in 2009[12] met with little success. In 2014 multiple candidates to treat the Ebola virus were given orphan drug designation, but this does not guarantee the drug will be developed as some companies were hesitant to

[11] Rare diseases are defined as those that affect 200,000 patients or less, or those that affect more but for which drug development costs are unlikely to be recovered in the United States.

[12] To amend the Internal Revenue Code of 1986 to provide a credit against tax for expenses paid or incurred in non-clinical research for neglected diseases, H.R. 3156, 111th Congress. 2009–2010. See https://www.congress.gov/bill/111th-congress/house-bill/3156 (accessed April 9, 2017).

start the process until they had secured additional funding through a partnership or government (Lyon, 2015; Radke, 2014). This further highlights the need for sustainable, collaborative investment for neglected diseases.

Priority Review Voucher Program

The PRV program was established in 2007 and designed to reward innovators for developing novel treatments for diseases that would otherwise not attract development interest. While initially intended for neglected diseases, additional PRV programs have since been created to include rare pediatric diseases in 2012 (Gaffney et al., 2016) and medical countermeasures in 2016 (Brennan, 2016a). In exchange for producing drugs for such diseases, FDA grants manufacturers a voucher that allows them to designate another product in their pipeline for priority review (Aurora et al., 2016). If manufacturers have potential blockbuster drugs in their pipeline, the ability to enter market even 4 months in advance could translate into millions of dollars in profit. As of November 2016, 13 vouchers had been awarded—4 of which were for drugs treating neglected (or tropical) diseases (Gaffney et al., 2016). Furthermore, there are currently three products in the pipeline for this category—motivated by a PRV—targeting river blindness, tuberculosis, and dengue fever (Aurora et al., 2016).

While the PRV program has some novel aspects to incentivize drug development for neglected diseases, such as permitting FDA to add new pathogens to the list of eligible diseases "by order,"[13] there are concerns about its effectiveness and whether the program is being exploited. The first PRVs granted for neglected disease were either already developed or in late-stage of development, leading some to question whether it is indeed incentivizing development or just acting as a giveaway to companies who were already doing that type of work. Furthermore, PRVs have been sold to other companies, often commanding high prices. The first ever sale was valued at $67 million, with subsequent vouchers being sold as high as $350 million (Gaffney et al., 2016). The most recent voucher was sold for $125 million (Brennan, 2017). Other concerns raised about the PRV program include the uncertainty that the drug will be approved, taken to market, or taken to market at an affordable price (Aurora et al., 2016). Finally, there are limitations in the application as only novel ingredients are eligible, so innovations in delivery such as follow-up formulations that can be applied to resource poor settings would not qualify (Kesselheim,

[13] With the passing of Public Law 113-233 (December 16, 2014), FDA is now permitted to add new viruses to the list of voucher-eligible tropical diseases "by order" instead of "by regulation." This allows FDA to make changes more quickly, without going through the typical notice-and-comment provisions of federal regulation (Gaffney et al., 2016).

2008). These concerns notwithstanding, the PRV program should be seen as one beneficial tool in the "incentives toolbox," but would benefit from reevaluation, and assurance that FDA has the appropriate resources needed to optimally manage the program.

Generating Antibiotic Incentives Now Act

In contrast with the Orphan Drug Act and the PRV program, the GAIN Act does not address a rare or neglected disease, but still fills an unmet need. As discussed in Chapter 3, the dire health and economic challenges that antimicrobial resistance poses, in addition to the dwindling pipeline for new antimicrobials, makes it essential to spur development. This is compounded by the high cost of bringing a new medicine to market, especially when antimicrobials generate such small revenue compared to other drugs. The GAIN Act encourages the development of new products targeting "qualifying pathogens"[14] by awarding an additional 5 years of market exclusivity, priority review, and eligibility for fast-track designation. In addition, the GAIN Act requires FDA to provide clarity on the development pathway of these therapeutics (Pew Charitable Trusts, 2013). As of September 2016, 40 new antimicrobials are in clinical development for U.S. market, many of which address indications eligible for GAIN Act benefits (Pew Charitable Trusts, 2016).

Ensuring Supply

Enabling the efficient development of medical products and streamlining regulatory processes to facilitate a faster timeline is only half the challenge of ensuring drugs, vaccines, and devices reach people in a timely manner. There is a need in the latter stages of development to ensure adequate manufacturing capacity for these products to meet global demand. This is especially important for diseases that might threaten the global population, such as pandemic influenza (reviewed in Chapter 3). The Biomedical Advanced Research and Development Authority (BARDA) within the Office of the Assistant Secretary for Preparedness and Response

---

[14] Following a final rule July 7, 2014, the list of qualifying pathogens includes *Acinetobacter* species, *Aspergillus* species, *Burkholderia cepacia* complex, *Campylobacter* species, *Candida* species, *Clostridium* difficile, *Coccidioides* species, *Cryptococcus* species, *Enterobacteriaceae* (e.g., *Klebsiella pneumoniae*), *Enterococcus* species, *Helicobacter pylori*, *Mycobacteriumtuberculosis* complex, *Neisseria gonorrhoeae*, *N. meningitidis*, nontuberculous mycobacteria species, *Pseudomonas* species, *Staphylococcus aureus*, *Streptococcus agalactiae*, *S. pneumoniae*, *S. pyogenes*, and *Vibrio cholera*. See https://www.federalregister.gov/documents/2014/06/05/2014-13023/establishing-a-list-of-qualifying-pathogens-under-the-food-and-drug-administration-safety-and (accessed April 7, 2017).

understands this need and has been working through global partnerships to increase manufacturing capacity for threats within their mission, such as pandemic influenza. In 2005, there were fewer than 1 million doses of influenza vaccine available worldwide, which prompted a move to advance clinical development by at least 9 developing country vaccine manufacturers and licensure by at least 7 developing country manufacturers (Bright, 2013).

In 2006, the Global Action Plan for Influenza Vaccines was implemented to increase capacity for manufacture and access to vaccines in LMICs. From 2006 to 2013, seasonal vaccines production increased from 500 million to 1.5 billion doses and pandemic vaccines rose from 1.5 billion to 6.2 billion doses (McLean et al., 2016). In 2015, pandemic vaccine capacity continued to increase from 6.2 billion to 6.4 billion doses, but seasonal vaccine capacity dropped to below 1.5 billion doses, largely due to a shift toward more quadrivalent vaccine[15] production and increased use of adjuvants[16] (McLean et al., 2016).

Since the pathogen that will cause the next pandemic is unknown, it would not be prudent to maintain ongoing capacity for every possible pathogen with pandemic potential. Yet, due to severe consequences of a pandemic, unique models are required to ensure supply of needed drugs, vaccines, and diagnostics. To help address this issue, in 2012 BARDA established three Centers for Innovation in Advanced Development and Manufacturing (CIADMs) that can transition quickly and cost effectively between products. CIADMs are public–private partnerships that bring together small biotechnology companies, academia, and large pharmaceutical companies with continued focus on improving current initiatives and medical countermeasures to reduce risk, increase yield, and reduce life cycle costs through flexible manufacturing. These CIADMs support workforce development through training current and future industry and government scientists, and can also augment manufacturing surge capacity in a public health emergency (HHS, 2017). Acknowledging the need for a long-term commitment and outlook when developing and manufacturing medical products, government contracts with CIADMs can be renewed for up to 25 years. While this is a step in the right direction, they will not solve the problem entirely, and have yet to be tested by the next pandemic. Sustained commitment and awareness in this area is needed.

[15] A quadrivalent vaccine is one that works by stimulating an immune response against four different antigens, such as four different viruses or other microorganisms (NCI, n.d.).

[16] An adjuvant is a substance that is formulated as part of a vaccine to enhance its ability to induce protection against infection. Adjuvants help activate the immune system, allowing the antigens—pathogen components that elicit an immune response—in vaccines to induce long-term protective immunity (NIAID, 2015).

Creating Market Incentives

When working with the private sector, the global health community and governments need to understand that companies are required to demonstrate a rational allocation of capital that provides the highest return on investment. There are areas of mutual interest and the private sector is a necessary partner in global health R&D, but it cannot be expected to make investments without any expectation of a return. As far back as the 1997 IOM report *America's Vital Interest in Global Health*, experts have understood the need for public–private cooperation and development of incentives for the pharmaceutical, vaccine, and medical device industries to invest in R&D of products with risky or unfavorable markets. The 1997 report called for allowing multi-tiered pricing of drugs and vaccines, safeguarding intellectual property rights, and increasing incentives for product development (IOM, 1997). The world has seen a huge amount of progress in this area in the last 20 years, and with the creation of BARDA in 2006, many types of incentives have been explored for medical countermeasure development, though a mixture of push[17] and pull mechanisms.[18] However, because many incentives include payments from the government to pharmaceutical companies, there is often a challenge in securing trust and buy-in from the public because of the optics of this type of relationship.

There are general areas of consensus around pull incentives, such as the agreement on reducing market uncertainty by guaranteeing volumes and prices, and building in provisions for public health objectives. De-linkage models that separate price from R&D costs—either full or partial—are especially favored with regards to antibiotic development because it guarantees returns on investments and removes the motivation to oversell the product (Renwick et al., 2016). Challenges with pull mechanisms exist because the political commitment needs to be sustained for several years, which is difficult to guarantee when government leaders can change every few years. Additional barriers exist because pull mechanisms, administered through appropriation funds, guarantee that a product will be funded. Yet, if these products are funded and developed with U.S. taxpayer money and the disease that they address never manifests as a threat, Congress will be skeptical to fund future projects. Similarly, push mechanisms are difficult for the U.S. government to implement because of the extremely high costs of drug development; they would require a large infusion of money up front in order to incentivize involvement. In 2014 the President's Council

[17] Push mechanisms incentivize industry by reducing the cost of R&D. These can include product development partnerships and direct research grants (Dimitri, 2012).

[18] Pull mechanisms incentivize industry by creating a market demand, which can include tiered pricing, advanced market commitments, and prize funds (i.e., a payment conditional on producing the product) (Dimitri, 2012).

of Advisors on Science and Technology (PCAST) report recommended a significant increase in economic incentives for developing urgently needed antibiotics (PCAST, 2014). The report proposed the establishment of an antibiotic incentive fund to provide advanced market commitments, or market guarantee, and milestone payments to reward developers. One new approved antibiotic per year was estimated to require an annual investment of $800 million.

Tiered pricing continues to be explored as a mechanism to expand access to affordable drugs and other health products. It has proven critical to the success of global immunization programs and expanded access to affordable vaccines. This mechanism is more effective when market risk is low, for example, when there is an assured source of financing like Gavi, the Vaccine Alliance (Gavi); and when there is a competitive market with adequate production capacity. The success of tiered pricing also depends on a tacit agreement of high- and middle-income markets that poorest countries will receive lower prices. Finally, mechanisms that help ensure that the low tier prices are available only in those approved low-income countries and do not leak into higher-income markets are important. When these conditions can be met, tiered pricing is a valuable mechanism to maintain a viable market for industry while ensuring the critical product is still available to the poorest people (Moon et al., 2011).

A Suite of Approaches

Overall, an important takeaway for incentives is that there is no magic bullet solution, as different approaches will be necessary for different shortcomings in the market. As a result, there is a need to articulate and test a suite of options and incentive models with multiple key stakeholders, as market shaping often requires partnership and coordination, since different options will appeal differently based on company characteristics (USAID, 2014). The U.S. Agency for International Development (USAID) has conducted market shaping for vital global health issues such as the latest Zika virus outbreak. To lower the risk and incentivize the private sector to accelerate the development of Zika diagnostics, USAID partnered with the United Nations International Children's Emergency Fund (UNICEF) to create an advanced purchase commitment valued at $10 million (USAID, 2017). Considerations for incentive development will vary by stakeholder involved (i.e., large pharmaceutical companies vs. small biotechnology companies), and the product or process being targeted (i.e., emerging infectious diseases versus classic drug development). Regardless of the incentive used, it is important for stakeholders to act soon and adapt, as markets fluctuate constantly (USAID, 2014). Multiple other studies and reports have echoed the call for flexibility and diversity of incentives in order to be effective when there is no clear market for the product—especially to address antimicrobial resistance (BCG et al., 2015; PCAST, 2014; Renwick et al., 2016; Review on Antimicrobial Resistance, 2015).

Research and Development Capacity

There are many opportunities to accelerate drug development through regulatory and market incentives, more innovative trial design approaches, streamlined regulations, and adequate supply. Yet, building local capacity to conduct clinical trials in countries where these diseases are endemic is paramount. As the world faces new health threats that can more easily cross national borders, investing in global R&D will require expansion of local capabilities to anticipate new threats and augment opportunities for the development of novel vaccines and therapeutics. As the economies of the world continue to grow, and many once-recipient countries begin to develop their own capacities for R&D, the role of the United States should also adapt.

Why Invest in Foreign Country Capacity?

True collaboration is vital to the success of R&D partnerships. They must be conceived through a clear understanding of the mutually understood benefits, resulting in a truly reciprocal approach for all parties (Lucas, 2005). This model provides the basis for strong collaborations that will help to dually develop capacity in LMICs and support the United States' efforts to prevent global outbreaks. In their 2016 report on the U.S. government's role in R&D for global health, the Duke University's Global Health Institute also emphasized the need to build R&D capabilities in countries receiving development assistance for health (DAH). This 2016 report agreed with the *Lancet* Commission on Investing in Health that DAH funding should increasingly be spent on global functions for health (similar to the concept of global public goods discussed in Chapter 8). One way to achieve this, the Duke team reported, is to increase the amount of DAH that is directed to individual countries to develop their own R&D capabilities—and suggested using Fogarty International Center at the National Institutes of Health (NIH) as a mechanism (Yamey et al., 2017).

Continuing research capacity abroad will allow for the development of more drugs and therapeutics to address diseases that plague people in both the United States and LMICs. As an example, with the recent improvement in diplomatic relations with Cuba, the U.S. Department of Health and Human Services (HHS) and Cuba's Ministry of Public Health "signed an umbrella accord that promises to make health a cornerstone of the new era of cooperation between the two countries" (Keck, 2016). This concept is becoming tangible as Cuba has promising treatments that can prevent the need for amputation in patients with diabetes, which have been unavailable to Americans since 2006 due to a U.S. trade embargo. Cuba also has a promising lung cancer vaccine, CIMAvax, with early results suggesting improved survival and quality of life for many patients with non-small cell lung cancer (Keck, 2016). Only since last year, when the United States lifted a medical embargo, has this type of collaboration been allowed. There is much to be learned by each country, and extrapolating this example of partnership across the world, the United States has an opportunity to encourage information sharing and research collaboration among all health and medical researchers.

Developing the R&D Workforce

Often in response to an emergency, the international community deploys personnel from across the world to the emergency site. However, the labor pool that has experience working in the setting of the emergency can be sparse, which occurred during the Ebola response, making it difficult to integrate international responders without local and contextual understanding. As labor cannot be supplied from international sources indefinitely, developing the workforce capacity locally is a much-needed solution.[19] U.S.-based institutions can play a role in fostering the development of a strong R&D workforce in LMICs and greater country independence through academic partnerships. The more developed institution provides the laboratory skills and expertise not available at the less developed institution, and the less developed institution contributes the clinical and contextual knowledge (Lucas, 2005). For example, the Academic Model Providing Access to Healthcare (AMPATH), an Indiana University–led initiative, has developed a partnership with Moi University in Kenya to provide 30 percent of medical students with financial aid to increase the number of Kenyan medical professionals (AMPATH, n.d.). This partnership supports the development of a local workforce that will provide health care to their own people, and also creates long-term mentorship opportunities for students and faculty with an interest in global health.[20] Programs like this can strengthen the local workforce to operate more independently and become global partners in health with donor countries.

Although these types of partnerships can be costly to U.S.-based academic institutions, additional funding can be leveraged through the Fogarty International Center at NIH and USAID,[21] which ensures sustainability of

---

[19] Personal communication with Daniel Bausch, Tulane University, November 9, 2016.

[20] Personal communication with Robert Einterz, AMPATH, December 5, 2016.

[21] Personal communication with Troy Moon, Vanderbilt University, November 8, 2016.

current projects and encourages collaborations in future projects. For example, Troy Moon at Vanderbilt University has collaborated with the University of Zambia to train doctorate-level researchers with an NIH-sponsored grant (Snyder, 2015). The goal of the project is to improve partnerships and mentorships among scientists to encourage technical independence among researchers in partnering countries (Snyder, 2015). Through another NIH-sponsored grant, Vanderbilt University is working with Tulane University and the Kenema Government Hospital in Sierra Leone to build capacity and training programs for researchers in the recently Ebola-affected countries so that they can soon write grant proposals and conduct their own clinical trials. In addition to becoming primary researchers, these foreign trainees gain the technical expertise to become advisors to Ministers of Health for aid programs such as The U.S. President's Emergency Plan for AIDS Relief (PEPFAR), and can have much greater success in influencing policy than "outsider" research scientists and diplomats.[22] U.S. grants lower the barrier to entry for researchers who hope to collaborate with in-country universities in developing R&D workforce capacity sustainably. This type of capacity-building support through the Fogarty Center is widely used by many universities and provides learning and mentorship opportunities not otherwise available to U.S.-based institutions and depended on by international universities to help build the research component of their country's health system.

USAID has created multiple programs to leverage investments by U.S. government science agencies to strengthen the research ecosystem in LMICs. For example, the Partnerships for Enhanced Engagement in Research (PEER) funds international scientists who work in partnership with institutions supported by U.S. federal science agency funding (USAID, 2016b). Additionally, USAID's Higher Education Solutions Network (HESN) leverages the knowledge and assets of seven top U.S. universities to develop technological advancements and spur innovative local solutions by partnering with international academic institutions (USAID, 2016a). A 2017 National Academies report, *The Role of Science, Technology, Innovation, and Partnerships in the Future of USAID*, called for continued engagement with partner countries through innovative programs, such as PEER and HESN. Lessons should be gleaned and expanded on to sustain collaborations with in-country researchers and institutions (NASEM, 2017b).

With much success, PEPFAR has also explored methods for sustainable workforce training through the Medical Education Partnership Initiative and Nursing Education Partnership Initiative, also supported by the Fogarty International Center and Health Resources and Services Administration (explained in Chapter 4). These initiatives provide students with

[22] Personal communication with Troy Moon, Vanderbilt University, November 8, 2016.

technical and diplomatic expertise and, in a similar way to Moon's projects, build robust academic partnerships with in-country institutions, creating more formal networks for bidirectional information sharing.

Developing Laboratory Research Capacity

In addition to the workforce capacity needed for R&D in LMICs, building laboratory research capacity is another vital investment category. By increasing the ability to conduct research on endemic diseases, countries will be able to self-sufficiently implement appropriate solutions. Investments toward research capacity date back to 1974 when the World Health Organization (WHO) Special Programme for Research and Training in Tropical Diseases (TDR) was established. Its support has been instrumental for institution strengthening in LMICs. For example, TDR funding was able to create the Malaria Research and Training Center (MRTC) in Mali in 1998, which conducts extensive studies on vector biology, ecology, and genetics (Ogundahunsi et al., 2015). Owing to subsequent funding by USAID and NIH, the MRTC has since expanded and now is paired with multiple laboratories—one of which is a Biosafety Level 3 (BSL-3) lab (NIAID, 2014). To have ongoing benefits, both to the country and to the rest of the world, this laboratory capacity in LMICs must be sustained.

Building laboratory capacity is critical for outbreak response, as the health research system is a vital component of a country's health system (NASEM, 2017a). As a recent example, when Ebola hit West Africa in late 2013, poor laboratory research capacity hindered efforts to quickly identify the source of the outbreak. The initial investigation conducted by the Ministry of Health in Guinea concluded that the cause was cholera, which impeded a swift and appropriate public health response because of the delay in accurate diagnosis (NASEM, 2017a). Even as CDC and other organizations sought to improve surveillance as the outbreak was declared, the weak laboratory capacity was a major barrier to continued case identification and implementation of proper public health measures. Conversely, the importance of adequate laboratory capacity is illustrated by the African Center of Excellence for Genomics of Infectious Diseases in Nigeria, which was able to accurately diagnose the index case of the Nigerian Ebola outbreak and enable the government to contain the spread before the outbreak became out of control (NASEM, 2017a).

Additionally, the U.S. Department of Defense's Cooperative Biological Engagement Program (DoD–CBEP) deployed mobile laboratories in Sierra Leone and Guinea during the 2014 Ebola outbreak. In 2015 these laboratories analyzed more than 6,000 samples and quickly detected nearly 80 positive cases of Ebola in these 2 countries. As a step in capacity building, the laboratories increased diagnostic capabilities during the outbreak and are now being transitioned to the countries' government to support future outbreak detection and response efforts (GHSA, 2017). Considering these differing examples, there is a clear motivation for the U.S. government to continue its engagement in laboratory capacity-building for outbreak response.

Taken together—both workforce and laboratory capacity are essential to build a strong health system able to respond to infectious disease outbreaks before they lead to catastrophic consequences, and in a cost-effective manner. According to Costello and Zumla (2000), by helping to create an independent researching body in LMICs, researchers are trained in their home countries and are encouraged to stay there because of the existing infrastructure; in-country grants investigate the problems most of interest to the nation's people; and results have a higher likelihood of leading to policy changes as compared to research conducted by individuals from other, high-income countries (Costello and Zumla, 2000). Similarly, local mental health research conducted in LMICs is found to be much more easily adaptable to solve local problems as compared to research conducted by high-income countries that is based on evidence from high-income countries (Sharan et al., 2007). Past estimates have shown that implementing recommendations for increased research and development capacity would cost $1 billion per year, which is much less than the potential cost of a pandemic (discussed more in Chapter 3) (GHRF Commission, 2016). The committee agrees with the statement made by the Committee on Clinical Trials During the 2014–2015 Ebola Outbreak, that "What seems certain to us is that the actual options are to pay now and prepare in advance, or to pay later when an outbreak occurs, with the likelihood that the cost will be multiple times greater in the latter case" (NASEM, 2017a, p. 185).

SUMMARY AND RECOMMENDATION

Underpinning health innovations is the necessary human and institutional capacity in the United States and globally. Yet the market for many global health products is often too uncertain or risky for private-sector partners to invest their know-how and capital in the development and manufacture of these products (Pedrique et al., 2013). Considering the extremely costly development process and the paucity of products in the pipeline to address neglected diseases, the current trial designs, regulatory approval options, and product supply motivations seem inadequate (Pedrique et al., 2013). Examining each of these areas and the methods and mechanisms currently available can provide an opportunity for the U.S. government to find ways to reduce the costs and timeline to ensure more products make their way into development all the way to approval. Push and pull incentivizing mechanisms can also ensure that appropriate vaccines, therapeutics, diagnostics, and devices are in the development pipeline for global health priorities with weak markets, including neglected diseases (Dimitri, 2012). In the absence of these mechanisms, the United States and other governments risk spending far more as they work to prevent, respond to, and treat diseases using suboptimal tools.

To complement the development of safe and efficacious products requires R&D capacity in countries where outbreaks begin and disease burdens are high (NASEM, 2017a). Although there are some notable exceptions, the necessary research capacity is weak in many such countries, making it difficult to conduct clinical and field trials, becoming even more of a costly and chaotic undertaking during a public health emergency (NASEM, 2017a). By examining the stages along the pharmaceutical development value chain, the U.S. government has an opportunity to identify specific actions that can be taken to streamline processes, reduce costs, and create more appropriate incentives to enable industry, academia, and others to contribute to developing the priority innovations for global health. This could be accomplished through an interagency working group, but would require dedicated commitment from all involved agencies, as well as coordination across the public and private sectors.

Conclusion: Despite substantial efforts from the U.S. government and other global health players, the pipeline of innovations for addressing persistent global health threats is inadequate. The U.S. government has the ability to design and expand push and pull mechanisms that can catalyze industry, academia, and others to develop, license, and introduce needed technologies and avoid the catastrophic loss of life and economic burdens that result from the lack of these innovations.

Conclusion: Creating the capacity for low- and middle-income countries to conduct clinical trials where the burden of disease is highest, using their own workforces and facilities, is both more efficient and more cost-effective than relying on donor nations for these efforts. Creating this capacity will require investing in laboratory capacity, and an appropriately trained research-competent workforce.

Recommendation 10: Accelerate the Development of Medical Products

U.S. government agencies should invest in a targeted effort to reduce the costs and risks of developing, licensing, and introducing vaccines, therapeutics, diagnostics, and devices needed to address global health priorities by enabling innovative trial design ap-

proaches, streamlining regulation, ensuring production capacity, creating market incentives, and building international capacity for research and development. This effort should include the following:

- **Enabling innovative approaches for trial design:** The U.S. Food and Drug Administration (FDA), the Biomedical Advanced Research and Development Authority (BARDA), the U.S. Department of Defense (DoD), and the National Institutes of Health (NIH) should actively encourage public- and private-sector product development efforts using innovative product development approaches, including platform studies, adaptive trial designs, pragmatic trials, and improved biomarker development. BARDA should assess expanding its list of priority products for codevelopment with industry, taking into account global health priorities.
- **Streamlining regulation:** FDA should receive adequate resources to improve the tropical disease priority review voucher program and should assess the application of the provisions outlined in the Generating Antibiotic Incentives Now Act to neglected tropical diseases beyond those on the qualified pathogen list.
- **Ensuring production capacity:** BARDA should increase its efforts to promote adequate global manufacturing capacity for priority technologies (e.g., Centers for Innovation in Advanced Development and Manufacturing).
- **Creating market incentives:** The U.S. government should invest in generating and disseminating accurate and transparent market estimates and should use the purchasing power of U.S. government agencies and global partnerships such as Gavi, the Vaccine Alliance, and the Global Fund to Fight AIDS, Tuberculosis and Malaria, as well as such creative financing mechanisms as volume guarantees, to reduce market uncertainty for priority health products.
- **Building international capacity for research and development:** The U.S. Centers for Disease Control and Prevention, NIH, and DoD should increase the number of people and institutions in partner countries capable of conducting clinical trials for global health priorities (e.g., through funding partnerships with academic institutions). This effort should encompass providing support for sustainable core capacities such as drug, vaccine, and diagnostic research capabilities and building the skills of principal investigators.

ENABLING INNOVATION: DIGITAL HEALTH

Telecommunications and wireless multimedia have contributed to significant advances in global health in recent years. By taking advantage of wireless network penetration in LMICs, digital health technology has bypassed deficiencies found in traditional "brick-and-mortar" health care systems and provides a myriad of solutions ranging from education for new and expectant mothers through the Mobile Alliance for Maternal Action (MAMA)[23] (MAMA, 2013) to reminders for adherence to chronic disease management (Hamine et al., 2015). Although there have been many successful applications of digital health tools around the world, they have typically employed a shortsighted approach and a narrow perspective (Mehl and Labrique, 2014). While this was likely done to create a simpler process for faster and easier results, the current models fail to prevent unnecessary duplication and address broader health system needs. Finally, both U.S. global health programs and countries around the world have seen much progress in improved health outcomes stemming from technological advances and digital health tools. Although they will continue to face up-front costs of establishing the digital infrastructure and training a workforce to utilize the digital platforms, the long-term commitment to their use has the potential to reduce costs and improve efficiency of health care programs (MoH, n.d.; WHO, 2009). The committee believes that now is a time to pause, review all of the progress made and lessons learned, and chart a strategic path forward in digital global health, with an emphasis on systematic approaches, multidisciplinary public–private collaboration, and country ownership.

Applications of Digital Global Health

Many U.S. government agencies and their implementing partners, as well as private companies and other national governments, have employed digital health technology to facilitate elements of global health, whether for disease surveillance, patient tracking, inventory maintenance, or telemedicine. Though the applications of digital health technology are expansive, the committee has categorized them into three broad application areas for discussion: data systems creation, health care service optimization, and

[23] The Mobile Alliance for Maternal Action (MAMA) was launched in 2011 as a public–private partnership between USAID, Johnson & Johnson, the UN Foundation, and BabyCenter with the goal of catalyzing a global community to deliver vital health information to new and expectant mothers and their families through mobile phones. BabyCenter created a core set of messages for MAMA that is timed and targeted to pregnant women and infants through 3 years old. Over just 5 years the program reached more than 7.5 million women and families (MAMA, 2013).

research efficiency, explored below, with examples of each highlighted in Box 7-2.

Data Systems

A hallmark of digital health utilization has been its support of data systems in developing countries. Health information in developing countries has long been captured on paper, which must then be physically transported, and the data manually aggregated and reentered, then extracted for review by high-level officials (Mehl and Labrique, 2014). This includes routine health facility data and acute event data, such as disease outbreaks. Understandably, delays and errors are commonplace—creating inefficiencies in a health system. Digital health tools have revolutionized this process, allowing for data collection, reporting, and action to occur much more rapidly, and with fewer opportunities to introduce error (RTI, n.d.). Box 7-2 illustrates an example of data systems improvement in LMICs through Coconut Surveillance.

Health Care Service Optimization

Access to quality health care in LMICs is often hindered by workforce shortages and poor infrastructure (MoH, n.d.). Though long-term, complete solutions to both of these issues requires the scale-up of human resources and creation of adequate amounts and types of clinics, digital health tools have been able to provide effective interim solutions. The most well-known form of digital health used to optimize service delivery is telemedicine, an effective means of providing access to more specialized care to remote regions (or those lacking high-skilled health care workers) in a cost-effective manner (Green, 2016; WHO, 2009). Other widely utilized modalities of digital health in this area include SMS reminders and mobile protocols (Hamine et al., 2015; MAMA, 2013).[24] As a result, while the longer-term goal of increasing the number of high-level medical providers will still require lengthy timelines, patients can access high-level care now, through leveraging these technology tools. Box 7-2 illustrates an example of this type of innovation through Operation ASHA.

Research Efficiency

Biomedical research and clinical trials—especially for infectious diseases endemic to certain areas in LMICs, such as Lassa Fever, Ebola, or

---

[24] Mobile Protocols: These tools enable health care providers to efficiently deliver health solutions, such as daily nutritional supplement reminders or dosage reminders.

BOX 7-2
Applications of Digital Global Health Tools

Data Systems: Coconut Surveillance

Coconut Surveillance is an open-source, mobile-based tool used for malaria control and elimination currently being used in Zanzibar. Community health workers use tablets to collect data as they conduct case detection. The information is then dispatched to health officials at the Zanzibar Malaria Elimination Program. Data collected are synchronized with a cloud database (accessible on the web) in near real-time, allowing for rapid analysis and decision making for targeting program resources.

Health Care Service Optimization: Operation ASHA

Operation ASHA is an India-based nongovernmental organization that seeks to improve tuberculosis (TB) treatment, which in collaboration with Microsoft created a software called eCompliance that seeks to reduce lapses in TB treatment (thereby preventing the development of multidrug resistant [MDR]-TB). eCompliance registers patients and staff through fingerprints and sends text message updates of patient compliance to counselors and program managers. If a dose is missed, the program sends an alert to the patient, health worker, and supervisor. eCompliance also empowers health care providers to provide counseling to patients who lapse in treatment so the spread of MDR-TB is reduced. The program has been rolled out for nearly 9,000 TB patients thus far in Cambodia, the Dominican Republic, India, Kenya, and Uganda and has already recorded more than 400,000 transactions with very positive results. Many health and medical challenges encounter loss of patient follow-up as a barrier to success—regardless of the country or income level. The model of eCompliance has the potential to be expanded beyond TB, to areas such as consistent antenatal care, childhood vaccination documentation, or prevention of mother-to-child HIV transmission.

Research Efficiency: Clinical Ink

Clinical Ink is a technology company that offers a mobile solution to streamline clinical trials, called SureSource, which is currently the only platform that meets all U.S. Food and Drug Administration guidelines for electronic source data. SureSource can capture information from onsite electronic medical records and from data collected at the time of the patient/provider interaction, making data collection easier and efficient. Furthermore, SureSource allows clinical researchers to directly engage with patients through a mobile app. They can also use their own mobile devices, a practice which is typically not standard protocol for many studies, but contributes to improved user participation due to their familiarity with their own device. This enables researchers to monitor patients remotely and encourages patients to self-report data.

SOURCES: Clinical Ink, 2015; Operation ASHA, 2016; RTI, n.d.; Seguine, 2016; USAID, 2013.

Zika virus, depend on robust and capable sites in these same regions. Recruitment for trials is an arduous process as they require a large group of patients to comprise the study sample (Zimmer et al., 2010). Leaning on technology, databases of patients with particular diseases, or disease registries, have been positioned as a critical prelude to clinical trials and can help improve recruitment, identity patient cohorts, provide data for natural history studies, and stimulate new research (Groft, 2014). Furthermore, using digital health tools can also facilitate in-country trials. Typically, patients need to continuously return to a clinical trial site for periodic data collection, but this can be a barrier in remote or resource-poor areas where travel is lengthy and expensive. Having remote options for check-in and periodic follow-up can remove this barrier (Seguine, 2016). Additionally, having a disease registry in a city or country can allow for faster start-up for other studies on different diseases, making that area more attractive to researchers. See Box 7-2 for an example of a digital health solution for clinical trials.

A Need for a Paradigm Shift

The tremendous value and corresponding excitement that digital health provides has come at a cost, as the proliferation of interest and the variety of stakeholders involved has created a fragmented approach to the use of digital health tools in many countries. In fact, in 2012, Uganda issued a temporary moratorium on digital health pilots because its health system became overrun with them (Green, 2016). Aid programs, nongovernmental organizations, and private companies often create individual, disease-focused tools that fail to be interoperable with one another and are duplicative to in-country systems. Therefore, despite the large investment in digital health applications, these parallel structures often lead to inefficiencies because they cannot be used for other diseases or health priorities. Multiple donors and organizations may be funding and operating multiple surveillance systems for different diseases in the same country, instead of aligning themselves into one interoperable system, integrated with existing national health system infrastructure. The benefit of digital health applications notwithstanding, there is a clear need for a paradigm shift in digital health infrastructure investments. The global health community and U.S. global health programs need to move away from the current practice of single application solutions to a more strategic approach that acts holistically with both current country priorities and long-term goals (Mehl and Labrique, 2014). By better coordinating the development of digital health applications, stakeholders involved in digital health can reduce duplication and ensure that the platforms are more aligned with those priorities and goals.

The committee envisions not only digital tools for real-time collection of health and health-related data from anywhere in the world, but also connected systems that ensure the data can be aggregated and shared (when appropriate), instantly analyzed and intuitively visualized so that health professionals and policy decision makers at all levels—community, district, country, and global—can take action. The committee sees this occurring through the development of digital health platforms within countries. The hallmark of a digital health platform is that it must be adaptable to local health needs. However, it is neither efficient nor practical for each program or country to invest in developing a full suite of needed tools to support their health system. Therefore, a core characteristic of a common digital health platform would be that of an open innovation platform that holds and facilitates access to health care and health-related data for a multitude of applications. By building a digital health platform that is modular, countries can attract and engage third parties (including the private sector) to develop useful applications that can be customized to their unique context and then integrated sustainably. While such a platform would be useful for day-to-day health care delivery and operations, it would also revolutionize how surveillance and response for public health threats can be managed within and between countries. The committee sees a digital health platform revolutionizing the three broad areas of digital health: data systems, health care service optimization, and research efficiency, as described in the following sections.

Data Systems

Though some systems can collect data in remote areas and others offer near real-time data streams, they do not interact with each other and the data cannot be easily aggregated. This severely limits the potential of using such data to optimize health care service delivery or surveillance of potential emerging global health threats. The committee therefore advocates for a common digital health platform architecture that can create interoperability across existing or future data systems, but would not require each user to adopt a prescribed solution. Instead, data could be collected across disparate sites and systems and be aggregated for everyday health care needs, including delivery of services, payments for services, and global health threats. The digital financial sector has already made key advances in this area in LMICs, as evidenced by the success of m-Pesa[25] or other

[25] m-Pesa is a mobile money transferring system in Kenya that operates through users' cell phones. Safaricom, the cellular telecommunications company that started m-Pesa, generates $250,000,000 per year in revenues from m-Pesa alone (CBS News, 2015). For more information, see https://www.safaricom.co.ke/personal/m-pesa (accessed April 7, 2017).

electronic payment systems. The digital health sector can learn from these innovations as related to their interoperability and privacy and to avoid developing them from scratch.

Health Care Service Optimization

Though digital health tools have provided numerous solutions in terms of augmenting health care workforces, a digital health platform can maximize this capacity. Enhanced access to data and information through a common digital platform will improve communication between patients and health care workers across the care continuum, as well as increase the productivity and quality of the workforce. While this does not replace the longer-term need to educate and train a larger workforce, these technology capabilities can address the short-term needs and expand the scope of a health workforce to match the demand for more integrated health services.

Research Efficiency

The digitalization of clinical trials and general global health research can reduce the waste of duplicative technology in global health and allow for streamlined and remote collection of data, thereby resulting in potential cost savings. A digital health platform can improve on the efficiencies already gained through facilitation of data-sharing among investigators, potentially allowing for novel research inquiry. For example, if two similar clinical trials are occurring simultaneously, a digital health platform could enable controlled sharing of data (within the scope of research ethics) to investigate another separate study question. Additionally, a common platform would likely allow for more targeted studies and faster recruitment, as country disease trends and relevant health information would be aggregated from multiple data streams to highlight burdens and gaps in existing care and tools.

Looking Forward: A Role for the U.S. Government in the World of Digital Global Health

As many partners around the globe, both public and private, have been supportive and involved with the creation of digital health tools, a need emerged for standardization and coordination as well as assistance to move from policy to implementation. To help bring clarity and coherence to governments on digital technology investment for health, WHO and partner organizations are developing a Global Digital Health Index, a tool designed to track, monitor, and evaluate the applicability of any digital technology

BOX 7-3
Global Digital Health Index

The Global Digital Health Index will provide data on the update and use of information and communications technology across countries, providing valuable information for trend analysis and planning. The index will

- guide governments to develop national frameworks to monitor the effects of digital health investments and guide where investments are needed,
- act as a global clearinghouse on best practices in digital health,
- identify and promote ways that the public and private sector can engage with each other, and
- benefit people around the world by enabling the better creation and use of digital health technology.

SOURCE: HealthEnabled, n.d.-b.

solution for a community's or country's health (Mechael and Kay, 2016). The Global Digital Health Index is further described in Box 7-3.

In addition to a global index, there is also increasing recognition of the importance of frameworks to help prioritize investments in digital health technology and identify opportunities for collaboration and integration with local health systems (Mehl and Labrique, 2014). Many national governments have started to adopt national e-health strategies, including Ghana (MoH, n.d.), Nigeria (MoH, 2015), and Tanzania (MoHSW, 2013). The common aspects of these frameworks include an efficient use of resources, improved data and information flow, and reduced fragmentation (HealthEnabled, n.d.-a). Donors often lack methods for the coordination and alignment of funding of digital health investments, which has resulted in fragmentation and an inability to scale. The national e-health strategies that are emerging signal a shift in thinking and open the door for better aid coordination driven by country priorities.

As the global community moves toward a more harmonized approach to digital technology application, the United States has an opportunity to re-assess its current strategy and direct resources and expertise toward the growing momentum for global alignment in this space. The United States can likely see greater returns on investment through coordinating U.S. digital health investments with the needs of the country, and where possible assisting countries to develop their e-health strategies. Furthermore, this alignment in partnership could incentivize local government toward co-investment, thus facilitating better transition to country ownership and sustainability.

In 2015, 25 percent of Africa and 58 percent of Asia had an internet connection (Poushter, 2016), with this number expected to continue increasing. Additionally, many innovations and services have been created even without internet access, such as through the massive proliferation of cellular networks using simple mobile phones (e.g., m-Pesa, described previously). To facilitate further growth in connectivity, the United States recently passed, with bipartisan support, H.R. 600, the Digital Global Access Policy Act. This bill encourages efforts in developing countries to improve internet access to spur economic growth and improve health, in addition to ensuring effective use of U.S. foreign assistance.[26] The act specifically calls for USAID to integrate efforts to expand internet access into education, development, and economic growth programs, as well as use of information and communications technologies for disaster relief. To do so, the Act calls for the use of the build-once principle, which hopes to lower the cost of infrastructure development by minimizing the number and scale of excavation activities when installing telecommunications infrastructure. The committee sees a strong opportunity for the United States to build on this goal and rethink its global health strategies to join the global momentum toward harmonization of digital health approaches.

SUMMARY AND RECOMMENDATION

Decreases in the costs and increased demand of mobile technology have allowed for the integration of successful digital health efforts in the United States and around the globe (Mehl and Labrique, 2014; Steinhubl et al., 2013). However, many of these investments in global health have been siloed and shortsighted in their approach, often focusing on single diseases or sectors and missing opportunities to develop a sustainable, integrated platform (Mehl and Labrique, 2014). Prioritizing health systems innovation through technical assistance and public–private partnerships in digital health can lead to better care and service delivery at lower cost, especially in situations in which already established technology is utilized (Mehl and Labrique, 2014; WHO, 2009). With growing mobile and internet connectivity worldwide and rapid advances in information and communication technology, the United States has an opportunity to better integrate digital health efforts in countries to reduce fragmentation and improve coordination and efficiency (Mehl and Labrique, 2014; Poushter, 2016).

[26] Digital Global Access Policy Act of 2017, H.R. 600, 115th Congress.

Conclusion: Countries need cross-cutting digital health platforms that are adaptable to local requirements and sovereignty, and can provide real-time data and analytic insights to inform health-related decisions. Such platforms need to address each country's health care priorities during steady-state times, thereby incentivizing country co-investment and ownership, while also serving as a resilient system for facilitating controlled sharing of data across countries to enhance surveillance, coordinate responses, and deliver services during an emergency.

Conclusion: Achieving the global health goals outlined in this report will require that U.S. global health programs leverage the expertise and resources of the U.S. government in digital health and the strong U.S. information and communication technology industry through public–private partnerships and smart financing strategies (see Chapter 8).

Recommendation 11: Improve Digital Health Infrastructure

Relevant agencies of the U.S. government should convene an international group of public and private stakeholders to create a common digital health framework that addresses country-level needs ranging from integrated care to research and development.

- **The U.S. Agency for International Development (USAID) and the U.S. Department of State should incentivize and support countries in building interoperable digital health platforms that can efficiently collect and use health data and analytic insights to enable the delivery of integrated services within a country.**
- **USAID's Global Development Laboratory should provide technical assistance to countries in the development and implementation of interoperable digital health platforms co-funded by the country and adaptable to local requirements.**
- **U.S. agencies should expand on the "build-once" principle of the Digital Global Access Policy Act and align U.S. funding in digital health by multiple agencies to reduce fragmentation and duplication, as well as maximize the effectiveness of investments. The provision of this funding should employ methods that reflect smart financing strategies to leverage private industry and country cofinancing (see Recommendation 13).**

REFERENCES

AMPATH (Academic Model for the Prevention and Treatment of HIV). n.d. *Mwangaza scholarships*. http://ampathkenya.org/our-programs/education-partnerships/mwangaza-scholarships (accessed February 13, 2017).

Anderson, M. L., J. Griffin, S. F. Goldkind, E. P. Zeitler, L. Wing, S. M. Al-Khatib, and R. E. Sherman. 2015. The Food and Drug Administration and pragmatic clinical trials of marketed medical products. *Clinical Trials* 12(5):511-519.

Aronson, J. K. 2005. Biomarkers and surrogate endpoints. *British Journal of Clinical Pharmacology* 59(5):491-494.

Aurora, P., M. Romine, and G. Daniel. 2016. *Are Priority Review Vouchers the answer to incentivize drug development? Not so fast.* http://healthaffairs.org/blog/2016/06/15/are-priority-review-vouchers-the-answer-to-incentivize-drug-development-not-so-fast (accessed March 18, 2017).

BCG (Boston Consulting Group), Öpp Deutschland AG, and Technische Universität Berlin. 2015. *Breaking through the wall: Enhancing research and development of antibiotics in science and industry.* https://www.bundesgesundheitsministerium.de/fileadmin/Dateien/3_Downloads/G/G7/Qualitaetswettbewerb_Gesundheitssystem_Whitepaper_2015-10-02.pdf (accessed January 10, 2017).

Bhatt, D. L., and C. Mehta. 2016. Adaptive designs for clinical trials. *The New England Journal of Medicine* 375(1):65-74.

Brennan, Z. 2016a. *House E&C Committee clears new Priority Review Voucher program.* http://www.raps.org/Regulatory-Focus/News/2016/07/14/25336/House-EC-Committee-Clears-New-Priority-Review-Voucher-Program (accessed February 15, 2017).

Brennan, Z. 2016b. *Regulatory explainer: 21st Century Cures redux and what it will mean for FDA.* http://raps.org/Regulatory-Focus/News/2016/11/28/26242/Regulatory-Explainer-21st-Century-Cures-Redux-and-What-it-Will-Mean-for-FDA (accessed March 18, 2017).

Brennan, Z. 2017. *Sarepta sells Priority Review Voucher for $125m to Gilead.* http://www.raps.org/Regulatory-Focus/News/2017/02/21/26898/Sarepta-Sells-Priority-Review-Voucher-for-125M-to-Gilead (accessed March 8, 2017).

Bright, R. 2013. "BARDA International Influenza Vaccine Manufacturing Capacity Building Program." Presentation at 6th Meeting with International Partners on Prospects for Influenza Vaccine Technology Transfer to Developing Country Vaccine Manufacturers. Dubai. March 18-19, 2013. http://www.who.int/phi/Day1_3_Bright_BARDA_PM_Dubai2013.pdf (accessed May 4, 2017).

CBS (Columbia Broadcasting System) News. 2015. *Want to text money? Kenya's been doing it for years.* http://www.cbsnews.com/news/want-to-text-money-kenya-has-been-doing-it-for-years (accessed March 15, 2017).

Chow, S.-C., and R. Corey. 2011. Benefits, challenges and obstacles of adaptive clinical trial designs. *Orphanet Journal of Rare Diseases* 6(1):79-88.

Ciociola, A. A., L. B. Cohen, and P. Kulkarni. 2014. How drugs are developed and approved by the FDA: Current process and future directions. *American Journal of Gastroenterology* 109(5):620-623.

Clinical Ink. 2015. *Introduction to SureSource.* http://www.clinicalink.com/wp-content/uploads/2015/04/Clinical-Ink_SureSource-Overview-Final_042815.pdf (accessed January 16, 2017).

Costello, A., and A. Zumla. 2000. Moving to research partnerships in developing countries. *BMJ: British Medical Journal* 321(7264):827-829.

Danzis, S. D. 2003. The Hatch-Waxman act: History, structure, and legacy. *Antitrust Law Journal* 71(2):585-608.

DiMasi, J. A., H. G. Grabowski, and R. W. Hansen. 2016. Innovation in the pharmaceutical industry: New estimates of R&D costs. *Journal of Health Economics* 47:20-33.

Dimitri, N. 2012. R&D incentives for neglected diseases. *PLOS ONE* 7(12):e50835.

FDA (U.S. Food and Drug Administration). 2004. *Innovation and stagnation: Challenges and opportuinty on the critical path to new medical products.* Silver Spring, MD: U.S. Food and Drug Administration, U.S. Health and Human Resources.

FDA. 2010. *Guidance for industry: Adaptive design clinical trials for drugs and biologics.* Silver Spring, MD: U.S. Food and Drug Administration, U.S. Health and Human Resources.

FDA. 2014a. *Breakthrough therapy.* http://www.fda.gov/ForPatients/Approvals/Fast/ucm405397.htm (accessed February 13, 2017).

FDA. 2014b. *Fast track.* http://www.fda.gov/ForPatients/Approvals/Fast/ucm405399.htm (accessed February 13, 2017).

FDA. 2014c. *Priority review.* http://www.fda.gov/ForPatients/Approvals/Fast/ucm405405.htm (accessed February 13, 2017).

FDA. 2016a. *Adaptive designs for medical device clinical studies: Guidance for industry and Food and Drug Administration staff.* https://www.fda.gov/downloads/medicaldevices/deviceregulationandguidance/guidancedocuments/ucm446729.pdf (accessed April 25, 2017).

FDA. 2016b. *Designating an orphan product: Drugs and biological products.* http://www.fda.gov/ForIndustry/DevelopingProductsforRareDiseasesConditions/HowtoapplyforOrphanProductDesignation/default.htm (accessed February 13, 2017).

FDA. 2017. Search orphan drug designations and approvals. Silver Spring, MD: U.S. Food and Drug Administration, U.S. Health and Human Resources.

Ford, I., and J. Norrie. 2016. Pragmatic trials. *New England Journal of Medicine* 375(5):454-463.

Franco, P. 2013. Orphan drugs: The regulatory environment. *Drug Discovery Today* 18(3-4):163-172.

Gaffney, A., M. Mezher, and Z. Brennan. 2016. *Regulatory explainer: Everything you need to know about FDA's Priority Review Vouchers.* http://www.raps.org/Regulatory-Focus/News/2015/07/02/21722/Regulatory-Explainer-Everything-You-Need-to-Know-About-FDA%E2%80%99s-Priority-Review-Vouchers/ (accessed February 13, 2017).

GHRF Commission (Commission on a Global Health Risk Framework for the Future). 2016. *The neglected dimension of global security: A framework to counter infectious disease crises.* doi: https://doi.org/10.17226/21891.

GHSA (Global Health Security Agenda). 2017. *Advancing the Global Health Security Agenda: Progress and early impact from U.S. investment.* Washington, DC: Global Health Security Agenda.

Green, A. 2016. *A new era in digital health.* https://www.devex.com/news/a-new-era-in-digital-health-88327 (accessed December 15, 2016).

Groft, S. 2014. *Patient registries as a prelude to clinical trials and post-approval studies.* http://www.fda.gov/downloads/MedicalDevices/NewsEvents/WorkshopsConferences/UCM381523.pdf (accessed February 13, 2017).

Hamine, S., E. Gerth-Guyette, D. Faulx, B. B. Green, and A. S. Ginsburg. 2015. Impact of mHealth chronic disease management on treatment adherence and patient outcomes: A systematic review. *Journal of Medical Internet Research* 17(2):e52.

HealthEnabled. n.d.-a. *Country dashboards.* http://healthenabled.org/index.php/healthe-africa/country-dashboards/ (accessed December 15, 2016).

HealthEnabled. n.d.-b. *Global Digital Health Index.* http://www.healthenabled.org/index.php/our-work/digitalhealthindex (accessed December 15, 2016).

HHS (U.S. Department of Health and Human Services). 2017. *Department of Health and Human Services Centers for Innovation in Advanced Development and Manufacturing (HHS-CIDAM).* https://www.medicalcountermeasures.gov/barda/core-services/ciadm.aspx (accessed February 13, 2017).

Hills, B., and B. Zegarelli. 2017. *21st Century Cures Act requires FDA to expand the role of real world evidence.* https://www.martindale.com/health-care-law/article_Mintz-Levin-Cohn-Ferris-Glovsky-Popeo-PC_2239128.htm (accessed April 10, 2017).

IOM (Institute of Medicine). 1997. *America's vital interest in global health: Protecting our people, enhancing our economy, and advancing our international interests.* Washington, DC: National Academy Press.

Keck, C. W. 2016. The United States and Cuba—turning enemies into partners for health. *New England Journal of Medicine* 375(16):1507-1509.

Kesselheim, A. S. 2008. Drug development for neglected diseases—the trouble with FDA review vouchers. *New England Journal of Medicine* 359(19):1981-1983.

Lucas, A. O. 2005. International collaboration in health research. *Bulletin of the World Health Organization* 82(7).

Lyon, K. 2015. ZMapp is granted orphan medicinal product designation by the EMA. In *Status May Enable Faster Approval of ZMapp*. San Diego, CA: LeafBio.

Mahajan, R., and K. Gupta. 2010. Adaptive design clinical trials: Methodology, challenges and prospect. *Indian Journal of Pharmacology* 42(4):201-207.

MAMA (Mobile Alliance for Maternal Action). 2013. *Mobile Alliance for Maternal Action (MAMA).* http://www.mobilemamaalliance.org (accessed February 13, 2017).

McLean, K. A., S. Goldin, C. Nannei, E. Sparrow, and G. Torelli. 2016. The 2015 global production capacity of seasonal and pandemic influenza vaccine. *Vaccine* 34(45):5410-5413.

Mechael, P., and M. Kay. 2016. *Unlocking the potential of digital health.* https://www.devex.com/news/unlocking-the-potential-of-digital-health-88274 (accessed December 15, 2016).

Mehl, G., and A. Labrique. 2014. Prioritizing integrated mHealth strategies for universal health coverage. *Science* 345(6202):1284.

Merrill, R. A. 1996. The architecture of government regulation of medical products. *Virginia Law Review* 82(8):1753-1866.

Millennium Project. 2006. *What they are.* Washington, DC: The United Nations Millennium Project. http://www.unmillenniumproject.org/goals (accessed March 10, 2017).

MoH (Nigerian Ministry of Health). 2015. *National health ICT stratgic framework.* Abuja, Nigeria: Federal Ministry of Health. http://www.uspf.gov.ng/images/files-temp/National_Health_ICT_Strategic_Framework2015-2020-DRAFT.pdf (accessed January 5, 2017).

MoH (Ghana Ministry of Health). n.d. *Ghana e-Health strategy.* Accra, Ghana: Ministry of Health. https://www.isfteh.org/files/media/ghana_national_ehealth_strategy.pdf (accessed January 5, 2017)

MoHSW (Ministry of Health and Social Welfare). 2013. *Tanzania national eHealth strategy 2012-2018.* Dar es Salaam, Tanzania: Ministry of Health and Social Welfare. http://www.who.int/goe/policies/countries/tza_ehealth.pdf (accessed January 5, 2017).

Moon, S., E. Jambert, M. Childs, and T. von Schoen-Angerer. 2011. A win-win solution?: A critical analysis of tiered pricing to improve access to medicines in developing countries. *Globalization and Health* 7(1):39.

NASEM (National Academies of Sciences, Engineering, and Medicine). 2017a. *Integrating clinical research into epidemic response: The Ebola experience.* Washington, DC: The National Academies Press.

NASEM. 2017b. *The role of science, technology, innovation, and partnerships in the future of USAID.* Washington, DC: The National Academies Press.

NCI (National Cancer Institute). n.d. NCI Dictionary of Cancer Terms. https://www.cancer.gov/publications/dictionaries/cancer-terms?cdrid=752982 (accessed April 24, 2017).

NIAID (National Institute of Allergy and Infectious Diseases). 2014. *Mali ICER program.* https://www.niaid.nih.gov/about/mali-icer-program (accessed April 10, 2017).

NIAID. 2015. What is a vaccine adjuvant? https://www.niaid.nih.gov/research/what-vaccine-adjuvant (accessed April 24, 2017).

NLM (National Library of Medicine). 2017. *Glossary of common site terms: Clinicaltrials.gov* https://clinicaltrials.gov/ct2/about-studies/glossary#C (accessed April 24, 2017).

Ogundahunsi, O. A. T., M. Vahedi, E. M. Kamau, G. Aslanyan, R. F. Terry, F. Zicker, and P. Launois. 2015. Strengthening research capacity—TDR's evolving experience in low- and middle-income countries. *PLOS Neglected Tropical Diseases* 9(1):e3380.

Operation ASHA. 2016. *Ecompliance biometric tracking system.* http://www.opasha.org/2016/09/20/ecompliance-biometric-tracking-system (accessed April 10, 2017).

Pammolli, F., L. Magazzini, and M. Riccaboni. 2011. The productivity crisis in pharmaceutical R&D. *Nature Reviews Drug Discovery* 10(6):428-438.

Patsopoulos, N. A. 2011. A pragmatic view on pragmatic trials. *Dialogues in Clinical Neuroscience* 13(2):217-224.

PCAST (President's Council of Advisors on Science and Technology). 2014. *Report to the president on combating antibiotic resistance.* Washington, DC: Executive Office of the President.

Pedrique, B., N. Strub-Wourgaft, C. Some, P. Olliaro, P. Trouiller, N. Ford, B. Pécoul, and J.-H. Bradol. 2013. The drug and vaccine landscape for neglected diseases (2000-11): A systematic assessment. *The Lancet Global Health* 1(6):e371-e379.

Pew Charitable Trusts. 2013. *Gain: How a new law is stimulating the development of antibiotics.* http://www.pewtrusts.org/en/research-and-analysis/issue-briefs/2013/11/07/gain-how-a-new-law-is-stimulating-the-development-of-antibiotics (accessed February 13, 2017).

Pew Charitable Trusts. 2016. *Antibiotics currently in clinical development.* http://www.pewtrusts.org/~/media/assets/2016/12/antibiotics_datatable_201612.pdf?la=en (accessed February 13, 2017).

Poushter, J. 2016. *Smarthphone ownership and internet usage continues to climb in emerging economies—but advanced economies still have higher rates of use.* Washington, DC: Pew Research Center.

Radke, J. 2014. Ebola drug given orphan designation—company seeking partners to develop. RareDiseaseReport. http://www.raredr.com/news/Another-Ebola-Drug-Orphan-Designation (accessed March 8, 2017).

Renwick, M. J., D. M. Brogan, and E. Mossialos. 2016. A systematic review and critical assessment of incentive strategies for discovery and development of novel antibiotics. *Journal of Antibiotics* 69(2):73-88.

Review on Antimicrobial Resistance. 2015. *Securing new drugs for future generations: The pipeline of antibiotics.* https://amr-review.org/sites/default/files/SECURING%20NEW%20DRUGS%20FOR%20FUTURE%20GENERATIONS%20FINAL%20WEB_0.pdf (accessed December 20, 2017).

RTI (RTI International). n.d. *Coconut surveillance: Open source mobile tool designed to take on malaria, other infectious diseases.* https://www.rti.org/impact/coconut-surveillance (accessed February 13, 2017).

Sachs-Barrable, K., J. Conway, P. Gershkovich, F. Ibrahim, and K. M. Wasan. 2014. The use of the United States FDA programs as a strategy to advance the development of drug products for neglected tropical diseases. *Drug Development and Industrial Pharmacy* 40(11):1429-1434.

Saville, B. R., and S. M. Berry. 2016. Efficiencies of platform clinical trials: A vision of the future. *Clinical Trials* 13(3):358-366.

Seguine, E. 2016. Innovation to build capacity and improve health. Paper read at Global Health and the Future of the United States: A Changing Landscape of Global Health, Washington, DC. http://www.nationalacademies.org/hmd/~/media/Files/Activity%20 Files/Global/USandGlobalHealth/Global-Health-and-The-Future-of-the-US/Meeting-2-Files/Ed-Seguine-Presentation.pdf (accessed December 12, 2016).

Sharan, P., I. Levav, S. Olifson, A. de Francisco, and S. Saxena. 2007. *Research capacity for mental health in low- and middle-income countries: Results of a mapping project*. Geneva, Switzerland: World Health Organization & Global Forum for Health Research.

Sherman, R. E., S. A. Anderson, G. J. Dal Pan, G. W. Gray, T. Gross, N. L. Hunter, L. LaVange, D. Marinac-Dabic, P. W. Marks, M. A. Robb, J. Shuren, R. Temple, J. Woodcock, L. Q. Yue, and R. M. Califf. 2016. Real-world evidence—what is it and what can it tell us? *New England Journal of Medicine* 375(23):2293-2297.

Snyder, B. 2015. *Grants bolster HIV-focused research capacity*. https://news.vanderbilt.edu/2015/08/20/grants-bolster-hiv-focused-research-capacity (accessed February 13, 2017).

Steinhubl, S., E. Muse, and E. Topol. 2013. Can mobile health technologies transform health care? *JAMA* 310(22):2395-2396. doi:10.1001/jama.2013.281078.

Strimbu, K., and J. A. Tavel. 2010. What are biomarkers? *Current opinion in HIV and AIDS* 5(6):463-466.

Sugarman, J., and R. M. Califf. 2014. Ethics and regulatory complexities for pragmatic clinical trials. *JAMA* 311(23):2381-2382.

Thaul, S. 2012. *How the FDA approves drugs and regulates their safety and effectiveness*. Washington, DC: Congressional Research Service.

Thomas, D. W., J. Burns, J. Audette, A. Carroll, C. Dow-Hygelund, and M. Hay. 2015. *Clinical development success rates 2006-2015*. Washington, DC: BIO, Biomedtracker, Amplion.

Trusheim, M., A. Shrier, Z. Antonijevic,, Beckman, R. Campbell, C. Chen, K. Flaherty, J. Loewy, D. Lacombe, S, Madhavan, H. Selker, and L. Esserman. 2016. PIPELINEs: Creating comparable clinical knowledge efficiently by linking trial platforms. *Clinical. Pharmacology and Therapeutics*, 100:713-729.

USAID (U.S. Agency for International Development). 2013. *Development innovation ventures: Investment portfolio*. Washington, DC: United States Agency for International Development.

USAID. 2014. *Healthy markets for global health: A market shaping primer*. Washington, DC: Center for Accelerating Innovation and Impact, United States Agency for International Development.

USAID. 2016a. *About the Higher Education Solutions Network*. https://www.usaid.gov/hesn/about (accessed February 13, 2017).

USAID. 2016b. *Partnerships for Enhanced Engagement in Research (PEER)*. https://www.usaid.gov/what-we-do/GlobalDevLab/international-research-science-programs/peer (accessed April 10, 2017).

USAID. 2017. *CII 2017 impact brief*. Washington, DC: Center for Accelerating Innovation and Impact, United States Agency for International Development.

Villa, S., A. Compagni, and M. R. Reich. 2009. Orphan drug legislation: Lessons for neglected tropical diseases. *International Journal of Health Planning and Management* 24(1):27-42.

Warshaw, R. 2015. *The economics of orphan drugs: The effectiveness of Priority Review Vouchers on the development of drugs to combat neglected tropical diseases*. Philadelphia: University of Pennsylvania.

WHO (World Health Organization). 2001. *Biomarkers in risk assessment: Validity and validation*. http://www.inchem.org/documents/ehc/ehc/ehc222.htm (accessed March 10, 2017).

WHO. 2009. *Telemedicine: Opportunities and developments in member states: Report on the second global survey on eHealth*. Geneva, Switzerland: World Health Organization.

Williams, C. T. 2016. Food and Drug Administration drug approval process: A history and overview. *Nursing Clinics of North America* 51(1):1-11.

Woodcock, J., and R. Woosley. 2008. The FDA Critical Path Initiative and its influence on new drug development. *Annual Review of Medicine* 59:1-12.

Yamey, G., A. Thoumi, J. Gonzalez-Smith, C. Binanay, I. Bharali, Z. Johar, D. Ridley, and N. Chapman. 2017. *Strengthening the United States government's role in research and development for global health.* Durham, NC: Duke Global Health Institute, Duke Margolis Center for Health Policy.

Zimmer, L. O., T. L. Nolen, S. Pramanpol, D. Wallace, M. E. Walker, P. Pappas, and P. Chetchotisakd. 2010. International collaboration between US and Thailand on a clinical trial of treatment for HIV-associated cryptococcal meningitis. *Contemporary Clinical Trials* 31(1):34-43.

Zwarenstein, M., and A. Oxman. 2006. Why are so few randomized trials useful, and what can we do about it? *Journal of Clinical Epidemiology* 59(11):1125-1126.

8

Smart Financing Strategies

As nations allocate more domestic funds to health and private-sector companies and multilateral organizations contribute more to global aid, the United States has an opportunity to reconsider its strategy for providing foreign assistance for health. Investments need to reflect a globalized world in which the commercial sector, nonprofit and faith-based organizations, and recipient governments all have a partnership role to play. Without this global collaboration and appropriately structured financing mechanisms, further global health progress will be difficult to realize. This chapter discusses several approaches for global health investment, including broad and cross-cutting goals such as global public goods, health system strengthening, and long-term visioning. Also explored are several creative and nontraditional mechanisms of financing global health programs and projects that have emerged in recent years. Finally, with the previous areas as context, this chapter concludes with priorities for U.S. global health investment approaches and mechanisms.

KEY APPROACHES FOR GLOBAL HEALTH INVESTMENT

In addition to the specific areas of focus outlined in the early sections of this report: global health security; continuous communicable diseases; saving and improving the lives of women and children; and the promotion of cardiovascular health and prevention of cancer, there are clear benefits to investing in global public goods, health systems strengthening, and long-term programs that lead to lasting change. Although the majority of global health investments are typically in single, vertical disease programs, these cross-cutting areas can produce large returns and long-term benefits. Future allocations of foreign assistance for health by the United States should consider investments focused on the greatest return, and also those that require strong leadership and commitment where the United States could play a role, such as the examples described below.

Contributing to Global Public Good

As countries transition out of bilateral aid, donor governments have an opportunity to think more strategically about investing in global public goods instead of direct country assistance (also discussed in Chapter 2). Global public goods are those that require too many resources for one country to create alone, such as research and development advancements in medical products or digital health technologies that can be shared with other entities. There is no "global government" to address these challenges and ensure provision of needed services or products (WHO, 2017), and there is little market incentive to motivate private-sector investment. Unfortunately, the benefits are not always immediately apparent and convincing government leaders to dedicate money to these collaborative goals can be challenging. Furthermore, it is demanding to report and measure concrete progress of the funds and programs dedicated to global public goods, which makes it difficult to directly attribute success to individual investments (Birdsall and Diofasi, 2015). However, returns on investment for global public goods are positive and sustainable. For example, the rotavirus vaccine, developed jointly by India and the United States, has significantly reduced the disease burden of rotavirus in India, translating to improved health and increased economic benefits (see Box 8-1).

As stated above, measurement of global efforts has been difficult, but is not impossible, and new tools are emerging. The Organisation for Economic Co-operation and Development (OECD) recently proposed a new measure, called the total official support for sustainable development (TOSSD), which aims to capture donor spending on global public goods and can facilitate learning exchange, track progress on global challenges, and inform policy discussions using empirical evidence (DAC, 2016). With international collaboration among donors, providers, civil society, multilateral organizations, and the private sector, OECD hopes to drive the operationalization of this measurement framework to have TOSSD enable the international community to monitor resources supporting the Sustainable Development Goals (SDGs) beyond overseas development aid (DAC, 2016). This could also be applied to many global public good efforts involving multiple countries.

BOX 8-1
Case Study: 116E Rotavirus Vaccine

Low- and middle-income countries (LMICs) face a significant burden of rotavirus gastroenteritis in the under-5 population. Prior to the global roll-out of rotavirus vaccines, this illness was responsible for 450,000 under-5 deaths each year, more than 95 percent of which occurred in Gavi, the Vaccine Alliance–eligible countries.

In India alone, about 113,000 children under 5 die of rotavirus every year, and Indians spend between $37.4 million and $66.8 million on direct medical costs for diarrhea hospitalizations and outpatient treatments. Acknowledging this glaring problem, the United States and India launched a bilateral vaccine action program and developed India's first indigenous rotavirus vaccine. Economic research in this area suggests that introducing the rotavirus vaccine with the already-established vaccine regimens avoids 34.7 deaths and $215,569 out-of-pocket expenses per 100,000 children under 5. Increasing vaccine coverage to 90 percent in India, including against rotavirus, prevents an additional 22.1 deaths and $45,914 out-of-pocket expenditures per 100,000 children under 5.

SOURCES: Bennett et al., 2016; Megiddo et al., 2014; NIAID, 2015; Tate et al., 2012.

Health Systems Strengthening

U.S. global health programs have often been designed and funded with a singular, vertical disease focus, such as The U.S. President's Emergency Plan for AIDS Relief (PEPFAR) and the President's Malaria Initiative (PMI). Though they have concrete and specific targets and have a positive impact, they do not sufficiently enable many of the cross-cutting elements necessary to build resilient and robust health systems. To address this in part, previous chapters in this report call for broadening workforce training and task-shifting for community health workers into established platforms like PEPFAR clinics and integrating services in maternal and child health services centers to better incorporate awareness and management of noncommunicable diseases (NCDs). As evidenced during the 2014 Ebola outbreak in West Africa, weak health systems and capabilities—including disease detection or response—contributed to the increased severity of the outbreak in Guinea, Liberia, and Sierra Leone (GHRF Commission, 2016). Building resilient health systems allows countries to better respond to global health security threats while simultaneously providing the necessary elements and workforce skills to effectively deliver everyday services such as surveillance, antenatal, well-child, and hypertension services. However, similar to resource mobilization for global public goods, there are often barriers to funding health system strengthening activities (i.e., financing design, workforce capacity building, and infrastructure building) without clear pathways for attribution or immediate results. Yet, as evidenced in Nigeria during the 2014 Ebola outbreak (see Chapter 3), developing fundamental capabilities can also contain emerging outbreaks and indirectly provide lasting benefits to surrounding populations.

Long-Term Investment for Long Lasting Change

In global health, programs that promise straightforward service delivery or quick results are often able to take precedence over long-term investments that take a much greater time period to demonstrate return on investments (IOM, 2014). For many health and development programs, change is gradual, and social and economic benefits often lag behind the costs and can even occur decades after an initial investment (Stenberg et al., 2014). For countries with scarce resources, it is challenging to make the case for investment in projects or programs that have long-term benefits. For example, building a hospital in a district to prevent the need to travel for health care is an important but costly venture. While it may take 1 year or more to build, the benefits of reducing premature mortality and the resulting demographic dividend may not be realized for decades. Conversely, if that same district has a high burden of malaria, it would be more politically feasible to spend money on quickly procuring mosquito nets with proven effects in malaria prevention—a less costly investment with more short-term, concrete benefits. As a result, best value investments may be ignored as success takes too long to be observed.

By working with other countries to look at the long-term investments, the United States has an opportunity to design efforts that will not only build capacity but also complement global public goods spending. The eradication of smallpox serves as an important success story from this type of investment (see Box 8-2). Though not endemic in many high-income countries in the 1960s, there was still a constant need to vaccinate citizens—including those in high-income countries such as the United States—which was a costly endeavor. The global decision to eradicate smallpox resulted in these costs being avoided, and returns on that moderate investment are still realized each year by the United States and the world (Barrett, 2013; Brilliant, 1985). Similarly, even though only a handful of polio cases are diagnosed each year, continued investment toward polio eradication will be imperative, especially when conflict zones and fragile states continue to enable environments for polio to survive (discussed in Chapter 3). The investment in the Global Polio Eradication Initiative in 1988 has already generated net returns of $27 billion, and is projected to reach $40–$50

BOX 8-2
Long-Term Investment and Payoff: Smallpox Eradication

Smallpox, once a truly global disease, was endemic to 59 countries in the 1950s and caused 50 million new cases per year. Using a strategy of surveillance and containment, the World Health Organization (WHO) was able to eradicate (a term used to signify a total absence of human cases) smallpox by 1977. This was a landmark achievement in public health and signified the first time a disease was successfully fought on a global scale. Estimates place the expenditures of the campaign at roughly $200 million for endemic countries and $98 million for nonendemic countries through international aid.

The cost of smallpox in endemic countries (including cost of care and loss of economic productivity) was estimated to be at least $1 billion per year at the start of the campaign. While industrialized countries were nonendemic at the start of the eradication effort, they still needed to maintain population-wide immunity to protect against the possibility of imported cases. The annual cost (both direct and indirect) in these countries was approximately $350 million. This places the global costs of smallpox in the 1960s at $1.35 billion per year. Though these costs could be avoided through eradication, the long-term benefits were difficult to convey to endemic countries due to other short-term needs taking precedence.

But, once eradication was achieved, the benefits of avoided infections outweighed the costs at a rate of 119:1 in low-income endemic countries, and as high as 178:1 in industrialized nonendemic countries, resulting in 159:1 globally. The United States, as the largest contributor to the campaign, saves the one-time expenditures it invested every 26 days that the world is free from smallpox, making smallpox eradication one of the best public health investments in history.

SOURCES: Barrett, 2013; Brilliant, 1985; Fenner et al., 1988; Miller et al., 2006; Seymour, 2004; WHO, 2010.

billion by 2035 (Duintjer Tebbens et al., 2010; GPEI, 2014). Continued support to achieve polio eradication could have as much, if not greater, long-term returns on investment as those realized for smallpox eradication.

Finding: Global public goods, health systems strengthening, and long-term investments in global health are three approaches that prove difficult to procure funds for, due to the challenges associated with attribution and the lack of immediate and clear benefits. Yet, when structured well, these types of investments can have robust and sustainable returns.

CHANGES TO GLOBAL HEALTH FINANCING METHODS

As reviewed in Chapter 2, the growing economies of several low-income countries will propel them toward middle-income status in coming years, which will allow for increased recruitment of domestic sources of financing to support their health programs. The United States can advise these growing economies on best practices for crafting stable tax bases, developing innovative tax initiatives, and restructuring debt ratios as they build up health systems. Through this technical assistance, the United States has a chance to begin to reduce its spending on development assistance for health (DAH). According to a 2016 development cooperation report from OECD, the United States already has begun to reexamine development assistance in order to more effectively achieve sustainable and transformational global health outcomes in light of the financing transitions occurring in global health. The United States has mobilized funds by increasing private capital flow, incorporating more private-sector and nongovernmental organization (NGO) partners, and investing in more science, technology, and innovation (OECD, 2016). As an example, the U.S. Agency for International Development (USAID) strengthened its Development Credit Authority (DCA) to unlock larger sources of capital. Furthermore, the Overseas Private Investment Corporation found that the United States was able to mobilize $10 billion from the private sector through guarantees in 2012–2014 to facilitate participation in the development of low- and middle-income countries (LMICs) (OECD, 2016). To help achieve the SDGs by 2030, as well as maintain its role as a global health leader and home to numerous multinational businesses, the committee believes that the United States is positioned to tackle global health in a more nimble and flexible way by unlocking additional capital and exploring alternative market strategies. This can be done through assisting countries in their transitions to domestic financing, exploring catalytic financing with the private sector, and creating value in financial structure—all discussed below.

Transitioning to Domestic Financing

Government health expenditure as a source (GHE-S)[1] in low-income countries rose 8.5 percent annually from 2000 to 2013 (IHME, 2016). Moreover, middle-income countries' use of GHE-S actually exceeded external DAH nearly 80 times in 2013 (IHME, 2016), indicating potential for targeted transition for those countries that are ready for more sustain-

[1] GHE-S is defined as expenditures on health from domestic government sources (IHME, 2016).

able sources of funding through domestic resource mobilization (DRM). It will be important to understand that while DRM is playing a larger role globally, this transition will vary based on individual country status. Low-income countries will still need continued DAH from donors to support their health programs, and approaches for middle-income countries will demand a focus on sustainability. Gavi, the Vaccine Alliance is well known for its long-term strategy of phasing its partner countries out of support through co-financing. First implemented in 2008, Gavi's policy designates the size of the domestic contribution based on the country's ability to pay and has been found to contribute to country ownership and sustainability (Gavi, 2014). Thus far, 2015 has been their most successful year for co-financing, with countries increasing their spending on vaccines per child by 47 percent in just 1 year (2013–2014) (Gavi, 2015). This policy was also included in Gavi's 2016–2020 strategy, which recognizes the need to integrate sustainability into country engagement at the beginning of the relationship (Gavi, 2015).

Recognizing this trend, many donors are hoping to help recipient governments transition health programs to domestic sources of financing. Tax revenues are often the main sources of funds that governments have to finance their health systems, and in LMICs tax revenues make up approximately 65 percent of total revenues (IMF, 2011). However, the majority of revenue in LMICs often comes from consumption taxes, which may not create a stable tax base (Reeves et al., 2015). LMICs need a more balanced approach to revenue mobilization, which includes corporate and capital gains taxes. Imposing higher corporate taxes can have important benefits to health, and in countries with particularly low tax revenues (<$1,000 per capita per year), the benefits are substantial (Reeves et al., 2015). Although LMICs have the most to gain from corporate taxes, many countries do not receive adequate revenues from them because they offer low rates to attract businesses (Birn et al., 2017). This trend frequently occurs with the natural and extractive resources industries, robbing governments of much-needed revenue (DanWatch, 2011) and needs to be considered during these transitions.

Catalytic Financing for Leveraging Social and Financial Returns

Global changes have already prompted global health players to find ways to make their investments more productive, and several modalities have emerged and been tested in recent years. There are smaller-scale innovations such as development impact bonds, or models like the Development Innovation Ventures through USAID's Global Development Lab (GDL). The private sector has also become an active global health player in the past decade, shifting their interests from "corporate social responsibility" line items to becoming sustainable partners because they see a true return on investment for their business. While it is clear the U.S. government investment in global health should be sustained, the committee sees an opportunity for reshaping investments to be more targeted and catalytic, and leverage more of the existing funds from other sources and mechanisms. Several examples of potential methods are reviewed below.

Small-Scale Innovations

Development Innovation Ventures The GDL within USAID has contributed to nimble and responsive innovative efforts since its creation in 2012. The Development Innovation Ventures initiative was created to find, test, and scale up ideas that could radically improve global prosperity. It invests in ideas across three stages of growth: Stage 1 (Proof of Concept), Stage 2 (Testing at Scale), and Stage 3 (Widespread Implementation) (USAID, 2017), with funding awards increasing as the projects grow. The Development Innovation Ventures model blends best practice strategies in a development approach that includes tiered risk management, economics research, and nonprofit and government development expertise. Hundreds of their projects across the world focus on health at various stages.

Debt buy-downs Debt buy-downs, or conversions, have been used in many low-income countries to decrease country debt and free up resources to fund domestic health programs (Policy Cures, 2012). In a buy-down, a third-party donor such as the Bill & Melinda Gates Foundation pays part of a loan on behalf of a country, allowing that country to spend more of their money on the health program. This can also be tied to performance, where the donor will only pay off their portion of the loan if specific indicators are met (Policy Cures, 2012). One example of this conversion is a bilateral debt swap called "Debt2Health" through the Global Fund to Fight AIDS, Tuberculosis, and Malaria (Global Fund) that increases both resources for global health and local investment in health (UN Integrated Implementation Framework, n.d.). Similarly, debt swaps allow countries to exchange debt, typically at a discount, for equity or counterpart domestic currency funds to finance a project (Kamel and Tooma, 2005). These can be structured to favor investments in priority sectors, often using them as incentives to encourage privatization or facilitate the return of flight capital (Moye, 2001). While these swapping mechanisms should not be a substitute for current foreign aid, they can be used as an additional tool for mobilizing domestic resources (Kamel and Tooma, 2005).

Social and development impact bonds Social impact bonds (SIBs) offer governments a smart way to deliver desired, measurable changes to their populations by leveraging multiple payers to achieve results. In a traditional model, service providers often cannot afford to make a large investment in a program, conduct a performance assessment, and then receive payment for the successful services offered (Harvard Kennedy School, 2017). The SIB model, which is better characterized as a loan from private funders than an actual bond, minimizes some of the risk associated with the investment in a service program (Harvard Kennedy School, 2017). As described in Figure 8-1, investors provide the upfront investment to a third-party, external organization for a desired government intervention provided by a service provider. Following a successful intervention, the government agency only repays the investor an agreed-upon return on investment for the outcomes (Shah and Costa, 2013). Service providers and governments, therefore, are not punished when interventions fail.

While SIBs are often used for local or state government development, development impact bonds (DIBs) are used for international development. Although DIBs bear many similarities to SIBs, external funders, rather than national governments, repay outcome payments (Shah and Costa, 2013). One example is the Mozambique Malaria Performance Bond (Saldeinger, 2013), sponsored by Nando's restaurant chain. Several years ago, leaders at Nando's recognized a lack of creativity in reaching the populations most vulnerable to malaria in Mozambique (Devex Impact, 2017). In response, they collaborated with the Ministry of Health in Mozambique to offer financial support in an effort to increase efficiency of malaria interventions (Devex Impact, 2017) with a goal of reducing malaria incidence by 30 percent or more after year 3. If this target is achieved, the Mozambique Malaria Performance Bond will repay the entire principal from Nando's and other investors with 5 percent interest. If the interventions are unsuccessful, the investors will be repaid 50 percent of their principal, with no interest (Devex Impact, 2017).

SIBs and DIBs have important limitations. First, because the success of these partnerships is contingent on a specific and measurable goal, sufficient historical data are required in order to create the goal (Shah and Costa, 2013). Second, SIBs and DIBs should not be used for essential services or for programs in which cessation would harm a population (Shah and Costa, 2013). Finally, the SIB process involves many steps, and therefore the partnership requires a large investment of time and resources to ensure success (Shah and Costa, 2013). Given that understanding, if executed successfully, SIBs and DIBs can be very helpful to governments.

Finding: Many small-scale innovations exist that can be replicated and used more widely to create more opportunities in global health.

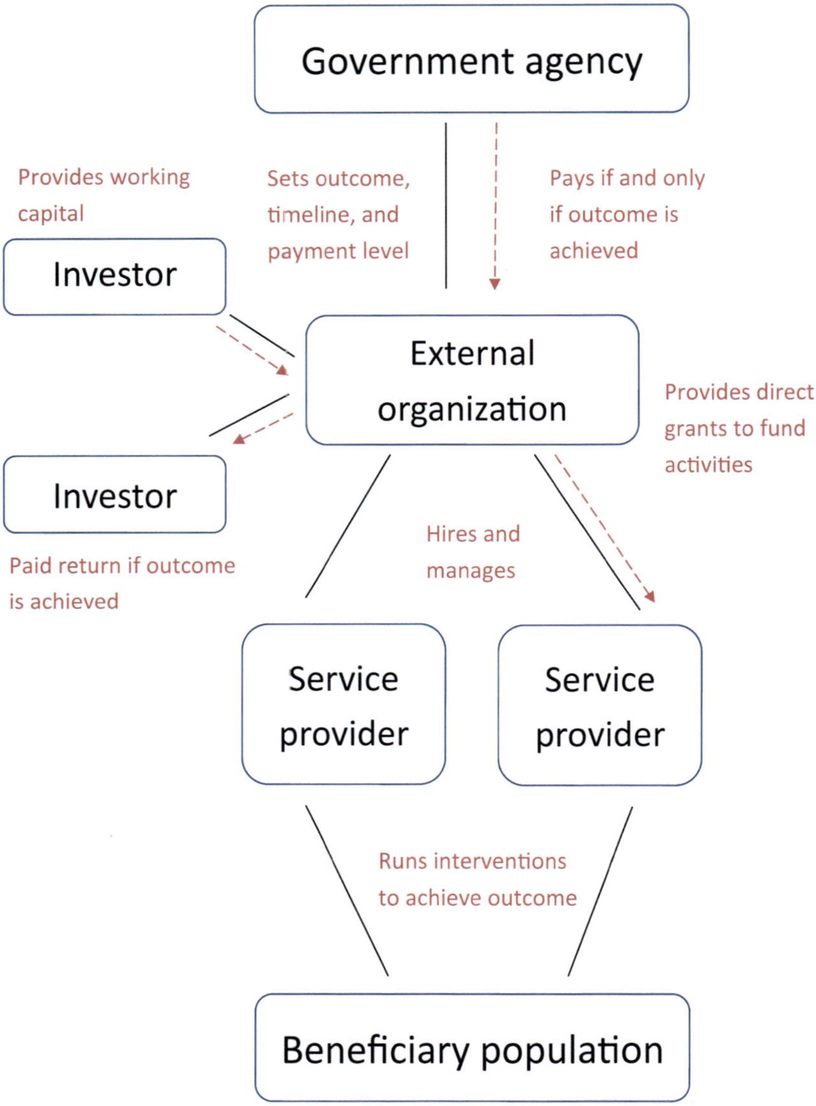

FIGURE 8-1 Social impact bond flow diagram.
SOURCE: This material [Social Finance: A Primer] was published by the Center for American Progress (www.americanprogress.org).

Private Corporations and Investors

The private sector has increasingly become a more active funding partner in global health projects in recent years. Their growing role will be critical in order to achieve many of the SDGs, in particular SDG 17, which calls for revitalizing global partnerships for sustainable development. Because of the inherent desire of the private sector to constantly improve their bottom line, people in every country may have a difficult time trusting private companies to make decisions that will improve outcomes for people living in poverty. However, encouraging private companies to use their skills and resources to both improve their markets and future business trajectories, while simultaneously contributing to social good, can be a sustainable strategy to improving global health outcomes. The private sector has a clear interest in preventing deaths and improving living conditions for populations, both of which promote economic development, create new markets, and contribute to better operating conditions for businesses (Sturchio and Goel, 2012). A notable example of private engagement in the global health space is the rise of product development partnerships, which use public and philanthropic funds to incentivize research and development. These have become more common in recent years and have been able to provide much-needed drugs at an affordable level (Mahoney, 2011). With 82 percent of capital that reaches the developing world coming from the private sector, it is imperative to ensure that these funds, in addition to the private sector's expertise, bolster the development agenda effectively (Nathan, 2017).

While private companies' philanthropic efforts have historically been categorized as corporate social responsibility, the last decade has seen a shift toward global health investment as a way to create shared value in their efforts. The shared value management strategy seeks to generate economic value while also addressing social problems (Porter and Kramer, 2011). Through linking social and business impact, companies can then move toward greater innovation and value creation. Notable methods of shared value that companies can use include reconceiving products and markets, redefining productivity in the value chain, and enabling local cluster development (Porter and Kramer, 2011). Greater collaboration among corporations, NGOs and governments for shared value will be important for further success (FSG, 2016), with a specific focus on leveraging the data collected by nonprofits and the public sector to bridge the gap between a shared value intervention and detecting evidence of benefits—though benefits will take time to be realized. However, this term of shared value may be too narrow to encompass the many efforts by companies to seek and obtain sustainable commercial returns in LMICs while also providing health products and needed services. For example, once generic alternatives were approved by the U.S. Food and Drug Administration (FDA) in 2006, the PEPFAR program and the World Health Organization (WHO) began increasing demand for inexpensive but quality antiretroviral drugs, leading to a competitive market that transformed the prospects for a number of generic companies (Waning et al., 2010).

Business models that are fit for purpose like many found in resource-constrained settings are more likely to be sustainable over the long run. Some companies have employed the "triple bottom line" strategy as a core element of their business to consider social, financial, and environmental factors when making important decisions. This focus on more comprehensive investment results has been growing across businesses and nonprofit organizations, with an eye for improved sustainable growth (Slaper and

BOX 8-3
Case Studies of Private Investment in Global Health

Novo Nordisk has taken a multifaceted approach, fulfilling their **triple bottom line** mission by adopting a patient-centered focus in Indonesia in 2006, where general awareness and access to diabetes care was poor, but the burden was high. In 2013, 7.6 million people in Indonesia had diabetes, and another 12.6 million had prediabetes. To improve awareness and understanding of diabetes, Novo Nordisk has contributed to community-based programs and increased clinical trials sponsorship. To increase access to care, Novo Nordisk trained about 2,000 internists through their INSPIRE program and increased knowledge of diabetes screening and care by 11 percent. Expansion of the program to general practitioners resulted in a 34 percent increase in knowledge among participants and found significant HbA1c reductions in their patients after 12 weeks of insulin therapy (as compared to 17 percent among not specially trained practitioners). All of Novo Nordisk's programs have helped to create a valuable, long-term relationship with Indonesian stakeholders and people, along with the potential to supply a major portion of the insulin market over the next several years. Finally, employees at Novo Nordisk reported a 21 percent increase in job satisfaction between 2008 and 2012, and employee turnover decreased by 7 percent during that same time frame.

The **Healthy Heart Africa** program was launched by **AstraZeneca** in 2014 to increase access to medicines that prevent and treat cardiovascular disease by 10 million people by 2025. In Africa, cardiovascular disease is the third-leading killer in the region; the number of deaths to cardiovascular disease increased more than any other condition between 2000 and 2012. Healthy Heart Africa has integrated blood pressure screening and hypertension diagnosis and treatment into the PEPFAR platforms built for human immunodeficiency virus/acquired immunodeficiency syndrome (HIV/AIDS) and maternal and child health, has strengthened the supply chain to ensure access, and worked at the community level to raise aware-

Hall, 2011). To more clearly illustrate some of these concepts and how they can fit into global health, the United Nations Global Compact and KPMG produced a matrix that examines opportunities for the private sector for alignment of core competencies of their business with social good or engagement within each of the SDGs (KPMG and United Nations Global Compact, 2015). See Box 8-3 for various examples of private-sector involvement in global health, including shared value, triple bottom line approaches, and alignment of core competencies.

Healthy workforce overlap For multinational companies that depend on a workforce in LMICs, the motivation to become more involved in global

ness of hypertension and the need for screening to drive demand. Working with local partners and the Mission for Essential Drugs, AstraZeneca re-engineered their supply chain to ensure medicines are always available to patients of their implementing partners, which enable up to 90 percent reduction in the cost of its medicines. In 2016, the Healthy Heart Africa program established new partnerships to continue to test approaches in Kenya and other countries in the region, specifically enhancing services for men ages 25–50 who typically access HIV/AIDS testing far less frequently than women. There will also be an independent impact evaluation of the program to provide further insight about how Healthy Heart Africa can be expanded and scaled up to other countries.

In 2015, **Sanofi** joined the International Telecommunication Union's **Be He@lthy, Be Mobile** program, a mobile phone-based service to improve the prevention of and treatment and care for NCDs in eight priority countries. Through partnerships with WHO, public–private partnerships, national governments, and the United Nations, this program has initiated an SMS message program to provide advice and support for patients with diabetes to improve communications with their health care providers and the overall continuum of care.

Novartis sought to address the growing issue of access to health care—focusing on rural India—and in 2007 launched an initiative called **Arogya Parivar**. This offered a portfolio of affordable medicines designed to meet common regional issues and were sold in a manner that made them affordable to daily wage earners. Furthermore, Novartis partnered with microfinance organizations to improve access to capital for patients. Arogya Parivar now reaches 72 million people and has increased health seeking behavior. Furthermore, Arogya Parivar became profitable 31 months after its initiation and its sales have increased 25-fold since 2007.

SOURCES: KPMG and United Nations Global Compact, 2015; Novo Nordisk, 2013; Ogola, 2015; Shared Value Initiative, 2017.

community health is even clearer. As mentioned in Chapter 4, the private sector has played a particularly important in role in malaria control and elimination, with the much direct financing and in-kind donations being provided by the oil/gas and mineral industries. For example, the AngloGold Ashanti mining company faced a significant problem of a 24 percent malaria incidence rate affecting its workforce across multiple African countries. Worker absenteeism and low productivity came with serious costs to the company. In response, AngloGold Ashanti implemented integrated malaria control programs in Ghana in 2005 that led to a 72 percent decrease in disease burden in the first 2 years; the reduction in treatment costs saved the company around $600,000 per year by 2013 (FSG, 2017). At another mine in Tanzania, AngloGold Ashanti developed a public–private partnership (PPP) with international development organizations and the National Medical Research Institute of Tanzania to build on the program. The first phase focused only on employees and achieved a 50 percent reduction in malaria, but expansion to other mining operations was able to cover more than 90 percent of the mine's employees and 100,000 community members (AngloGold Ashanti, 2013).

An example with a multi-country focus, the Lubombo Spatial Development Initiative (LSDI) was a PPP formed in 2000 to address malaria control in southern Africa including Mozambique, South Africa, and Swaziland (Moonasar et al., 2016) and improve the health and economic viability of the region. BHP Billiton, a large resource company with 17,000 employees in South Africa and Mozambique and one of the founding partners of LSDI, had a keen interest as their workforce was continually threatened by malaria (WEF, 2006). Since the majority of the new malaria cases in northeastern South Africa and Swaziland, both wealthier middle-income countries, were imported from neighboring Mozambique, LSDI understood that to truly eliminate malaria there was a need to take a targeted approach at control measures in Mozambique. Following the implementation of control measures in Mozambique alone, Swaziland saw a 95 percent reduction in malaria cases between 2000 and 2004 (Laxminarayan, 2016).

U.S. public–private partnerships in research and development As discussed in Chapter 7, the Biomedical Advanced Research and Development Authority (BARDA) appreciates that the pervasive challenges of medical countermeasure development and antimicrobial resistance require a global effort. They use PPPs to recruit skilled institutions and companies of all sizes to solve this global problem of medical product development in an uncertain market. The Combating Antibiotic-Resistant Bacteria Biopharmaceutical Accelerator, or CARB-X, was created in 2016 as the world's largest global antibacterial public–private partnership focused on preclinical discovery and early stage development of new antimicrobial products (HHS, 2016).

CARB-X is a collaboration between National Institute of Allergy and Infectious Diseases, BARDA, and four life science accelerators, with each partner playing a unique role in their shared goal to set up a diverse portfolio with more than 20 high-quality antibacterial products—dozens more than a single company would normally pursue. CARB-X plans to accomplish their goals, and get more innovative products into clinical testing by leveraging $250 million from BARDA in the first 5 years, with matching funds from the Wellcome Trust and the AMR Centre.

In addition to the CARB-X partnership, BARDA is also pursuing a pipeline of new antibiotics through a mechanism called the Other Transaction Authority (OTA), which allows BARDA and partners to diversify their investment across a portfolio of compounds. Traditional federal contracting often requires significant costs and time, but with more flexibility to change directions mid-course within the portfolio, OTA offers time-saving benefits as well. All strategic decision making is done jointly with BARDA and the senior staff at the companies involved. The portfolio model enables the partnership to adjust plans according to the most promising candidates with the cost and risk shared between the parties, something that was not possible through more traditional funding mechanisms (Houchens, 2015). The Blue Ribbon Study Panel on Biodefense recommended further use of this mechanism by BARDA, but has only found one instance of use since October 2015 (Blue Ribbon Study Panel on Biodefense, 2016). The committee supports expanded use of this type of flexible funding mechanism, also called for by the Senate Committee on Appropriations.[2]

Pandemic Emergency Financing Facility

Launched by the World Bank in May 2016 at the G7 Ministers of Finance meeting, the Pandemic Emergency Financing Facility (PEF) is designed as a pandemic emergency response mechanism (World Bank, 2016). This mechanism is only to be used in emergency response; it is not a substitute for preparedness investments. The World Bank understands that quality, resilient health systems and strong public health capabilities are crucial, but once an emergency event occurs, there is also a need to act quickly. The PEF accelerates and improves emergency response immediately, and similar to the Public Health Emergency Fund in the United States, described in Chapter 3, the PEF fills a gap in the current global financing architecture and is activated once an outbreak triggers a pre-designated level of severity. It is financed through an insurance window, with funding provided by resources from the reinsurance market combined with catastrophe bond

[2] U.S. Departments of Labor, Health and Human Services, and Education, and Related Agencies Appropriations Bill. Report 114-74. Senate. 2016.

proceeds, as well as a cash window, providing more flexible funding to address a larger set of emerging pathogens with uncertain consequences. Japan provided the first $50 million in funding commitment in 2016, and the World Bank expects the PEF to be active in 2017.

> **Finding: The private sector has grown as an active global health stakeholder in recent years to go beyond simply involvement through corporate social responsibility to aligning their core business competencies with social good and improvement of health outcomes. As evidenced by the number of companies investing their own resources, the private sector can be leveraged as a sustainable partner for governments in the future of global health.**

Value in Financial Structure

The traditional aid model that provides a scheduled stream of funds does not produce the best incentives or results and is often too highly focused on short-term outcomes or inputs into their system instead of long-term outcomes or outputs. As part of the reevaluation of the U.S. global health enterprise strategy to sustainably provide aid and achieve the goals set in this report in a cost-effective manner, the U.S. government could turn to successful multilateral organizations such as Gavi for new mechanisms. These organizations have successfully engaged in partnerships and market-shaping models to make their money go farther. For example, the Global Fund only finances programs when there is assurance that they do not replace or reduce other sources of health funding, and it actively seeks opportunities to catalyze additional donor and recipient investment through grants and other supportive structures (Brenzel, 2012). Additionally, the World Bank and other development banks have pursued better ways of putting money toward development, and tying results to financing, with much success. The committee identified front-loading investments and results-based financing as two alternative financing mechanisms that bring more value for money to U.S. global health spending.

Front-Loading Investments

Front-loading an investment allows more resources to be used initially while maintaining the level of investment over time. The theoretical benefit of this is that having a larger pool of resources upfront will enable a program to achieve its goals faster (Barder and Yeh, 2006). For example, in the context of an advanced-purchase agreement for vaccines, a front-loaded payment would increase the incentive for a manufacturer to bring products to market quickly (Berndt and Hurvitz, 2005) and provide a more efficient use of resources over time (Barder and Yeh, 2006).

Gavi employs these types of various alternative financing models to avoid defaulting, and ensuring sustainability of services provided in the countries involved in their partnership. As an example, their Advanced Market Commitment (AMC) generates incentives for vaccine manufacturers to produce affordable vaccines for the world's poorest countries. Following the launch of its pneumococcal conjugate pilot in 2007, accelerated immunization coverage against pneumococcal disease was documented across 53 Gavi countries, with 49 million children found to be fully immunized (BCG, 2015). The AMC secures lower prices for vaccines and increases access for the world's poorest children more quickly than before. Recommendations for future AMCs or other innovative financing mechanisms noted that successful engagement with the pharmaceutical industry is critical to improve sustainability of initiatives and enable manufacturers to shift from a corporate social responsibility-based approach to a more commercially viable strategy (BCG, 2015) as highlighted in the previous sections of this chapter.

Through another front-loading investment strategy called the International Finance Facility for Immunization (IFFIm), established in 2006, Gavi accelerates the availability and predictability of funds to support immunization programs by issuing bonds in the capital markets and converting long-term donor pledges into immediate cash resources (Bilimoria, 2016). This type of mechanism, and others like it, was encouraged for replication by the Action Agenda at the Financing Conference for Development in Addis Ababa, Ethiopia, in 2015 (UN, 2015). Through an independent evaluation in 2011, findings demonstrated that IFFIm was financially efficient, had achieved supranational status in capital markets, and was a robust and flexible model in challenging environments. Most importantly, it was credited with saving at least 2.75 million lives (Pearson et al., 2011).

Results-Based Financing

Results-based financing (RBF) programs for health transfer money or goods—either to patients when they take health-related actions or to health care providers when they achieve performance targets (Morgan, 2009). Currently, the RBF model is being supported by the World Bank through the Health Results Innovation Trust Fund, which was launched in 2007 with a special focus to achieve the women's and children's health-related Millennium Development Goals (MDGs). Following smaller-scale pilot grants, the RBF activities and relevant network have grown in both supply and demand. In fact, RBF programs around the world have demonstrated evidence-based transformational effects to maternal and child health. For example, the probability of in-hospital neonatal mortality of babies whose mothers enrolled in Plan Nacer, a RBF program, dropped by 74 percent in Argentina; in Nigeria, the rate of modern contraceptive use in RBF areas was approximately twice that of non-RBF areas at 21.5 percent and 10 percent, respectively (World Bank, 2014). The researchers were also able to show that the quality of care improved in these areas that implemented RBF practices.

RBF programs can also improve in-country harmonization of comprehensive strategies for targeted sector services, such as maternal and child health. For example, the government of Rwanda directs its alignment efforts underneath its RBF program, inviting donors to provide support for indicators that they have already designated (World Bank, 2014). This method of harmonization allows for reduced transaction costs and improved efficiency in reporting and verification for partners. Importantly, this method also provides a solution to the problem of poor alignment of donor goals and national priorities that has emerged in recipient countries.

Global Financing Facility Following this trend of increased progress and successful results through RBF, the World Bank Group and the governments of Canada, Norway, and the United States announced in September 2014 the creation of the Global Financing Facility (GFF) to mobilize support for developing countries' plans to accelerate progress on the MDGs and end preventable maternal and child deaths by 2030 (Claeson, 2017; GFF, 2016a). The GFF, the financing arm of Every Woman Every Child,[3] is a multi-stakeholder partnership that supports country-led efforts to improve the health of women, children, and adolescents by focusing on a specific set of challenges—including health financing and health systems. The main aim of the GFF is to close the $33 billion financing gap to meet these challenges in 63 target countries, with the national governments leading the process through their own country platform of stakeholders (GFF, 2016b). Thus far, 16 "front runner" countries have begun piloting the GFF process.[4] The first step is the creation of an Investment Case, which establishes a unique set of evidenced-based interventions for a national government. Of the 16 countries that have initiated the GFF process, 7 have begun to implement their

[3] Every Woman Every Child is a global movement that puts into action WHO's Global Strategy for Women's, Children's, and Adolescents' Health. Launched by the UN Secretary-General in 2010, Every Woman Every Child aims to mobilize national governments, international organizations, the private sector, and civil society to solve the health issues that women, children, and adolescents face around the world (Every Woman Every Child, 2016).

[4] The countries include Bangladesh, Cameroon, the Democratic Republic of the Congo, Ethiopia, Guatemala, Guinea, Kenya, Liberia, Mozambique, Myanmar, Nigeria, Senegal, Sierra Leone, Tanzania, Uganda, and Vietnam (Claeson, 2017).

cases. To help countries successfully do so, GFF strives to move away from traditional development assistance, by using four smart financing pathways: improved efficiency, increased domestic resource mobilization, increased and better aligned external financing, and leveraged private-sector resources (Claeson, 2017). The first two pathways are especially useful given that 20 to 40 percent of health expenditures are lost due to inefficiency and that GFF modeling suggests that the combination of economic growth, tax base increases, and increased prioritization of health would close 71 percent of the $33 billion financing gap (Claeson, 2017). Though the majority of GFF's efforts are aimed at national governments, it also supports efforts at the subnational level.

Finding: Creating value in financial structure, through mechanisms like front-loading investments and results-based financing can secure lower prices for commodities, save lives, and encourage sustainability of programs and health outcomes.

PRIORITIES FOR U.S. GLOBAL HEALTH PROGRAMS

Moving into the next decade of global health, it is clear that the aspirational global health goals set across many sectors will demand more than the previous DAH structures can offer. The questions then become, how can U.S. government programs support growing economies of middle-income countries to take on more ownership of their health programs? How can all governments continue to attract investment and technical expertise from private companies as sustainable partners? What do these private companies need in order to feel comfortable investing their own resources? And finally, what can the United States do differently to make investments in global health more efficient and cost-effective?

Supporting Domestic Resource Mobilization

For countries with burgeoning economies and middle-classes, the economic case can be made to ministers of finance that investments in health infrastructure and personnel can be critical for building ownership and driving returns. Investment in community health workers results in a return on investment as high as 10:1 according to the WHO report *Strengthening Primary Health Care through Community Health Workers* (2015). The report also recommended that bilateral donors "allow for and actively promote the use of disease-specific funding for integrated . . . community health worker plans" (Dahn et al., 2015, p. 25). As countries do shift to domestic financing, the United States can advise nations in ways to structure their debt ratios and tax bases, and develop tax initiatives in order to create new revenue streams or make better use of existing donor funds to strengthen their health systems. Other types of support could include engagement with ministries on system design and financing to assist in plan design, model refinement and expansion, return on investment analysis and financial plan execution. Further nontraditional support could include intellectual property and knowledge management such as case studies on financing pathways, documenting funding flows, and South-South capacity building functions (Qureshi, 2016).

This advisory role is beginning to take shape, with the Sustainable Finance Initiative (SFI) for HIV/AIDS, an interagency partnership among the Bureau for Economic Growth, Education and Environment at USAID, PEPFAR, and the U.S. Treasury. SFI works through other countries' ministries of health and finance to help national governments examine methods of increasing their funding commitment to HIV/AIDS (USAID, 2016). Five countries already have representatives from the U.S. Treasury working in the USAID mission office to ensure this is done correctly and sustainably from the outset. As an example, SFI's impact in Kenya has contributed to an increase of $30–$40 million in new domestic spending being allocated to HIV response in each of the next 5 years. Finally, creating more flexibility for innovative finance can better support this transition to domestic resource mobilization. As an example, USAID could allow development credit authority greater latitude to apply certain restrictions where the ultimate outcome will catalyze additional private-sector resources and the capital markets. These restrictions could include limited ability to guarantee sovereigns, or caps on total amount of risk guaranteed in a development credit authority structure (Qureshi, 2016).

Attracting Investment from Private Companies

To continue to attract new money and maintain the interest of the private sector, U.S. programs need to increase their flexibility in developing innovative financing products and modalities. Examples could include working with the finance sector to push the envelope on innovative sources of financing, or crowding-in[5] private-sector capital (Qureshi, 2016). Governments can crowd-in additional funding sources by increasing the demand for goods through public funds and sharing risk in various ways, which then catalyzes private investment that would not have otherwise taken place (Powers and Butterfield, 2014). Additionally, to provide more certainty for the private sector in investing, U.S. government global health

[5] Crowding-in is an economic principle in which private investment increases as debt-financed government spending increases. This is caused by government spending boosting the demand for goods, which in turn increases private demand for new output sources.

programs could include a provision to provide matching funds for public–private partnerships, which have proven to be effective in encouraging companies to invest through other programs such as PEPFAR, Power Africa, and the Millennium Challenge Corporation (Sturchio and Schneider, 2017). For countries that the United States will continue to support through DAH, current investments can be made more effective and efficient, thus helping to stretch farther the dollars being spent. This could be accomplished through integration of services as discussed in Chapter 6 and through the many PPPs highlighted in this report, so an established platform like PEPFAR can be used to address additional health burdens without much increase in cost.

Stressing Increased Efficiency and Cost-Effectiveness

Overall, many viable tools, including debt buy-downs, social impact bonds, and other mechanisms not discussed in this chapter such as impact investing, microfinance schemes, traditional equity investments can improve the accessibility of funds and efficiency of global health programs (Sturchio and Schneider, 2017). The historical challenges and limitations of traditional bilateral aid from the U.S. government make the contracting process slow and dated, and the outcomes not as effective as they could be. These new methods, though not risk-free, offer a fresh perspective to aid disbursement and new opportunities. Many experts have reviewed and assessed various innovative financing mechanisms in much more detail than is called for in this report, but these expert analyses should be consulted when designing changes to global health investments to ensure fit-for-purpose and avoid re-creation of mechanisms (Atun et al., 2012; de Ferranti et al., 2008; Sturchio and Schneider, 2017). Encouraging more cooperation between U.S. development finance tools can also maximize impact when multiple agencies are brought together to work across sectors.

SUMMARY AND RECOMMENDATIONS

Current U.S. global health financing is focused largely on immediate disease-specific priorities such as HIV/AIDS or malaria. This financial support is seen as development and humanitarian assistance for strategic partner countries, rather than as a means of achieving long-term goals of building global health systems and platforms that are disease-agnostic and can respond rapidly and flexibly to emerging diseases that threaten the entire world, including the United States. However, these cross-cutting systems and platforms can produce large returns and long-term benefits. For example, smallpox eradication saves the United States the one-time expenditures it invested every 26 days, and the global benefits of avoided infections outweigh the global costs 159:1 (Barrett, 2013). Similarly, efforts toward polio eradication are projected to generate net returns of up to $50 billion by 2035 (Duintjer Tebbens et al., 2010), but even more returns will remain out of reach if the handful of polio cases diagnosed each year continue and annual funding is still required.

As countries continue to grow economically, their needs will change from direct support for drugs, diagnostics, and other commodities to technical support and sustainable financing from multiple sources. Additionally, current investments in global health also can be made more effective and efficient. For example, existing programs such as PEPFAR or the work of BARDA can be augmented through public–private partnerships to have a greater impact on health outcomes in countries. Furthermore, there are opportunities for working with the finance sector to allow more flexibility and innovation in financing mechanisms for programs. Given the limitations of traditional federal bilateral aid from the U.S. government, new methods such as impact investing, microfinance schemes, and equity investments could improve the accessibility of funds and efficiency of global health programs (Sturchio and Schenider, 2017).

Finally, the private sector has a clear interest in preventing deaths and improving living conditions for many international populations—both of which promote economic development, create new markets, and contribute to better operating conditions for businesses (Sturchio and Goel, 2012). As 82 percent of capital reaching LMICs comes from the private sector, there are many opportunities for both donors and national recipient governments to bolster the health and development agenda more effectively (Nathan, 2017).

Conclusion: The U.S. government needs to conduct more strategic and systematic assessments with an eye toward making long-term investments in global health instead of focusing on short-term expenditures.

Conclusion: Increased financial gains in middle-income countries and a plethora of new and committed global health partners have created an opportunity for the United States to take smarter and more creative directions when financing global health programs. A variety of innovative financing mechanisms are being employed around the world, and there is a need for expansion and diversification of current U.S. financing methods.

Conclusion: Thinking more strategically about how to help countries transition out of bilateral aid programs and optimize their use of domestic resources in a sustainable way is an important future role of the United States. Providing assistance to low- and middle-income countries in structuring debt ratios and tax initiatives in ways that can build stronger and more holistic health systems can provide multiple returns on investments, and is a next step for donor governments.

Recommendation 12: Transition Investments Toward Global Public Goods

The U.S. Agency for International Development, the U.S. Department of State, and the U.S. Department of Health and Human Services should, together, systematically assess their approach to global health funding with an eye toward making long-term investments in high-impact, country-level programs. The focus should be on programs that both build national health systems and provide the greatest value in terms of global health security (to prevent pandemics), as well as respond to humanitarian emergencies and provide opportunities for joint research and development for essential drugs, diagnostics, and vaccines that will benefit many countries, including the United States.

Recommendation 13: Optimize Resources Through Smart Financing

Relevant agencies of the U.S. government should expand efforts to complement direct bilateral support for health with financing mechanisms that include results-based financing; risk sharing; and attracting funding from private investment, recipient governments, and other donors.

- **The U.S. Agency for International Development (USAID) and The U.S. President's Emergency Plan for AIDS Relief (PEPFAR) should structure their financing to promote greater country ownership and domestic financing. Assistance should be provided in developing innovative financing products/modalities and in working with the finance sector to push the envelope on innovative sources of financing, crowding in private-sector capital.**
- **USAID and PEPFAR should engage with ministries on system design and financing to assist in plan design, model refinement and expansion, return-on-investment analysis, and financial plan execution.**
- **USAID should expand the use and flexibility of such mechanisms as the Development Credit Authority, and the U.S. Treasury, the U.S. Department of State, and USAID should motivate the World Bank; the International Monetary Fund;**

the Global Fund to Fight AIDS, Tuberculosis and Malaria; and Gavi, the Vaccine Alliance, respectively, to promote transitioning to domestic financing, assist countries in creating fiscal space for health, leverage fiscal policies to improve health, and attract alternative financing sources.

REFERENCES

AngloGold Ashanti. 2013. *Creating a sustainable solution for malaria in Continental Africa region*. http://www.anglogoldashanti.com/en/Media/Our-Stories/Pages/Creating-a-sustainable-solution-for-malaria-in-Continental-Africa-Region.aspx (accessed February 13, 2017).

Atun, R., F. M. Knaul, Y. Akachi, and J. Frenk. 2012. Innovative financing for health: What is truly innovative? *The Lancet* 380(9858):2044-2049.

Barder, O. M., and E. Yeh. 2006. *The costs and benefits of front-loading and predictability of immunization*. Washington, DC: Center for Global Development.

Barrett, S. 2013. Economic considerations for the eradication endgame. *Philosophical Transactions of the Royal Society B: Biological Sciences* 368(1623):20120149.

BCG (Boston Consulting Group). 2015. *The Advance Market Commitment pilot for pneumococcal vaccines: Outcomes and impact evaluation*. Boston, MA: Boston Consulting Group.

Bennett, A., N. Bar-Zeev, and N. A. Cunliffe. 2016. Measuring indirect effects of rotavirus vaccine in low income countries. *Vaccine* 34(37):4351-4353.

Berndt, E. R., and J. A. Hurvitz. 2005. Vaccine advance-purchase agreements for low-income countries: Practical issues. *Health Affairs* 24(3):653-665.

Bilimoria, N. 2016. Gavi, the Vaccine Alliance. Paper read at Global Health and the Future of the United States: A Changing Landscape of Global Health, December 6, 2016, Washington, DC. http://www.nationalacademies.org/hmd/~/media/Files/Activity%20Files/Global/USandGlobalHealth/Global-Health-and-The-Future-of-the-US/Meeting-2-Files/Bilimoria Presentation.pdf (accessed December 10, 2016).

Birdsall, N., and A. Diofasi. 2015. Global public goods that matter for development: A path for US leadership. *The White House and the world: Practical proposals on global development for the next US president*, edited by N. Birdsall and B. Leo. Washington, DC: Center for Global Development.

Birn, A.-E., Y. Pillay, and T. H. Holtz. 2017. *Textbook of global health*. Oxford, England: Oxford University Press.

Blue Ribbon Study Panel on Biodefense. 2016. *Biodefense indicators: One year later, events outpacing efforts to defend the nation*. Arlington, VA: Blue Ribbon Study Panel on Biodefense.

Brenzel, L. 2012. Global and donor financing. In *MDS-3: Managing access to medicines and health technologies*, edited by M. Ryan. Arlington, VA: Management Sciences for Health.

Brilliant, L. B. 1985. *The management of smallpox eradication in India*. Ann Arbor: University of Michigan Press.

Claeson, M. 2017. The Global Financing Facility: Towards a new way of financing for development. *The Lancet*. 389(10079):1588-1592.

DAC (Development Assistance Committee). 2016. TOSSD: A new statistical measure for the SDG era. Washington, DC: The Development Assistance Committee, Organisation for Economic Co-operation and Development.

Dahn, B., A. T. Woldemariam, H. Perry, A. Maeda, D. von Glahn, R. Panjabi, N. Merchant, K. Vosburg, D. Palazuelos, C. Lu, J. Simon, J. Pfaffmann, D. Brown, H. Austin, P. Heydt, and C. Qureshi. 2015. *Strengthening primary health care through community health workers: Investment case and financing recommendation.* http://www.who.int/hrh/news/2015/CHW-Financing-FINAL-July-15-2015.pdf?ua=1 (accessed January 10, 2017).

DanWatch. 2011. *An investigation of tax payments and corporate structures in the mining industry of Sierra Leone: Not sharing the loot.* http://www.resourcegovernance.org/sites/default/files/Not_Sharing_the_Loot.pdf (accessed March 20, 2017).

de Ferranti, D., C. Griffin, M. L. Escobar, A. Glassman, and G. Lagomarsino. 2008. *Innovative financing for global health: Tools for analyzing the options.* Washington, DC: Brookings Institution.

Devex Impact. 2017. *Goodbye malaria: Mozambique Malaria Performance Bond.* https://www.devex.com/impact/partnerships/goodbye-malaria-mozambique-malaria-performance-bond-362 (accessed February 13, 2017).

Duintjer Tebbens, R. J., M. A. Pallansch, S. L. Cochi, S. G. Wassilak, J. Linkins, R. W. Sutter, R. B. Aylward, and K. M. Thompson. 2010. Economic analysis of the global polio eradication initiative. *Vaccine* 29(2):334-343.

Every Woman Every Child. 2016. *About.* https://www.everywomaneverychild.org/about (accessed April 15, 2017).

Fenner, F., D. A. Henderson, I. Arita, Z. Jezek, and I. D. Ladnyi. 1988. *Smallpox and its eradication, history of international public health no. 6.* Geneva, Switzerland: World Health Organization.

FSG. 2016. *Competing by saving lives: Pushing the frontier for shared value in health: Report to participants.* New York: Frontier Strategy Group.

FSG. 2017. *Anglogold Ashanti malaria program.* https://sharedvalue.org/groups/anglogold-ashanti-malaria-program (accessed February 13, 2017).

Gavi (Gavi, the Vaccine Alliance). 2014. *Co-financing policy evaluation.* http://www.gavi.org/results/evaluations/co-financing-policy-evaluation (accessed February 13, 2017).

Gavi. 2015. *Keeping children healthy: The Vaccine Alliance progress report 2015.* Geneva, Switzerland: Gavi, the Vaccine Alliance.

GFF (Global Financing Facility). 2016a. *Global Financing Facility partners.* https://www.globalfinancingfacility.org/about/partners (accessed March 17, 2017).

GFF. 2016b. *Global Financing Facility introduction.* https://www.globalfinancingfacility.org/introduction (accessed March 17, 2017).

GHRF Commission (Commission on a Global Health Risk Framework for the Future). 2016. *The neglected dimension of global security: A framework to counter infectious disease crises.* doi: https://doi.org/10.17226/21891.

GPEI (Global Polio Eradication Initiative). 2014. *Economic case for eradicating polio.* Global Polio Eradication Initiative.

Harvard Kennedy School. 2017. *Pay for success: Social impact bonds.* http://govlab.hks.harvard.edu/social-impact-bond-lab (accessed February 13, 2017).

HHS (U.S. Department of Health and Human Services). 2016. *CARB-X: Combating Antibiotic Resistant Bacteria Biopharmaceutical Accelerator.* https://www.phe.gov/about/barda/CARB-X/Pages/default.aspx (accessed February 13, 2017).

Houchens, C. 2015. *Innovative partnerships support antibiotic development.* https://www.phe.gov/ASPRBlog/pages/BlogArticlePage.aspx?PostID=157 (accessed February 13, 2017).

IHME (Institute of Health Metrics and Evaluation). 2016. *Financing global health 2015: Development assistance steady on the path to new global goals.* Seattle, WA: Institute for Health Metrics and Evaluation.

IMF (International Monetary Fund). 2011. *Revenue mobilization in developing countries.* Washington, DC: International Monetary Fund.

IOM (Institute of Medicine). 2014. *Investing in global health systems: Sustaining gains, transforming lives.* Washington, DC: The National Academies Press.

Kamel, S., and E. A. Tooma. 2005. *Exchanging debt for development: Lessons from the Egyptian debt-for-development swap experience.* Giza, Egypt: Economic Research Forum.

KPMG (Klynveld Peat Marwick Goerdeler) and United Nations Global Compact. 2015. *SDG industry matrix: Healthcare & life sciences.* https://www.unglobalcompact.org/library/3111 (accessed February 13, 2017).

Laxminarayan, R. 2016. Trans-boundary commons in infectious diseases. *Oxford Review of Economic Policy* 32(1):88-101.

Mahoney, R. T. 2011. Product development partnerships: Case studies of a new mechanism for health technology innovation. *Health Research Policy and Systems* 9(1):33-41.

Megiddo, I., A. R. Colson, A. Nandi, S. Chatterjee, S. Prinja, A. Khera, and R. Laxminarayan. 2014. Analysis of the universal immunization programme and introduction of a rotavirus vaccine in India with Indiasim. *Vaccine* 32 (Suppl 1):A151-A161.

Miller, M., S. Barret, and D. A. Henderson. 2006. Control and eradication. In *Disease control priorities in developing countries.* Vol. 2, edited by D. T. Jamison, J. G. Breman, A. R. Measham, G. Alleyne, M. Cleason, D. B. Eavns, P. Jha, A. Mills, and P. Musgrove. Washington, DC: World Bank.

Moonasar, D., R. Maharaj, S. Kunene, B. Candrinho, F. Saute, N. Ntshalintshali, and N. Morris. 2016. Towards malaria elimination in the MOSASWA (Mozambique, South Africa and Swaziland) region. *Malaria Journal* 15(1):419.

Morgan, L. 2009. *Performance incentives in global health: Potential and pitfalls.* https://www.rbfhealth.org/sites/rbf/files/RBF_FEATURE_PerfIncentivesGlobalHealth.pdf (accessed February 13, 2017).

Moye, M. 2001. *Overview of debt conversion.* London, UK: Debt Relief International Ltd.

Nathan, T. 2017. *5 ways to make blended finance work.* https://www.weforum.org/agenda/2017/01/ways-to-make-blended-finance-work (accessed February 13, 2017).

NIAID (National Institute of Allergy and Infectious Diseases). 2015. *Indo-U.S. vaccine action program overview.* https://www.niaid.nih.gov/research/indo-us-vaccine-action-program-overview (accessed February 13, 2017).

Novo Nordisk. 2013. *Where economics and health meet: Changing diabetes in Indonesia.* Novo Nordisk.

OECD (Organisation for Economic Co-operation and Development). 2016. *Development co-operation report 2016: The sustainable development goals as business opportunities.* Paris, France.

Ogola, E. N. August 2015. *Healthy Heart Africa: The Kenyan experience.* Paper presented at Pan-African Society of Cardiology Hypertension Task Force Meeting, London, United Kingdom. http://www.pascar.org/uploads/files/HEALTHY_HEART_AFRICA_Elijah_Ogola.pdf (accessed February 18, 2017).

Pearson, M., J. Clarke, L. Ward, C. Grace, D. Harris, and M. Cooper. 2011. *Evaluation of the International Finance Facility for Immunization (IFFIm).* London, UK: Health and Life Science Partnership.

Policy Cures. 2012. *Policy brief 6: Debt buydowns or conversions.* Paper presented at Asia-Pacific Development Summit, Jakarta, Indonesia. http://policycures.org/downloads/Policy%20Brief%206%20-%20Debt%20Conversion.pdf (accseed March 5, 2017).

Porter, M., and M. Kramer. 2011. Creating shared value. *Harvard Busisness Review.* https://hbr.org/2011/01/the-big-idea-creating-shared-value (accessed April 15, 2017).

Powers, C., and W. M. Butterfield. 2014. Crowding in private investment. In *Frontiers in development: Ending extreme poverty*, edited by R. Shah and N. Unger. Washington, DC: U.S. Agency for International Development.

Qureshi, C. 2016. Financing community health: Briefing for the National Academies of Sciences, Engineering, and Medicine. Paper read at Global Health and the Future of the United States: A Changing Landscape of Global Health, Washington, DC. http://www.nationalacademies.org/hmd/~/media/Files/Activity%20Files/Global/USandGlobalHealth/Global-Health-and-The-Future-of-the-US/Meeting-2-Files/Claire-Qureshi-Presentation.pdf (accessed December 15, 2016).

Reeves, A., Y. Gourtsoyannis, S. Basu, D. McCoy, M. McKee, and D. Stuckler. 2015. Financing universal health coverage—effects of alternative tax structures on public health systems: Cross-national modelling in 89 low-income and middle-income countries. *The Lancet* 386(9990):274-280.

Saldeinger, A. 2013. *How a restaurant chain pioneered a social impact bond to fight malaria.* https://www.devex.com/news/how-a-restaurant-chain-pioneered-a-social-impact-bond-to-fight-malaria-82212 (accessed February 13, 2017).

Seymour, J. 2004. Eradicating smallpox. In *Millions saved: Proven successes in global health.* Vol. 1, edited by R. Levine and The What Works Working Group. Washington, DC: Center for Global Development.

Shah, S., and K. Costa. 2013. *Social finance: A primer.* https://www.americanprogress.org/issues/economy/reports/2013/11/05/78792/social-finance-a-primer (accessed February 13, 2017).

Shared Value Initiative. 2017. *Novartis delivers healthcare and education to remote communities.* https://sharedvalue.org/examples/arogya-parivar-local-healthcare-delivery-and-education (accessed March 20, 2017).

Slaper, T. F., and T. J. Hall. 2011. The triple bottom line: What is it and how does it work? *Indiana Business Review* 86(1):4-8.

Stenberg, K., H. Axelson, P. Sheehan, I. Anderson, A. M. Gülmezoglu, M. Temmerman, E. Mason, H. S. Friedman, Z. A. Bhutta, J. E. Lawn, K. Sweeny, J. Tulloch, P. Hansen, M. Chopra, A. Gupta, J. P. Vogel, M. Ostergren, B. Rasmussen, C. Levin, C. Boyle, S. Kuruvilla, M. Koblinsky, N. Walker, A. de Francisco, N. Novcic, C. Presern, D. Jamison, and F. Bustreo. 2014. Advancing social and economic development by investing in women's and children's health: A new global investment framework. *The Lancet* 383(9925):1333-1354.

Sturchio, J. L., and A. Goel. 2012. *The private-sector role in public health: Reflections on the new global architecture in health.* Washington, DC: Center for Strategic and International Studies.

Sturchio, J. L., and M. Schneider. 2017. *Strengthening partnerships with the private sector: Supporting universal coverage of women's and family health.* Washington, DC: Center for Strategic and International Studies.

Tate, J. E., A. H. Burton, C. Boschi-Pinto, A. D. Steele, J. Duque, and U. D. Parashar. 2012. 2008 estimate of worldwide rotavirus-associated mortality in children younger than 5 years before the introduction of universal rotavirus vaccination programmes: A systematic review and meta-analysis. *Lancet Infectious Diseases* 12(2):136-141.

UN (United Nations). 2015. *Addis Ababa action agenda of the third international conference at financing for development.* Addis Ababa, Ethiopia: United Nations.

UN Integrated Implementation Framework. n.d. *Debt2Health.* http://iif.un.org/content/debt2health (accessed March 16, 2017).

USAID (U.S. Agency for International Development). 2016. Mobilize domestic resources for health. https://www.usaid.gov/what-we-do/global-health/health-systems/goals/mobilize-domestic-resources-health (accessed April 24, 2017).

USAID. 2017. *Development innovation ventures.* https://www.usaid.gov/div (accessed March 16, 2017).

Waning, B., M. Kyle, E. Diedrichsen, L. Soucy, J. Hochstadt, T. Bärnighausen, and S. Moon. 2010. Intervening in global markets to improve access to HIV/AIDS treatment: An analysis of international policies and the dynamics of global antiretroviral medicines markets. *Globalization and Health* 6:9.

WEF (World Economic Forum). 2006. *Global health initiative: Public-private partnership case example.* Geneva, Switzerland: World Economic Forum.

WHO (World Health Organization). 2010. *The smallpox eradication campaign—SEP (1966-1980).* http://www.who.int/features/2010/smallpox/en (accessed February 14, 2017).

WHO. 2017. *Global public goods for health (GPGH).* http://www.who.int/trade/resource/GPGH/en (accessed February 13, 2017).

World Bank. 2014. *A smarter approach to delivering more and better reproductive, maternal, newborn, and child health services.* Washington, DC: World Bank.

World Bank. 2016. *Pandemic emergency facility: Frequently asked questions.* http://www.worldbank.org/en/topic/pandemics/brief/pandemic-emergency-facility-frequently-asked-questions (accessed March 17, 2017).

9

Global Health Leadership

"Medical diplomacy must be made a significantly larger part of our foreign and defense policy. . . . America has the best chance to win the war on terror and defeat the terrorists by enhancing our medical and humanitarian assistance to vulnerable countries."

—Former Secretary of Health and Human Services Tommy Thompson (2005 Boston Globe *editorial)*

Throughout this report the committee has reiterated the need to understand the changing landscape of health, which is strongly influenced by globalization, climate change, increased travel and trade, and increased life expectancies around the globe. Despite these global changes, history has proven that advancing foreign policy and national security can be achieved through and by health. Global health itself has long been used as a tool to advance foreign policy interests, including security and influence (Feldbaum and Michaud, 2010). The scope of global health in diplomacy was greatly expanded with the creation of the World Health Organization (WHO) in 1948, and since then, by the advent of the International Sanitary Regulations in 1951 (with subsequent updates to become the International Health Regulations [IHR] in 1969 and 2005). The involvement of the United States in the creation of the Global Fund to Fight AIDS, Tuberculosis and Malaria (Global Fund) in 2002, the rollout of The U.S. President's Emergency Plan for AIDS Relief (PEPFAR) in 2003, and the development of the Global Health Security Agenda (GHSA) in 2014, shows the continuing need for a U.S. role in global health diplomacy has not abated.

To maintain the status of the United States as a global health leader and ensure safety for its people, the committee argues it will be essential to stay engaged and involved in international agencies, collaborations, and partnerships. A strong connection to the many multilateral organizations involved in global health and development is critical to maintain situational awareness and a keen recognition of when a small-scale problem could erupt into a global emergency. Consider the example of the involvement of U.S. diplomats in the international response in Nigeria in 2003. At the time northern Nigerian states banned polio immunization campaigns, which lead to a global outbreak and ended hopes of eradicating the disease in that decade (Kaufmann and Feldbaum, 2009). Though it was difficult for U.S. health officials to understand the diplomatic tools they had, together with the Global Polio Eradication Initiative and the United Nations (UN), U.S. diplomats were able to raise the issue on multiple state visits to the Middle East. Furthermore, by working through the U.S. Embassy in Nigeria, the U.S. was able to influence other countries to put pressure on Nigeria to restart the vaccination campaign (Kaufmann and Feldbaum, 2009). This is just one example demonstrating the benefits of taking a strategic approach to U.S. efforts in global health diplomacy.

This chapter opens with a review of the definitions and needs for global health governance, including the recent calls for reform of WHO following the 2014–2015 Ebola outbreak in West Africa, and newly established multilateral organizations. Next, it offers suggestions for the U.S. approach to global health diplomacy, including coordinated roles for the U.S. Department of State and the U.S. Department of Health and Human Services, and then describes how health could be integrated into the foreign service system. Finally, this chapter discusses the creation of a workforce pipeline to support this proposed approach, and closes with conclusions and recommendations.

GLOBAL HEALTH ARCHITECTURE AND GOVERNANCE

The international architecture for global health governance is complex, cross-cutting, and often driven by political motives. Many definitions of global governance put *interdependence* in the center (Kickbusch and Szabo, 2014), perhaps illustrating the reasons that global health governance has become so challenging and important in the last few decades. Kickbusch and Szabo (2014) explain the complex interplay of global health governance along three political spaces (see Figure 9-1). Though *global health governance* refers to institutions with an explicit health mandate, such as WHO, it is now well understood that *global governance for health* extends to organizations that may have direct or indirect effects on health, such as the UN and its agencies, including the UN International Children's Emergency Fund (UNICEF), UN Population Fund, and UN Development Programme; the World Trade Organization; or the World Bank (Kickbusch and Szabo, 2014). Finally, *governance for global health* refers to mechanisms and institutions that contribute to global health governance and governance for global health, including regional strategies for global health (Kickbusch and Szabo, 2014).

Kickbusch and Szabo argue that just as public health challenges can no longer be effectively addressed only within the health sector and at the

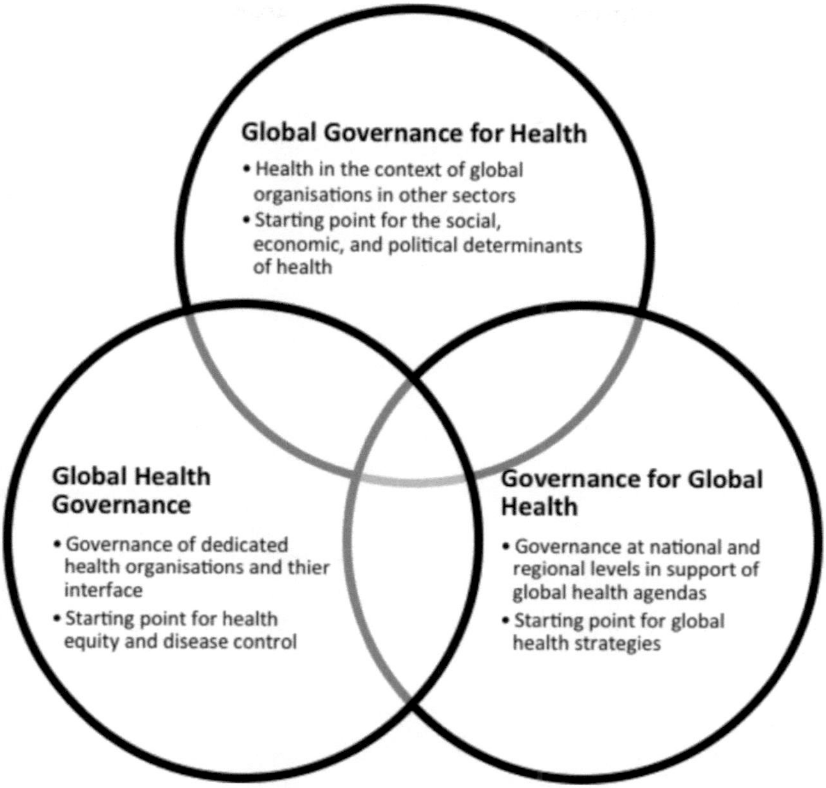
Global Governance for Health
• Health in the context of global organisations in other sectors
• Starting point for the social, economic, and political determinants of health
Global Health Governance
• Governance of dedicated health organisations and thier interface
• Starting point for health equity and disease control
Governance for Global Health
• Governance at national and regional levels in support of global health agendas
• Starting point for global health strategies

FIGURE 9-1 Global health governance along three political spaces.
SOURCE: Kickbusch and Szabo, 2014.

national level, WHO can no longer be the sole manager of these types of intergovernmental health challenges. Despite many criticisms, there is still a need for WHO, its strong convening power to coordinate the many new global health players, and its ability to set norms and standards in global health care (The *PLOS Medicine* Editors, 2007). Yet, the response to the 2014 Ebola outbreak demonstrated that the current state of global health governance is not adequate to manage and respond to the health needs of all countries, and that there is an urgent need for reform.

Calls for WHO Reform

The 2014 Ebola outbreak exposed major vulnerabilities in the WHO emergency response capabilities and leadership structure, such as poor IHR compliance, lack of technical capacity, unstable financing and lack of accountability (Moon et al., 2017). To address those vulnerabilities, several commissions were convened in the year after the height of the outbreak to discuss areas of WHO governance and outbreak response improvement.[1] Each of the commissions emphasized the need for reforms in WHO outbreak response and global governance (Gostin et al., 2016).

The Ebola response was hindered by poor coordination at global, national, and subnational levels; therefore, the commissions recommended that outbreak preparedness at all levels be refocused as the core of WHO's work. Overall, the commissions recommended the creation of a Centre for Emergency Preparedness and Response to integrate and strengthen WHO's preparedness, response, and humanitarian activities (Gostin et al., 2016). With the understanding that WHO has cut nearly two-thirds of its emergency response unit, this new governing body would fill a much-needed gap that will declare public health emergencies of international concern (PHEICs) and coordinate responses more quickly. The commissions also recommended WHO lead the assessments of countries' implementation of the core capacities outlined in the IHR (Gostin et al., 2016). While nations must be held responsible for developing their own infrastructure to respond to emerging health threats, the commissions argued that WHO must coordinate global preparedness and hold nations accountable for its maintenance.

The legitimacy and ability of WHO to respond in an outbreak are contingent on strong governance at all levels. Described as suffering from a "crisis of confidence," WHO was asked to make a number of reforms by the commissions to ensure it remains a global leader in health (Gostin et al., 2016). Specifically, the commissions recommended that to prepare for outbreaks, WHO should partner with countries to ensure they have the technical support required to implement the core capacities necessary to comply with IHR, with the ultimate goal of having every government develop and publish concrete plans to achieve these core capacities by 2020 (Gostin et al., 2016). Additionally, the commissions recommended that WHO take the role of watchdog in ensuring that restrictions on travel and trade set by nations during outbreaks are justified, so that countries experiencing outbreaks are not unjustly punished (Moon et al., 2017). Possible solutions, including "naming and shaming" countries that impose unjusti-

[1] Commissions for WHO reform included (1) the World Health Organization (WHO) Ebola Interim Assessment Panel (WHO Interim Assessment); (2) the Harvard University and the London School of Hygiene & Tropical Medicine's Independent Panel on the Global Response to Ebola (Harvard/LSHTM); (3) the Commission on a Global Health Risk Framework for the Future (CGHRF) convened by the U.S. National Academy of Medicine; and (4) the United Nations High-Level Panel on the Global Response to Health Crises (UN Panel) (Gostin et al., 2016).

fied restrictions or encouraging the creation of enforcement mechanisms for the enactment of travel and trade restrictions (Moon et al., 2017), would allow WHO to take on an aggressive role of being the authoritative voice in times of PHEICs. Finally, the commissions recommended that WHO reform its internal structure through better management of human resources, increased transparency and accountability through a freedom of information policy, creation of an inspector general role, and marshaling of more effective leadership (Moon et al., 2017).

Up to the release of this report, the work to implement the recommended changes has begun, but is far from finished, and the success of these reforms is contingent on sustainable funding. Multiple assessments and commissions have called for improved funding for WHO (Gostin et al., 2016; Ebola Interim Assessment Panel, 2015); to ensure that countries have the capacity to implement and maintain the IHR, WHO has leveraged additional funding to help countries that need assistance. The Group of Seven (G7) has committed to assisting 76 countries at the 2015 and 2016 summits (Moon et al., 2017). The United States has committed $1 billion for building capacities in 31 countries, largely through the GHSA. South Korea has pledged an additional $100 million to support the GHSA in 13 countries. Additionally, in an effort to find better methods to mobilize both domestic resources and development assistance, the World Bank has "sought funding to assist at least 25 countries with pandemic preparedness plans in its latest financing round and established an international working group on financing preparedness in November 2016" (Moon et al., 2017, p. j281). Despite the financial support for improvements, no formal programs or new guidelines have been announced for travel and trade restrictions for those that do not follow the IHR, and "WHO has not initiated any major institutional reforms since the Ebola outbreak" (Moon et al., 2017, p. j283). While the improvements in financing and engagement from member countries is encouraging, ensuring reforms that improve transparency will be of vital importance for the organization to continue to be the lead authority in global health.

Finding: WHO performs essential functions for the global community, including the setting of international standards, such as the International Health Regulations, and the provision of technical advice and guidance to national health authorities.

Finding: Multiple calls have been made for management and operational reforms of WHO to improve future responses to public health emergencies of international concern.

Strong and Promising International Organizations

While many countries look to WHO as an authoritative leader in global health, several other multilateral organizations and partnerships that have been created in the last 15 years now play extremely important roles in global health governance. Organizations such as the Global Fund and Gavi, the Vaccine Alliance, have constituency-based models of governance and narrowly defined missions that enable more flexibility and support to accomplish their goals.

As multiple infectious disease outbreaks have immediately threatened global health security in the past several years, newer partnerships have been formed just since 2014, including the Coalition for Epidemic Preparedness Innovation (CEPI) and the GHSA. CEPI, supported by the governments of Germany, Japan, and Norway, the Bill & Melinda Gates Foundation, and the Wellcome Trust, is initially investing $540 million to finance and coordinate the development of new vaccines to protect against infectious diseases (CEPI, 2017). While new, CEPI has shown strong commitment from supporters through engagement and funding, and holds promise for accelerating capacity building and critical medical product development. Because GHSA was launched as a partnership by the United States, and has received positive feedback thus far on its progress, the committee has included more detailed examples of its successes.

Global Health Security Agenda

As introduced in Chapter 3, the U.S. government undertakes a significant number of activities within GHSA, but the agenda is a global one. Currently, GHSA has a membership of 55 countries, as well as WHO, the World Organisation for Animal Health, and the Food and Agriculture Organization of the UN (GHSA, 2016), and has endorsements from the G7 and Group of 20 (HHS, 2017). Furthermore, the GHSA's unique operating style allows the United States to maintain a leadership role in global health security while encouraging shared responsibility with partner countries through its 10-country steering group (GHSA, 2016). This work is also supported by a roundtable of several private-sector partners that strives to mobilize industry to help countries prepare for emergencies and strengthen health systems. The Private Sector Roundtable also aims to be a clearinghouse for industry to respond to health emergencies in collaboration with governments and multilateral stakeholders (GHSA, n.d.). The roundtable has even set up working groups aligning with member capabilities across the action packages, including Supply Chain and Logistics; Policy Development and Advocacy; Workforce Development; Partnerships, Technology and Analytics; and Antimicrobial Resistance.

Because of its convening of multisectoral actors and coordination at both the White House and in-country levels, GHSA has shifted the U.S. government health security approach from a fragmented strategy—a characterization of many global health programs—to a more coherent and cohesive one. In bringing multiple organizations and sectors to the table, including the United States, GHSA provides a different, more innovative approach to answering the world's global health security issues through comprehensive assessments and technical assistance. Additionally, in part because of increased accountability and partnership, the abilities of countries to prevent, detect, and respond to outbreaks have improved. For example, the United States has strengthened the public health laboratory and surveillance systems in Uganda, in addition to supporting the creation of a public health emergency operating centers (EOCs). The first test of this occurred in March 2016 when an outbreak of yellow fever was contained by the Uganda Ministry of Health through the quick activation of the EOC and improved lab capacity (GHSA, 2017). In 2015 alone, GHSA was able to produce measurable improvements in national capacities to prevent, detect, and respond to infectious disease threats: 9 countries established or strengthened mechanisms to limit animal-to-human spillover; 17 countries participated in Field Epidemiology Training Programs (FETPs); and 12 countries activated EOCs (GHSA, 2017).

The United States can capitalize on this momentum for global health security. By continuing to provide technical and financial assistance and collaborate with partners to help countries assess and improve their national health security capacities, together the world can more effectively contain outbreaks, as well as promote evidence-based plans for limiting the global spread of disease (Nuzzo and Shearer, 2017).

Finding: Many international agencies, organizations, and partnerships are now critical parts of the global health architecture and also carry out essential global functions.

U.S. APPROACH TOWARD GLOBAL HEALTH DIPLOMACY

American foreign policy has long been the "three-legged stool" of defense, development, and diplomacy. Though the defense leg has been the main driver, it will continually be important for the United States to be able to tell its story in ways that do not include military force. The military needs civilian partners in the battle against extremism. This idea of soft power—the ability to attract others without force or coercion through development efforts, including in health—is supported by a rationale that it reinforces American values, improves how the United States is viewed by the rest of the world by promoting peace and prosperity, and contributes to U.S. security at home by building stability abroad (Armitage and Nye, 2007). Consider the example of the falling of the Berlin Wall, where U.S. diplomacy shared a central role in bringing an end to the cold war, and encouraging American values of free speech and democratic governance to citizens in other countries (Kuo, 2016). This can also be applied to fighting terrorism. A RAND study in 2008 examined more than 600 terrorist groups since 1968 and found that the majority of them have ended because they either joined the political process or because key members were arrested or killed by local police and intelligence (Jones and Libicki, 2008). The RAND authors found that rarely has military force been the reason for the ending of terrorist groups. Many opportunities like this still exist to protect American interests through development and soft-power diplomacy initiatives, and if the United States fails to act through the other two legs of the foreign policy stool, other countries are likely to fill this role instead.

In the last few decades, China has quietly increased many of its health and development programs around the world, asserting itself as a powerful and committed leader both through bilateral programs and taking a leadership role in multilateral organizations. China's flexibility and lack of conditionality in its aid programs has generated large amounts of good will and political capital in the world (Armitage and Nye, 2007). Furthermore, China has sent more than 15,000 doctors to Africa and has treated nearly 180 million African patients, which has helped to ensure its long-term foreign policy interests in energy and food security (McGiffert, 2009). Additionally, Cuba has sent medical staff and medical diplomats to about 70 countries and provided free medical training in return for various benefits, including oil from Venezuela (Fieinsilver, 2009). How countries spend their money overseas directly reflects their priorities. People on the receiving end understand this notion, and in turn often base their opinions on these aid and development decisions, setting the stage for how various wealthy countries are viewed globally (Armitage and Nye, 2007).

As evidenced through previous chapter discussions about globalization, the growing economies of many low- and middle-income countries, and the proliferation of private-sector players in the global health sphere, there is a clear need to change the way the United States engages in foreign policy and development assistance. Specifically, as countries mobilize domestic resources, develop health systems, structure fiscal policies, and build surveillance systems, the U.S. government could transition away from the provision of bilateral aid toward the sharing of technical assistance. Doing so will allow the United States to maintain close relationships with partner countries and an awareness of health issues they face, while allowing funds typically allocated to foreign aid to be spent on other global goods. However, there are a limited number of countries in this position, and those low-income countries will still depend on donor governments like the United States for foreign aid until they can advance their economies. These countries, sometimes also afflicted by conflict or poor governance, can also be a source of insecurity and instability for global health, so a continued commitment of direct aid will still be critical. Currently, a number of U.S. agencies, including the U.S. Department of State and U.S. Department of Health and Human Services, coordinate global health interests abroad. But there is a need to better coordinate the activities of these agencies, with long-term strategic vision and cross-cutting approaches in order to maximize efforts and efficiency.

Finding: The role of the United States in global diplomacy has proven useful in events ranging from the fall of the Berlin Wall to the resuming of Nigeria's polio vaccination campaign.

Finding: Other countries, such as China and Cuba, have increased their participation in global health and development around the world, positively affecting how they are viewed globally.

The Role of the U.S. Department of State

The U.S. Department of State is the primary agency responsible for foreign affairs, and global health is interwoven into its structure and activities in both its regional bureaus and functional bureaus. Table 9-1 provides an overview of the functional bureaus and their offices, which explicitly conduct activities that relate to global health. The Office of International Health and Biodefense is the primary office responsible for global health issues (U.S. Department of State, 2017b),[2] but the other offices listed offer pockets of knowledge and work in a variety of domains that include biological weapons control and nonproliferation, biosecurity, GHSA, finance, and migration (ISAB, 2016). Given the range of offices within the U.S. Department of State that work on global health, it is apparent that the department considers global health a vital, cross-cutting issue. However, the strengths within these bureaus on global health are not mirrored by similar strengths at U.S. embassies, which often lack personnel with global health expertise.

A Sustainable Career Track

Almost every U.S. embassy has foreign service officers (FSOs) that are assigned to work on global health issues, with some selected to become

[2] The Office of International Health and Biodefense leads the U.S. Department of State's efforts for pandemic response, and ensures that global health issues, such as emerging infectious diseases, global health security and antimicrobial resistance, are incorporated into U.S. foreign policy.

TABLE 9-1 Bureaus and Offices in the U.S. Department of State That Explicitly Work on Global Health-Related Issues

Undersecretary for Economic Growth, Energy, and the Environment		Undersecretary for Arms Control and International Security		Undersecretary of Civilian Security, Democracy, and Human Rights		Undersecretary for Political Affairs	
Bureau of Economic and Business Affairs	Bureau of Oceans and International Environmental and Scientific Affairs	Bureau of Arms Control, Verification and Compliance	Bureau of International Security and Nonproliferation	Bureau of Democracy, Human Rights, and Labor	Bureau of Population, Refugees, and Migration	Regional Bureaus	Bureau of International Organizations
Office of International Finance and Development	Office of International Health and Biodefense	Office of Chemical and Biological Weapons	Office of the Biological Policy Staff				
			Office of Cooperative Threat Reduction				
			Office of Missile, Biological, and Chemical Nonproliferation				
			Office of Threat Reduction				

SOURCES: ISAB, 2016; U.S. Department of State, 2016, n.d.

environment, science, technology, and health (ESTH) officers. Although health is a component of ESTH officers' portfolios (ISAB, 2016), it is not the strongest part of their training (NASEM, 2015). Not only do ESTH officers receive inadequate health training (a mere 1.5 hours in global health at the Foreign Service Institute) (ISAB, 2016), there is a sentiment that ESTH postings are outside the mainstream FSO career track. Due to the up-or-out promotion system within the U.S. Department of State (OIG, 2002), FSOs reportedly lack interest to pursue such postings (NASEM, 2015). In embassies that lack ESTH officers, the health portfolio is managed by economic officers.[3] The neglect of global health in the Foreign Service career track system (which includes consular, economic, management, political, and public diplomacy) (U.S. Department of State, 2017a) means that the U.S. Department of State's workforce lacks the requisite skills for sustainable approaches to global health, which can result in the development of ad hoc solutions and policy.

Although the lack of this specific workforce capacity is not always evident, it comes into sharp focus in the midst of a large-scale global health event. Consider the example of the U.S. response to the 2014–2015 Ebola outbreak in West Africa, where the U.S. Department of State formed an Ebola coordination unit using "ambassadorial leadership and staff borrowed from across the department" (ISAB, 2016, p. 20). The unit was comprised almost entirely of FSOs, but only two had a background in science. This issue was also notable in an analysis of the previously mentioned polio vaccination response in Nigeria in 2003, where public health professionals were found to lack the skills needed to approach ministries of foreign affairs. Similarly, diplomats required greater training on the role of health in foreign policy (Kaufmann and Feldbaum, 2009). If more staff members had public health or global health backgrounds, stronger alliances could have been built during the relief effort (Chen, 2015). These ad hoc, stand-alone groups, like the now-defunct Avian Influenza Action Group, do not allow for learning or the development of institutional knowledge for future events because they often disband immediately after the crisis ends (ISAB, 2016).

Strategizing for Downstream Effects

While many global health programs are measured in terms of direct health outcomes and perhaps cost-effectiveness, appropriately designed programs can also have multiple downstream effects on other sectors of society. These downstream effects can affect poverty, education, or employment, and in turn provide diplomatic advantages for the donor government (Feldbaum

[3] Personal communication Matthew Brown, NIH, November 9, 2016.

and Michaud, 2010; Kevany, 2015). PEPFAR is one of the most robust and well-known U.S. global health programs, has had measured success in several nonhealth areas, as discussed in Chapter 4, and is overseen by the Office of Global AIDS Coordinator at the U.S. Department of State. This position also leads the Office of Global Health Diplomacy (OGHD) at the U.S. Department of State, though since its creation in 2013, the OGHD has not been as targeted and effective with its efforts as many had hoped. Moving forward, OGHD could offer an opportunity for the United States to be more strategic about its soft power development and diplomacy initiatives, and to align them with the ongoing critical investments in health across the U.S. government that have been made in the last decade. If adequately funded, a central office such as OGHD could guide U.S. global health policy through a more coherent approach, and elevate the issues of health and development worldwide while giving them greater credence within the U.S. government. Importantly, part of the success of the PEPFAR program and the whole-of-government approach is the important work that is implemented by other government agencies such as the U.S. Agency for International Development (USAID) and the U.S. Centers for Disease Control and Prevention (CDC). With their technical competence and established in-country networks, these two organizations significantly contribute to the health diplomacy of the United States. If the health programs were designed and measured for indicators beyond just health outcomes, their use and knowledge generation could be attractive to foreign policy experts and decision makers (Kevany, 2015). Accordingly, having FSOs with global health expertise would be important to complement the work of implementing agencies, and support the U.S. Department of State's day-to-day functioning and its responses to health emergencies as they occur. Building on lessons learned from the failed Global Health Initiative (described in Chapter 1), in order for this to be successful OGHD would require funding, accountability, and authority.

The Role of the U.S. Department of Health and Human Services

The U.S. Department of Health and Human Services (HHS) and its agencies, such as CDC, the U.S. Food and Drug Administration, and the National Institutes of Health (NIH), also play a vital role in global health, including global health diplomacy. These agencies are responsible for U.S. health program implementation, technical advisory actions, and health workforce training programs. HHS also engages at a high level of diplomacy with partner countries by using a specialized cadre of workers known as health attachés, the definition and roles of which are presented in Box 9-1 (Brown et al., 2014).

Health attachés, though officially working at U.S. embassies abroad, are typically on-loan from HHS agencies. Often populated by employees

BOX 9-1
Definition and Role of Health Attachés

Health attachés are defined as diplomats "who collect, analyze, and act on information concerning health in a foreign country or countries and provide critical links between public health and foreign affairs stakeholders." They work in the realm of *core* global health diplomacy, and because of their role in conducting policy negotiations on behalf of the U.S. government, health attachés must have sound technical skills in public health as well as skills in the conventional diplomatic fields of political, economic, and public affairs.

SOURCE: Brown et al., 2014.

with field experience serving from CDC or NIH, placement and support of health attachés is coordinated by the HHS Office of Global Affairs (OGA) (HHS, 2016b), which acts as the central leadership for all of HHS's global activities (Bliss, 2014). As a result, health attachés report to OGA at the headquarters level,[4] but they also report directly to the U.S. ambassador of the embassy to which they are assigned (U.S. Department of State and USAID, 2010). The United States currently has six health attachés posted in Brazil, China, India, Mexico, South Africa, and Switzerland. While the first five support U.S. embassies in direct country to country relationships, the health attaché posted in Geneva, Switzerland, offers support to the U.S. mission to the UN (HHS, 2016b).

Health attachés have played a critical role at U.S. missions. A notable example was the bilateral negotiation that took place between the United States and China during the 2003 Severe Acute Respiratory Syndrome outbreak. The health attaché posted in Beijing brokered a memorandum of understanding between the Chinese Ministry of Health and HHS to form the U.S.–China Collaboration of Emerging and Reemerging Infections (U.S. Department of State, 2010).[5] Although the agreement itself was positive for health-related outcomes at the time, the ongoing relationship that was developed served as a platform for collaboration in the subsequent H5N1 and Ebola epidemics. During the H5N1 pandemic in 2005, this agreement enabled smoother sharing of information, and during the Ebola outbreak in 2014, the agreement clarified roles each country would play in the response (in which China built a treatment center in Liberia and a 60-bed hospital

[4] Personal communication with Matthew Brown, NIH, January 5, 2017.
[5] Personal communication Matthew Brown, NIH, November 9, 2016.

in Sierra Leone).[6] This partnership has since been renewed for 5 years in 2015 (Huang, 2016).

Creating an International Workforce

Despite the clear value of the expertise brought by health attachés, there is limited placement of health attachés at U.S. missions. This is partly because of inadequate funding, as the annual cost of placement can be close to $500,000 per year.[7] Yet more importantly, the limited placement of health attachés is due to a lack of appropriately experienced personnel to draw from—resulting from limitations in how HHS can hire for overseas positions. For new employees or outside hires, HHS uses term appointments to hire and deploy personnel abroad. While this in itself is not a problem, the lack of a global health career track in HHS and the temporary, ad hoc nature of the available positions makes these positions one-off and not attractive to a talented pool of candidates. At the conclusion of their term, employees often leave the U.S. government to seek a career in global health elsewhere, taking with them critical cross-cultural, management, leadership, and scientific skills that can take years or decades to acquire. However, HHS's workforce abroad has expanded between 2000 and 2015 from less than 50 to more than 500 in more than 70 countries. Despite this expansion though, HHS has an average standing vacancy rate of more than 30 percent for its overseas positions.[8] As a result, many positions go unfilled or have large gaps between incumbents, which create deficits in HHS's ability to ensure the safety and security of the U.S. population.[9] Furthermore, due to the lack of a predictable and unified process of rotating HHS employees in and out of overseas positions, the department is unable to maintain institutional knowledge of overseas operations and is not flexible enough to meet its expanding global mandate.[10]

HHS has acknowledged this weakness, and in an *American Journal of Tropical Medicine and Hygiene* editorial, Nils Daulaire (former Assistant Secretary for OGA) stated that OGA is working to "establish a global health career track within HHS to formalize career opportunities and training for our staff working in global health, both domestically and internationally" (Daulaire, 2012). In August 2015, a pilot project was conducted with support from HHS Idea Lab to develop the Global Bidding and Assignment System (GBAS), a specialized system for department-wide recruitment,

[6] Personal communication Matthew Brown, NIH, November 9, 2016.

[7] Personal communication with David Hohmann, formerly Office of Global Affairs (HHS), November 8, 2016.

[8] Personal communication with Matthew Brown, NIH, November 9, 2016.

[9] Personal communication with Matthew Brown, NIH, March 28, 2017.

[10] Personal communication with Matthew Brown, NIH, March 28, 2017.

assessment, bidding, and deployment for overseas positions (HHS, 2016a). More than 200 HHS employees applied to GBAS and 90 were selected to be matched to U.S. missions. As of November 2016, 23 percent of the selected HHS employees seeking overseas placements have been matched and are in the process of being deployed.[11] However, as of the release of this report, GBAS has not been renewed or taken to scale.

Finding: The limited number of noncareer health appointments currently available abroad is an ad hoc system. It does not facilitate institutional knowledge across events or a promising career track for global health professionals.

A PLACE FOR HEALTH IN FOREIGN SERVICE

Between the U.S. Department of State and HHS, the U.S. government has an inadequate workforce to meet its global health needs. Owing to the neglect of global health in the Foreign Service career track system and limited knowledge of health by ESTH officers, the U.S. Department of State is unable to address global health in a concerted fashion across its embassies. Similarly, because of the inability to consistently deploy employees overseas, HHS is unable to build institutional knowledge on vital global health matters or develop a workforce that has global health experience. The latter is problematic as it limits the number of individuals with appropriate competencies that HHS can draw from to appoint health attachés and other needed positions. With the ever-changing landscape of global health, and the constant array of threats that have the potential to affect the health of Americans, a constant standing workforce deployed abroad that is well versed in global health would benefit the United States. Current efforts to address this issue, which include courses and certificates in diplomacy and science and technology, are not able to address competency issues in the workforce in a scalable and real-world fashion. Furthermore, current mechanisms to inject global health expertise into the U.S. Department of State, such as the limited noncareer appointments, while useful in filling workforce deficiencies for programs like PEPFAR (U.S. Department of State, 2017c) are short-term solutions and fail to address the loss of institutional knowledge and the need for the creation of a true global health career track.[12]

Establishing a global health career track in the U.S. Department of State would address the workforce deficiencies described above. However, this would require a strong commitment by State to build global health as a career path and elevate it as a critical issue. This could happen simi-

[11] Personal communication with Matthew Brown, NIH, November 9, 2016.
[12] Personal communication with Matthew Brown, NIH, January 9, 2017.

larly to how the U.S. Department of State elevated economic diplomacy by increasing training in economics, establishing a chief economist, and creating a role of an Undersecretary for Economic Growth, Energy, and the Environment—as was described in the 2010 Quadrennial Diplomacy and Development Review (U.S. Department of State and USAID, 2010). Creating a global health track would first involve establishing a skill code for public health in the Foreign Service and more thoroughly introducing global health into the School of Professional and Area Studies, perhaps by creating a dean at the Foreign Service Institute.[13] This would establish a solid foundation for global health within the Foreign Service, but it would need to be supplemented by designating positions for global health at all levels within the department to align with the promotion system. Though this would be resource intensive, it could lead to a sustainable and proactive approach to addressing global health issues throughout the world within the U.S. Department of State's purview.

Enabling Knowledge Sustainment

Because it will take time for the U.S. Department of State to establish the global health career track, an integrated system with HHS and the U.S. Department of State would enable HHS employees (who have a full depth of expertise in health-related issues, such as disease surveillance and research) to populate positions in the U.S. Department of State as the track gets developed, and can lead to cooperation during outbreaks and global health emergencies in the future. An amendment of the Foreign Service Act by Congress to authorize HHS to use the Foreign Service Personnel System[14] would also be a first step to developing a foreign service arm of HHS. As the U.S. Department of State itself has called for more collaboration and workforce mobility between it and other departments and agencies to foster a whole-of-government approach to diplomacy (U.S. Department of State and USAID, 2010), allowing HHS to access the Foreign Service Personnel System could help to foster this collaboration. Additionally, during public health emergencies, this foreign service arm designation would facilitate a rapid injection of knowledgeable people from HHS into the U.S. Department of State to meet temporary needs (U.S. Department of State and USAID, 2010), providing the U.S. government much needed agility and a more cohesive approach to responding to urgent threats.

The need for a Foreign Service arm of HHS, namely at CDC, was echoed by multiple respondents from this committee's information gather-

[13] Personal communication with Matthew Brown, NIH, February 6, 2017.

[14] This would be similar to that of the Foreign Agricultural Service and the Foreign Commercial Service.

ing solicitation (described in Chapter 1). With CDC's leading role in GHSA and the clear effects of emerging infectious disease threats on national security, it is evident that the current ad hoc approach is insufficient and such an arm is needed. By using the Foreign Service Personnel System, HHS can enable employees to pursue a career in global health in the short term. In the long term, this would systematically build a global health workforce—a necessary prerequisite for HHS to develop a pool from which to draw future health attachés to support U.S. embassy missions.

Creating the Workforce Pipeline

To create a sustainable U.S. workforce with these types of health and foreign diplomacy skills, it is important to think about the education and skills needed. Universities are already creating environments that support interdisciplinary education and research and blending majors to ensure cross-sector thinking and interaction. This is particularly relevant to the field of global health, with nearly 250 North American universities now offering global health education. This reflects the growing interest from American students in global health as well as a trend of funding agencies turning to universities as problem solvers for global health. These networks of interdisciplinary collaboration and culture of reciprocity make universities great environments for innovation. Pushing the feedback loop even further are entities like USAID's Higher Education Solutions Network, which is using this built expertise to help solve global health problems. These universities are prime locations to start integrating diplomacy skills and leadership into global health curricula in a manner that reflects the necessary shared competencies (Brown et al., 2016). As centers of learning already supported by international partners (Hosseini Divkolaye et al., 2016), they can create a strong and dedicated workforce for the United States' global health diplomacy.

SUMMARY AND RECOMMENDATION

The developments described throughout this report have created an environment for a centralized and comprehensive strategy for global health diplomacy. For the United States to continue to be a leader in global health, as well as adequately protect U.S. citizens at home and abroad, continued engagement in the international global health architecture is paramount. Though there are many calls for management and operational reforms in WHO (Gostin et al., 2016), the functions that it performs will continue to be essential for global health security and prosperity. Additionally the increased number of other multilateral organizations focused on health, either directly or indirectly, provides an opportunity to synergize efforts toward achieving aligned global health goals more sustainably and efficiently (Nuzzo and Shearer, 2017).

The United States can maintain a health presence in countries in today's interconnected world while sustainably beginning to phase down direct aid programs. In the absence of a health career track in the Foreign Service, the demand for U.S. health expertise in host countries cannot be sustainably filled and those that are deployed often lack diplomacy skills. Similarly, during an international health emergency, the U.S. Department of State does not have historical experience and appropriate health knowledge networks to draw from, leading to ad hoc groups being formed for each new event that are much less effective than they could be (Chen, 2015; Kaufmann and Feldbaum, 2009).

Conclusion: While the committee agrees on the need for management and operational reform for the World Health Organization (WHO), it also recognizes that the organization is underfunded and that many functions it performs are essential. In addition, many other United Nations agencies and international organizations and partnerships formed in the last few decades are crucial in providing support around the world. The success of all these entities will help the U.S. government accomplish its global health goals and maximize its returns on investments.

Conclusion: Important priorities for the U.S. government, such as global health security, reduction of child mortality, research and development to create new tools and improve program delivery, and achievement of the goal of an AIDS-free generation, will depend on continued engagement with and strengthening of these established and emerging multilateral institutions.

Conclusion: With the changing landscape of global health, the U.S. government has an opportunity to be more strategic in its programs and diplomacy. There is a need for better bidirectional communication and partnership between health and diplomacy professionals.

Recommendation 14: Commit to Continued Global Health Leadership

To protect itself from global threats, benefit from successes achieved in global health programs, and maintain a strong research and development pipeline, the United States should commit to maintaining its leadership in global health and actively participating in global health governance, coordination, and collaboration. To

this end, the U.S. Department of State and the U.S. Department of Health and Human Services (HHS) should do the following:

- **Use their influence to improve the performance of key United Nations agencies and other international organizations important to global health, particularly the World Health Organization (WHO). WHO is in need of greater resources to address the health challenges of the 21st century, and many of its priorities align with those of the U.S. government. However, U.S. government financial contributions to WHO should come with a requirement that the organization adopt and implement the much-needed management reforms identified in recent reports.**
- **Remain involved in and firmly committed to innovative global partnerships that further U.S. global health goals, such as the highly successful Gavi, the Vaccine Alliance, and the Global Fund to Fight AIDS, Tuberculosis and Malaria, as well as promising new entities such as the Global Health Security Agenda and the Global Financing Facility.**
- **Implement a more strategic approach to achieving global health goals. This new approach should include the commitment of the U.S. Department of State to creating a global health career track and congressional action to enable the establishment of a cadre of global health experts within HHS through an amendment to the Foreign Service Act. This would create the environment necessary to expand the health attaché program, particularly in middle-income countries.**

REFERENCES

Armitage, R. L., and J. S. Nye Jr. 2007. *CSIS Commission on Smart Power: A smarter, more secure America.* Washington, DC: Center for Strategic and International Studies.

Bliss, K. E. 2014. *Global health within a domestic agency: The transformation of the Office of Global Affairs at HHS.* Washington, DC: Center for Strategic and International Studies.

Brown, M., J. Bergmann, T. Mackey, Q. Eichbaum, L. McDougal, and T. Novotny. 2016. Mapping foreign affairs and global public health competencies: Towards a competency model for global health diplomacy. *Global Health Governance* 10(2):3-49.

Brown, M. D., T. K. Mackey, C. N. Shapiro, J. Kolker, and T. E. Novotny. 2014. Bridging public health and foreign affairs: The tradecraft of global health diplomacy and the role of health attachés. *Science and Diplomacy* 3(3).

CEPI (Coalition for Epidemic Preparedness Initiative). 2017. *CEPI: New vaccines for a safer world.* http://cepi.net/sites/default/files/CEPI_2pager_03_Feb_17.pdf (accessed March 1, 2017).

Chen, J. F. 2015. Reinstituting the ESTH cone within the US foreign service. *Journal of Science Policy and Governance* 7(1).

Ebola Interim Assessment Panel. 2015. *Report of the Ebola Interim Assessment Panel.* Geneva, Switzerland: World Health Organization.

Daulaire, N. 2012. The importance of the global health strategy from the U.S. Department of Health and Human Services. *The American Journal of Tropical Medicine and Hygiene* 87(3):382-384.

Feldbaum, H., and J. Michaud. 2010. Health diplomacy and the enduring relevance of foreign policy interests. *PLOS Medicine* 7(4):e1000226.

Fieinsilver, J. 2009. Cuban medical diplomacy. In *The Cuba Reader: History, Culture, Politics*, edited by A. Chomsky, P. M. Smorkaloff and B. Carr. Durham, NC: Duke University Press. Pp. 590-594.

GHSA (Global Health Security Agenda). 2016. *Membership.* https://www.ghsagenda.org/members (accessed December 15, 2016).

GHSA. 2017. *Advancing the Global Health Security Agenda: Progress and early impact from U.S. investment.* Washington, DC: Global Health Security Agenda.

GHSA. n.d. *Global Health Security Agenda Private Sector Roundtable: Mobilizing industry for action.* https://www.ghsagenda.org/docs/default-source/default-document-library/ghsa-private-sector-roundtable-508.pdf (accessed February 20, 2017).

Gostin, L. O., O. Tomori, S. Wibulpolprasert, A. K. Jha, J. Frenk, S. Moon, J. Phumaphi, P. Piot, B. Stocking, V. J. Dzau, and G. M. Leung. 2016. Toward a common secure future: Four global commissions in the wake of Ebola. *PLOS Medicine* 13(5):e1002042.

Huang, Y. 2016. *China's healthcare sector and U.S.-China health cooperation.* Paper presented at the Hearing on China's 13th Five-Year Plan. Washington, DC: U.S.-China Economic and Securty Review Commission.

HHS (U.S. Department of Health and Human Services). 2016a. *Health attachés.* https://www.hhs.gov/about/agencies/oga/global-health-diplomacy/health-attaches/index.html (accessed December 15, 2016).

HHS. 2016b. *Global Bidding & Assignment System: Filling overseas global public health vacancies with a specialized system for global recruitment.* https://www.hhs.gov/idealab/projects-item/global-bidding-assignment-system (accessed December 15, 2016).

HHS. 2017. *Global health security.* https://www.hhs.gov/about/agencies/oga/global-health-security/index.html?language=es (accessed February 2, 2017).

Hosseini Divkolaye, N. S., M. H. Radfar, F. Seighali, and F. M. Burkle. 2016. When health diplomacy serves foreign policy: Use of soft power to quell conflict and crises. *Disaster Medicine and Public Health Preparedness* 10(5):724-727.

ISAB (International Security Advisory Board). 2016. *Report on international security and foreign policy implications of overseas disease outbreaks.* Washington, DC: International Security Advisory Board, U.S. Department of State.

Jones, S. G., and M. C. Libicki. 2008. *How terrorist groups end: Lessons for countering al qa'ida.* Arlington, VA: RAND Corporation.

Kaufmann, J. R., and H. Feldbaum. 2009. Diplomacy and the polio immunization boycott in northern Nigeria. *Health Affairs* 28(4):1091-1101.

Kevany, S. 2015. Diplomatic advantages and threats in global health program selection, design, delivery and implementation: Development and application of the Kevany Riposte. *Globalization and Health* 11(1):22.

Kickbusch, I., and M. M. C. Szabo. 2014. A new governance space for health. *Global Health Action* 7(1):25307.

Kuo, M. A. 2016. U.S.-China relations: Public diplomacy and soft power. *The Diplomat*, December 5. http://thediplomat.com/2016/12/us-china-relations-public-diplomacy-and-soft-power (accessed January 15, 2017).

McGiffert, C. 2009. *Chinese soft power and its implications for the United States: Competition and cooperation in the developing world: A report of the CSIS Smart Power Initiative*. Washington, DC: Center for Strategic & International Studies.

Moon, S., J. Leigh, L. Woskie, F. Checchi, V. Dzau, M. Fallah, G. Fitzgerald, L. Garrett, L. Gostin, D. L. Heymann, R. Katz, I. Kickbusch, J. S. Morrison, P. Piot, P. Sands, D. Sridhar, and A. K. Jha. 2017. Post-Ebola reforms: Ample analysis, inadequate action. *British Medical Journal* 356:j280-j288.

NASEM (National Academies of Sciences, Engineering, and Medicine). 2015. *Diplomacy for the 21st century: Embedding a culture of science and technology Throughout the Department of State*. Washington, DC: The National Academies Press.

Nuzzo, J. B., and M. P. Shearer. 2017. International engagement is critical to fighting epidemics. *Health Security* 15(1):33-35.

OIG (Office of the Inspector General). 2002. *Memorandum audit report: U.S. Department of State's Foreign Service "up-or-out" promotion system*. Washington, DC: Office of Inspector General, U.S. Department of Health and Human Services.

The *PLOS Medicine* Editors. 2007. How is who responding to global public health threats? *PLOS Medicine* 4(5):e197.

U.S. Department of State. 2010. *Momorandum of understanding for the collaborative program on emerging and re-emerging infectious diseases between the Department of Health and Human Services of the United States of America and the Ministry of Health of the People's Republic of China*. Washington, DC: U.S. Department of State.

U.S. Department of State. 2016. *Department of State organization chart: November 2016*. https://www.state.gov/r/pa/ei/rls/dos/99484.htm (accessed February 10, 2017).

U.S. Department of State. 2017a. *Career tracks for foreign service officers*. https://careers.state.gov/work/foreign-service/officer/career-tracks (accessed February 2, 2017).

U.S. Department of State. 2017b. *International health and biodefense*. https://www.state.gov/e/oes/intlhealthbiodefense (accessed February 2, 2017).

U.S. Department of State. 2017c. *Limited non-career appointments (LNAs)*. https://careers.state.gov/work/foreign-service/lna (accessed February 2, 2017).

U.S. Department of State. n.d. *What we do*. https://www.state.gov/whatwedo (accessed April 10, 2017).

U.S. Department of State and USAID (U.S. Agency for International Development). 2010. *Leading through civilian power: The first quadrennial diplomacy and development review*. Washington, DC: U.S. Department of State.

10

Summary of Conclusions and Recommendations

The global vision that has brought improved travel and trade and increased interdependency among countries also calls for a common vision of health around the world. All countries are vulnerable to the ever-present threats of infectious disease, outbreaks, and epidemics. At the same time, there are opportunities for shared innovation and universal purpose as many countries that suffer from similar disease burdens strive to develop best practices and strong health systems for their citizens.

Throughout this consensus study, the committee emphasized the need for a more holistic examination of problems and challenges in global health. Such an approach applies not only to issues of global health security but also to the external factors that influence health security, such as the building of general capacity in countries and the creation of strong societies that foster stability, healthy lifestyles, and accessible economic opportunities. Unless core capacities and strong health systems are developed around the world, the global risk of infectious disease will continue to threaten the health and security of the United States. Beyond the imperative of addressing infectious disease threats, it is necessary to understand the fundamental connection between health and economic prosperity. In addition to the economic costs of responding to infectious disease outbreaks, the increasing prevalence of chronic or noncommunicable diseases (NCDs) has negatively affected global economies—compromising societal gains in life expectancy, productivity, and overall quality of life (WEF, 2017).

Many countries currently face the dual burden of a rapid increase in NCDs, such as cardiovascular disease (CVD) and cancer, and the continuing need to eliminate infectious diseases, such as malaria and tuberculosis

(TB), in addition to the priority of reducing the burden of human immunodeficiency virus/acquired immunodeficiency syndrome (HIV/AIDS). Moreover, some countries are considered to bear a triple burden, as traumatic injury has been found to be the second leading cause of premature death in young men after HIV/AIDS (Marquez and Farrington, 2013). Combined, these three disease burdens can stall the progress of a country's development and significantly affect its ability to become a strong trading partner or a business or travel destination. The cost of productivity losses associated with disability, unplanned absences, and increased accidents can be as much as 400 percent higher than the cost of treatment (WEF, 2010). Research also shows that investors are less likely to enter markets where the labor force suffers a heavy disease burden (Bloom et al., 2004). Human capital clearly contributes significantly to economic growth, and it follows that having a healthy population is critical for economic prosperity. This point has been demonstrated in recent years: between 2000 and 2011, 24 percent of income growth in low- and middle-income countries (LMICs) resulted from improvements in health (Jamison et al., 2013).

The root causes of all three of these health burdens are often linked by such underlying social factors as poverty, education, and location (Frenk and Gómez-Dantés, 2016; Marmot, 2005). This commonality suggests that methods for prevention are linked as well, and the tools used to prevent one burden can help to prevent the others, emphasizing the need for holistic examination of programs. Over the last few decades, the United States has demonstrated remarkable leadership in global health. Notable progress has been achieved by such initiatives as The U.S. President's Emergency Plan for AIDS Relief (PEPFAR) and the President's Malaria Initiative (PMI), as well as the nation's commitment to such multilateral organizations as the Global Fund to Fight AIDS, Tuberculosis and Malaria (Global Fund); Gavi, the Vaccine Alliance; and, more recently, the Global Health Security Agenda (GHSA). Similarly, progress has been achieved by efforts to combat antimicrobial resistance (AMR) at the national and international levels. Against the backdrop of an influential legacy on the global health stage, the new U.S. administration faces the choice of whether or not to ensure that the gains won with billions of U.S. dollars, years of dedication, and strong programs are sustained and poised for further growth.

CHANGING THE WAY THE UNITED STATES ENGAGES

The committee has focused this report where it believes the United States can have the most immediate and substantial effect despite the limited resources available. Throughout the report, the committee has highlighted four priority areas that demand continued attention from U.S. global health investment within a two-pronged approach of securing against global threats (areas 1 and 2), and promoting productivity and economic growth in other countries (areas 3 and 4):

1. achieving global health security (including addressing pandemics and AMR)
2. maintaining a sustained response to the continuous threats of communicable diseases such as HIV/AIDS, TB, and malaria
3. saving and improving the lives of women and children
4. promoting cardiovascular health and preventing cancer

In addition, the committee has underscored the imperative to change the way the United States does business in global health, highlighting an immediate need to focus on ensuring protection against global threats and enhancing productivity and economic growth in all countries. To these ends, a more systematic, proactive, and integrated approach is needed that includes long-range planning and vision; greater application of rigor and measurement in achieving return on investment; and cooperation with all global health partners to leverage the respective strengths of each, including the advancement of innovation through the private sector and political commitment to achieving global goals on the part of national governments and multilateral partners. This shift in approach places the focus on prevention and preparedness, with a vision of investing in cross-cutting infrastructure in three areas: catalyzing innovation in health systems through medical product development and digital health, enabling more flexible financing mechanisms to fund global health programs, and maintaining U.S. global health leadership internationally. The outcome of this approach will be resilient countries with positive health outcomes, resulting in turn in robust trade partners, safer travel destinations, and more active collaborators in preventing and controlling global health problems that affect citizens in every country, at every income level.

SECURING AGAINST GLOBAL THREATS

Many laudable public health successes have been achieved at the global, regional, national, and community levels. However, the world continues to evolve, and public health measures must change accordingly. The global community is no safer from infectious disease today than it was 20 years ago when the Institute of Medicine report *America's Vital Interest in Global Health* (IOM, 1997) was written. The U.S. Army recently estimated that if a severe infectious disease pandemic were to occur today, the number of U.S. fatalities could be almost double the total number of battlefield fatalities sustained in all of the nation's wars since the American Revolution (GAO, 2017). Poverty and climate change have led to greater risk of mosquito-borne illness in the southern United States (Hotez et al., 2014); AMR has been elevated to a global crisis by the United Nations (UN) (UN, 2016); and the largest outbreak of influenza A (H7N9) to date is currently occurring in China (Iuliano et al., 2017). The risk of transnational outbreaks may be greater today than ever before given recent dramatic increases in international trade and travel, urbanization, and population density, as well as critical biodiversity loss worldwide. Strong public health infrastructure is essential to combat these threats successfully wherever they may emerge. While the burden of infectious diseases rests predominantly with low-income countries, where limited resources and weak health care systems are unable to control and prevent them, these are global threats that can significantly affect any country, including the United States, and that need to be understood as a threat to U.S. national security.

As noted above, the costs of infectious diseases extend beyond human suffering and mortality through indirect impacts on economies. In just a few short months, for example, the 2003 outbreak of severe acute respiratory syndrome (SARS) cost the world between $30 and $54 billion (Fan, 2003; World Bank, 2013). During the Ebola outbreak, which involved just four domestic cases, the United States spent $1.1 billion on domestic response (Epstein et al., 2015)—120 percent of the annual public health and health care preparedness budget for state and local health department and hospital capacity.[1] Between October 2014 and December 2015, $119 million was spent just on domestic migration and quarantine activities, such as airport screening and follow-up of potentially sick passengers, costing an average of more than $4,000 per passenger (CDC, 2016).[2] And direct costs for just two Ebola patients treated at the specialty center in Nebraska were estimated at more than $1 million (Gold, 2014).

Looking forward, a moderate influenza pandemic[3] is projected to cost the world $570 billion annually in terms of income loss and mortality (Fan et al., 2016) with some estimates as high as $2 trillion (Burns et al., 2008). Furthermore, the threat of AMR continues to grow because of poor stewardship, weak surveillance systems, and a lack of second-line therapeutics in the development pipeline. And in addition to naturally occurring threats is the potential for terrorist use of man-made biological weapons. Regardless of whether epidemics or biosecurity threats originate naturally or through

[1] This percentage was calculated by using fiscal year 2016 Public Health Emergency Preparedness program funding ($660 million) and Hospital Preparedness Program funding ($255 million) as the preparedness amounts. See Chapter 3 for more details.

[2] During this timeframe, 29,000 people were monitored following screening at five major U.S. international airports. The monitoring included follow-up for 21 days, and a check and report Ebola kit including a thermometer, a prepaid cell phone, and educational materials.

[3] A "moderate" influenza pandemic is defined as one in which global output is reduced by more than 2 percent.

human engineering, it is critical for the United States to recognize the severity of these threats and take proactive measures to build capacities and establish sustainable and cost-effective infrastructure to combat them.

Coordination of International Health Emergency Response

As experienced during the Ebola outbreak in 2014, the U.S. population's indifference to remote diseases can quickly turn to panic when even a single suspected case is reported within U.S. borders. The U.S. government implements extreme, government-wide responses to such occurrences—costing tremendous amounts of time and money—in a piecemeal, reactive fashion that can actually impede swift and efficient action, delaying response and discouraging private-sector involvement. While multiple agencies can bring unique expertise to a U.S. government–led response, it is difficult to execute a coordinated emergency plan in the midst of a crisis without a clear chain of command, a dedicated budget, and designated leadership. There is a need for a framework to guide international response to public health emergencies, similar to the domestic National Response Framework. While the Obama administration attempted this level of coordination on the fly with the creation of an Ebola czar, it would be more effective to consider the need for coordination in advance.

In addition to coordination, rapid access to funds during a response is of paramount importance to mobilizing assets and implementing needed interventions. After 7 months of disagreement and delay in fulfilling President Obama's request for $1.9 billion in Zika funding, Congress finally approved $1.1 billion with the passing of H.R. 5243[4] (Wexler et al., 2016). Before this approval was secured, agencies were forced to shift funds from other accounts for Zika-related activities, including by borrowing money from the Ebola supplemental funding and from the U.S. Centers for Disease Control and Prevention's (CDC's) state-level emergency public health care preparedness account (Epstein and Lister, 2016; Kodjak, 2016). While the appropriate focus is on prevention and preparedness, some level of response will always be necessary. To enable swift and rapid response when necessary, the committee supports the creation of a public health emergency response fund, to be used only in declared health emergencies.

Finally, the development of needed vaccines, therapeutic agents, and diagnostics is severely inadequate to enable the United States and the world to respond effectively to these global health threats. Currently, product development for response to pandemic and bioterror threats depends on the interagency Public Health Emergency Medical Countermeasures Enterprise, which is limited by annual appropriations and dependent on the goodwill

[4] Zika Response Appropriations Act, H.R. 5243. 2016.

of industry partners. Adequately protecting U.S. citizens requires long-term planning and vision that enables the development of strong and comprehensive capabilities to detect and diagnose pandemic threats wherever they occur, ensure the availability of needed medical products, reduce the risk of transmission, and properly treat and care for infected patients here in the United States. A critical medical product development fund supporting long-term, stable research and development through the engagement of industry, academia, and other partners would ensure the development of critical drugs, vaccines, and diagnostics.

Preparedness and Capacity Building for Global Health Security

Public health infrastructure in most countries, including the United States, is extremely underresourced or nonexistent, making levels of preparedness, even for everyday emergencies, decades behind where they should be and allowing for significant risks when a disaster does strike. Funding levels for U.S. health preparedness have been severely reduced since the Public Health Security and Bioterrorism Response Act was enacted in 2002. A dual focus on health preparedness at home and abroad is essential to reduce the risk of outbreaks and the transmission of infectious disease to U.S. citizens. To this end, it is necessary to build core preparedness capacities and public health infrastructure in the United States and in LMICs, supported by such partnerships as the GHSA.

While a portion of the Ebola supplemental funding was directed toward nonspecific capacity building over 5 years, the sustainability of funding thereafter is unclear. This sustainability is also vulnerable to new or reemerging diseases; Ebola funding was the first coffer proposed to be tapped upon the emergence of Zika (Epstein and Lister, 2016). By contrast, a sustained level of investment in multidisciplinary One Health systems[5] can result in $15 billion in annual expected benefits from the prevention of mild pandemics and other major outbreaks (World Bank, 2012). Assuming that improved systems could detect and control even half of incipient pandemics, the rates of return are well above those on nearly all other public spending and private capital markets (World Bank, 2012), making this capacity building a smart investment. Enabling the right institutional capacity to reduce health risks, respond to emergencies, and innovate to improve the actions taken can dramatically improve the prevention and control of and response to health threats. At the same time, it is essen-

[5] Defined as the funding needed to bring major zoonotic disease prevention and control systems in developing countries up to World Organisation for Animal Health and World Health Organization standards. The World Bank report estimates that the required investments range from $1.9 billion to $3.4 billion per year.

tial to remain engaged and coordinated with domestic and international stakeholders, including the World Health Organization (WHO), the UN Secretary-General's Committee on AMR, and the GHSA.

Recommendation 1: Improve International Emergency Response Coordination

The administration should create a coordinating body for international public health emergency response that is accountable for international and domestic actions and oversees preparedness for and responses to global health security threats. This body should have its own budget, experience with handling logistics, and the authority necessary to coordinate players across the government at the deputy secretary level. This coordinating body should do the following:

- **Oversee the creation of an International Response Framework to guide the U.S. response to an international health emergency. Through this framework, this body would coordinate and direct activities involved in international response and preparedness, but would not duplicate functions already established in the Office of the Assistant Secretary for Preparedness and Response, the U.S. Centers for Disease Control and Prevention, the U.S. Agency for International Development, or the U.S. Department of Defense.**
- **Oversee three separate funding streams, dedicated to investments in preparedness, emergency response, and critical medical product development. The Office of Management and Budget should conduct an analysis to determine the appropriate levels for these three funding streams, commensurate with the associated risk, understanding that predictable and timely funds for these three purposes are critical.**
- **Align and coordinate efforts with effective multilateral organizations to reduce duplication and promote efficiency in building capacity and resilience in other countries.**

Recommendation 2: Combat Antimicrobial Resistance

The U.S. Department of Health and Human Services, the U.S. Department of Defense, the U.S. Department of Agriculture, and the U.S. Agency for International Development (USAID) should continue to invest in national capabilities and accelerate the development of international capabilities to detect, monitor, report, and combat antibiotic resistance. Efforts to this end should include the following:

- **Enhance surveillance systems to ensure that new resistant microbial strains are identified as soon as they emerge.**
- **Assist low-income countries in improving infection control and antimicrobial stewardship.**
- **USAID should leverage current supply chain partnerships with other countries to strengthen antibiotic supply chains, thus reducing the use of illegitimate antimicrobials and improving drug quality.**
- **Incentivize the development of therapeutics (including alternatives to antibiotics), vaccines, and diagnostics for use in humans and animals.**

Recommendation 3: Build Public Health Capacity in Low- and Middle-Income Countries

The U.S. Centers for Disease Control and Prevention, the National Institutes of Health, the U.S. Department of Defense, and the U.S. Agency for International Development should expand training and information exchange efforts to increase the capacity of low- and middle-income countries to respond to both public health emergencies and acute mass casualty disasters. This training and information exchange should encompass core capacities such as surveillance, epidemiology, and disaster and injury care response, as well as enhanced capabilities to improve communication and information pathways for the dissemination of innovative findings.

Maintaining a Sustained Response to Continuous Threats: HIV/AIDS, Tuberculosis, and Malaria

Considerable successes have been achieved in slowing the advancement of HIV/AIDS, TB, and malaria worldwide, as evidenced by the millions of lives saved. However, these diseases are continuing health threats that can jeopardize global security and inflict a high cost on the economies of the countries in which they are prevalent. As of the end of 2015, there remained more than 36.7 million people living with HIV/AIDS globally (UNAIDS, 2015b), and there were more than 1.1 million deaths from AIDS (UNAIDS, 2015a). In 2015, 1.4 million people died from TB (WHO, 2016b), and 429,000 people died from malaria (WHO, 2016d). Complacency toward these diseases can lead to severe risk and harm for the entire global community, as all three are capable of developing strains resistant to currently available treatments. Should that occur, an even more lethal resurgence of these diseases would likely take place, threatening all progress made on these diseases in previous decades.

HIV/AIDS

PEPFAR has played a key role in successfully slowing the HIV/AIDS epidemic globally since 2003, reducing new infections, and helping to save millions of lives around the world (PEPFAR, 2017). In addition to this progress on its primary goal, studies have shown that the countries in which PEPFAR is active had better opinions of the United States (Daschle and Frist, 2015) and also saw 13 percent increase in employment rates among men compared to non-PEPFAR countries (Wagner et al., 2015).

As a truly bipartisan, collaborative program that has undergone transitions and shifts throughout the last 15 years, PEPFAR has adapted its focus to changes in the HIV/AIDS epidemic from that of a highly lethal, rapidly spreading emergency to one that requires sustaining care while targeting at-risk populations. Yet this work is far from finished, as 2 million new HIV infections still occur each year, and millions are without access to treatment (PEPFAR, 2017). The next phase of PEPFAR will continue to require cross-sector and data-driven efforts to dramatically reduce the number of new HIV infections and AIDS-related deaths globally by 2030. However it will also rely on continued and expanded partnerships with the private sector and communities. A promising example is PEPFAR's multidisciplinary Determined, Resilient, Empowered, AIDS-free, Mentored, and Safe women (DREAMS) partnership, which focuses on lowering rates of HIV infection in young women by addressing multiple factors outside of the health sector that affect rates of infection (e.g., enabling and encouraging them to stay in school, addressing gender-based violence, and changing community norms). Given the substantial reduction in the costs of drugs used to treat HIV/AIDS, the increased involvement of private-sector partnerships, and the effect of treatment on preventing new infections, program ownership should continue shifting to host countries where possible. PEPFAR also should leverage its existing structures and platforms to address other priority health issues for its HIV-infected patient population, based on country needs.

Recommendation 4: Envision the Next Generation of PEPFAR

With its next reauthorization, Congress should fund The U.S. President's Emergency Plan for AIDS Relief (PEPFAR) at current levels, and allow for more flexibility within the PEPFAR program by continuing to relax specific funding targets for all program areas. Continued accountability, efficiency, and measurement of results should be emphasized. In the future, moreover, PEPFAR should focus on the following key areas:

- **Ensure that national governments assume greater ownership of national HIV/AIDS programs through joint planning and decision making, and that they increase domestic funding to help cover the costs of prevention and treatment.**
- **Adapt its delivery platform to become more of a cost-effective, chronic care system that is incorporated into each country's health system and priorities.**
- **Continue to support the Global Fund to Fight AIDS, Tuberculosis and Malaria (Global Fund), and rely on it for specific functions where it has the comparative advantage. Such functions could include the Global Fund's efficient procurement of products and multipartner efforts to encourage countries to transition to domestic sources of funding.**
- **Enhance emphasis on primary prevention through multisector efforts, including strong interventions against gender-based violence, given that many new HIV infections are occurring in adolescent girls.**

Tuberculosis

Unfortunately, TB has not shown the same progress in treatment and prevention as HIV/AIDS and has been a historically underfunded disease. In 2015, there were 10.4 million new cases of TB and 1.4 million attributable deaths (WHO, 2016b). Further complicating efforts to combat this disease is the rapid rise of multidrug-resistant strains of TB (MDR-TB). The current available drug regimens for TB, MDR-TB, and a more severe extensively drug-resistant TB (XDR-TB) are lengthy and complex and frequently have low success rates (WHO, 2016b). Furthermore, treatment for MDR-TB and XDR-TB can cost 100 times as much as treatment for nonresistant TB (Laurence et al., 2015; Nieburg et al., 2015; Pooran et al., 2013). With few drugs available to treat MDR-TB and XDR-TB and little progress on new treatment options, TB and its drug-resistant strains pose a growing threat to the health and health security of all countries, including the United States. TB has been a priority for the United States since passage of the Foreign Service Act of 1961, and in 2010 the U.S. Agency for International Development (USAID) laid out a sweeping strategy[6] for combating global TB. Of the $4 billion authorized over 5 years to implement this strategy, however, only 40 percent was ever appropriated. The U.S. government's underprioritization of TB undercuts its capability to reduce the global burden of disease. Accordingly, the U.S. government should reevaluate its investment in and strategies for combating TB.

---

[6] See Lantos-Hyde United States Government Tuberculosis Strategy.

Recommendation 5: Confront the Threat of Tuberculosis

> **The U.S. Centers for Disease Control and Prevention, the National Institute of Allergy and Infectious Diseases, and the U.S. Agency for International Development should conduct a thorough global threat assessment of rising tuberculosis (TB) levels, including multidrug-resistant TB and extensively drug-resistant TB. They should then execute a plan of action, including governance structure and priority activities, for developing and investing in new diagnostics, drugs, vaccines, and delivery systems.**

Malaria

Commensurate with the dedicated investment in combating malaria by the global community are tremendous successes in preventing and controlling the disease, with an estimated 41 percent reduction in incidence since 2000 and a 62 percent reduction in mortality rates globally (WHO, 2016d). This progress has been possible in large part because of increases in programmatic and financial support—from $100 million in 2000 (WHO, 2013) to $2.9 billion in 2015 (WHO, 2016d;). Through PMI and the Global Fund, which accounted for an estimated 35 percent of global funding for malaria efforts in 2015, the United States has, both directly and indirectly, been a major contributor to this success (WHO, 2016d). While the investment in malaria may appear costly, a cost–benefit analysis modeling the effect of global reduction and elimination of the disease found that the net gains in economic output would be worth $208.6 billion (Purdy et al., 2013).

As a result of these investments, elimination of malaria has become a realistic goal for many countries. Some countries can now declare themselves malaria-free, a welcome status for not only healthier communities but also healthier economies. Additionally, since 2006, all 15 PMI countries have seen up to 50 percent reductions in child mortality due to malaria infection (USAID, 2014). However, malaria still imposes a major burden of disease, with 212 million cases occurring in 2015 (WHO, 2016d), further imposing a financial burden on families and country economies. Malaria can cost families 25 percent of their income through lost days of work and prevention and treatment costs, and since 2000, average annual costs to sub-Saharan Africa totaled nearly $300 million simply for case management (UNICEF, 2004; WHO, 2015a). Given these high costs to individuals and countries and the threat of drug-resistant strains, a sustained, dedicated focus on malaria should continue.

Recommendation 6: Sustain Progress toward Malaria Elimination

> **Relevant agencies of the U.S. government should continue their commitment to the fight against malaria through the President's Malaria Initiative and collaborative work with all partners toward elimination of the disease.**

ENHANCING PRODUCTIVITY AND ECONOMIC GROWTH

The general health and well-being of other countries, including their burden of NCDs such as CVD and cancer, may at first glance not appear to be the top priority of donor countries such as the United States. However, investing in countries' prosperity and stability can result in greater order and predictability in the world, as well as promote U.S. health and prosperity and create more reliable and durable global partners. Premature death and disability stemming from NCDs coalesce to contribute to decreased productivity, decreased gross domestic product, and overall higher costs of health care because existing health systems are not designed to care for chronic disease in an integrated and holistic fashion (OECD, 2011).

As prevention is always less costly than treatment, efforts to prevent premature death and disability from NCDs ideally begin at birth and continue across an individual's life course. Cost-effective investments made during a child's early years can mitigate deleterious effects of poverty and social inequality, often resulting in long-lasting gains through adulthood. Healthy behaviors formed during childhood also can have long-term effects. Interventions carried out during the very early years can even translate into lifelong benefits in terms of labor market participation, earnings, and economic growth, generating returns of up to 25 percent (Gertler et al., 2014). Furthermore, the private sector has a clear interest in preventing NCDs as globalization continues to encourage international travel and trade. Multinational companies have workforces in many regions of the world and have interests in a productive and capable employee base, which also results in societies that are attractive places to locate their businesses.

Saving and Improving the Lives of Women and Children

Remarkable strides have been made in reducing mortality among women and children worldwide. Through the launch of the Ending Preventable Maternal and Child Death initiative, USAID has saved the lives of 46 million children and 200,000 women since 2008 (USAID, 2017). Yet global mortality rates for both mothers and children under 5 are still unacceptably high, with maternal mortality at 216 deaths per 100,000 births and child mortality at 41 deaths per 1,000 live births. As a result, each year 5.9 million children die before their fifth birthday (WHO, 2016a), and an estimated 303,000 women die from causes related to pregnancy and childbirth (WHO, 2016c). The majority of these deaths are preventable through interventions whose effectiveness is supported by extremely strong evidence, but challenges remain around how to scale up these interventions. Accelerating investments in cost-effective, evidence-based interventions is critical to sustain the progress made thus far and further avoid preventable deaths of infants, children, adolescents, and pregnant and lactating women.

Recommendation 7: Improve Survival in Women and Children

> **Congress should increase funding for the U.S. Agency for International Development to augment the agency's investments in ending preventable maternal and child mortality, defined as global maternal mortality rates of fewer than 70 deaths per 100,000 live births by 2020 and fewer than 25 child deaths per 1,000 live births by 2030. Investments should focus on the most effective interventions and be supported by rigorous monitoring and evaluation. These priority interventions include**
>
> - **immunizations;**
> - **integrated management of child illness;**
> - **nutrition (pregnant women, newborns, infants, children);**
> - **prenatal care and safe delivery, including early identification of at-risk pregnancies, safe delivery, and access to emergency obstetrical care; and**
> - **access to contraceptives and family planning.**

The committee found that while continued investment in the survival agenda is critical, it is only part of the challenge. Without proper progress in development in the first 1,000 days of life, many adverse consequences resulting from disease and malnutrition can follow a child through life. Strong neurological evidence demonstrates long-term mental and physical effects of such early risk factors as poor nutrition, lack of nurturing care, and lack of immunizations (Sudfeld et al., 2015). In LMICs, extreme poverty and stunting causes 250 million children (43 percent) younger than 5 fail to reach their developmental potential (Black et al., 2017). Building empowering, nurturing, and cognitively enriching environments (which include responsive and emotionally supportive parenting, opportunities for play and learning, and support for early education) for vulnerable children under 5 and their mothers requires an agenda that incorporates the health, education, and social services sectors. Thus, a thrive agenda is an important focal point for investment in addition to the existing survival agenda.

Recommendation 8: Ensure Healthy and Productive Lives for Women and Children

The U.S. Agency for International Development, The U.S. President's Emergency Plan for AIDS Relief, their implementing partners, and other funders should support and incorporate proven, cost-effective interventions into their existing programs for ensuring that all children reach their developmental potential and become healthy, productive adults. This integration should embrace principles of country ownership, domestic financing, and community engagement. These interventions should include the following:

- **Provide adequate nutrition for optimal infant and child cognitive development.**
- **Reduce childhood exposure to domestic and other violence.**
- **Detect and manage postpartum depression and other maternal mental health issues.**
- **Support and promote early education and cognitive stimulation in young children.**

Promoting Cardiovascular Health and Preventing Cancer

NCDs such as CVD, chronic obstructive pulmonary disease, and lung cancer kill 40 million people globally each year, almost three-quarters of whom are in LMICs (WHO, 2015b). Of these deaths, 17 million are considered "premature." The annual global cost of CVD alone is estimated to rise to more than $1 trillion in 2030 (Reddy et al., 2016). Additionally, more people are dying from cancer in LMICs than from AIDS, TB, and malaria combined, with the total annual cost in 2010 approximated at $1.16 trillion[7]—more than 2 percent of total global gross domestic product (Stewart and Wild, 2014). Between 30 and 50 percent of cancer deaths are preventable through prevention, early detection, and treatment. This means that more than 2.4 million annual deaths are avoidable, with an approximate $100–$200 billion in global economic savings to be achieved (Stewart and Wild, 2014). Yet many health care systems in these countries are not designed to manage NCDs, and they have difficulty integrating various platforms across disease types. The lack of a properly trained workforce and of the effective population-level policies described in Chapter 6 is also a challenge for LMICs, and indeed for countries at all income levels. With

[7] This figure is the sum of the costs of prevention and treatment, plus the annual economic value of disability-adjusted life years (DALYs) lost as a result of cancer. This value fails to estimate longer-term costs to families and the costs that patients and families attribute to human suffering.

conditions across the NCD spectrum also affecting populations in the United States, this is a clear area for shared innovation to tackle common problems. Greater awareness of successful interventions and best practices for combating CVD, cancer, and other NCDs can reduce duplication and allow for more rapid information exchange, leading more quickly to solutions.

Unfortunately, many efforts to combat NCDs are incorporated into other programs as an afterthought, and there is no overall coordination mechanism or strategy for a global focus on these diseases. However, U.S. programs have established strong networks and knowledge bases in many countries through decades of global health efforts by various agencies, through such program areas as PEPFAR and maternal and child health efforts. These existing platforms can serve as opportunities in which to integrate prevention and treatment efforts for NCDs. Additionally, as noted earlier, recent years have seen strong interest from the private sector in addressing the global burden of these diseases because of their clear effects on workforce productivity; however, there is no synergy among private-sector efforts across countries or health systems. The knowledge base acquired by U.S. agencies and programs should be leveraged and paired with private-sector interest and community-level commitment to mobilize and coordinate high-impact, evidence-based interventions that can be applied in all countries. Absent such concerted efforts, these diseases will continue to result in high rates of premature death and lost productivity, reversing the recent gains in and trends toward improved economic growth and stability in many countries.

Recommendation 9: Promote Cardiovascular Health and Prevent Cancer

The U.S. Agency for International Development, the U.S. Department of State, and the U.S. Centers for Disease Control and Prevention, through their country offices, should provide seed funding to facilitate the mobilization and involvement of the private sector in addressing cardiovascular disease and cancer at the country level. These efforts should be closely aligned and coordinated with the efforts of national governments and should strive to integrate services at the community level. The priority strategies to ensure highest impact are

- **Target and manage risk factors (e.g., smoking, alcohol use, obesity) for the major noncommunicable diseases, particularly through the adoption of fiscal policies and regulations that facilitate tobacco control and healthy diets;**
- **Detect and treat hypertension early;**
- **Detect and treat early cervical cancer; and**

- **Immunize for vaccine-preventable cancers (specifically human papilloma virus and hepatitis B vaccines).**

MAXIMIZING RETURNS ON INVESTMENTS

The committee identified opportunities for changing the way the United States operates in the arena of global health and finances relevant programs to maximize the returns on U.S. investments through improved health outcomes and cost-effectiveness. If the United States can transition from its traditional siloed and reactive approach to global health to a more proactive, systematic, and sustainable approach, the committee believes U.S. investments will have an even more significant positive impact on the four priority areas outlined in this report—achieving global health security, maintaining a sustained response to the continuous threats of communicable diseases, saving and improving the lives of women and children, and promoting cardiovascular health and preventing cancer. To maximize the returns on investments in these four areas and achieve better health outcomes and more effective use of funding, the United States will need to

- catalyze innovation through the accelerated development of both medical products and integrated digital health infrastructure;
- employ more nimble and flexible financing mechanisms to leverage new partners and funders in global health; and
- maintain U.S. status and influence as a world leader in global health while adhering to evidence-based science and economics, measurement, and accountability.

Catalyze Innovation

Achieving the improvements in global health called for by numerous previous reports will require changing the way global health business is conducted to better enable innovation. Given the multisectoral nature of health, simply addressing individual challenges in a singular, siloed manner will never solve the overall problem. Challenges in the development process for vaccines and drugs to prevent and treat infectious and neglected diseases have plagued researchers and developers since before HIV/AIDS captured the world's attention in the 1980s. Additionally, health systems in LMICs are typically underresourced and lack basic infrastructure, making it difficult to provide all types of care and public health protections, such as surveillance or access to specialty care. Unless researchers, regulators, health providers, and private-sector partners are encouraged to think more creatively to solve these complex problems and enable changes in current processes, new and innovative models will be difficult to achieve. The committee believes that the creation of an environment that enables innovation can accelerate the development of critical medical products and make it possible to augment public health services through technology such that they can be provided in a more sustainable manner.

Development of Medical Products

Global health priorities will be difficult to achieve without safe and effective drugs, vaccines, diagnostics, and devices. The private sector is an essential player, together with academia, civil society, and government, in ensuring that required products are developed and manufactured. However, the markets for many global health products are uncertain or risky, making it difficult for private-sector development and manufacturing partners to justify their shareholders' investments. For example, industry considers investments in innovations to address unpredictable and fast-moving pandemics high-risk, especially given the experience of several firms with investing millions of dollars in the development of vaccines against SARS and Ebola only to find that the government was no longer interested in these products (Ebola Vaccine Team B, 2016; Osterholm and Olshaker, 2017). Through regulatory or market incentives, the U.S. government can reduce or share the burden of development costs and risks with industry, effectively "pushing" a product through the pipeline. Similarly, the U.S. government can reduce market risk (creating market "pull") by increasing the certainty, speed, or volume of the purchase of products. In the absence of these push and pull interventions, the United States and other governments risk spending far more than is necessary to prevent, detect, respond to, and treat disease outbreaks by using suboptimal tools.

In addition to market forces, human and institutional capacity for research and development (R&D) underpins the ability of the private sector, academia, civil society, and governments to develop priority technologies. This R&D capacity is needed in countries where outbreaks begin and disease burdens are high. Helping to build the capacity for LMICs to conduct clinical trials using their own workforces and facilities is both more efficient and more cost-effective than trying to export foreign human capacity and technical infrastructure for every disease outbreak. The necessary capacity includes laboratory capacity, the ability to collect baseline data on disease burden, and an appropriately trained research-competent workforce. Building this capacity also enables sustainability and encourages innovation by creating environments in which local researchers can solve local problems. The U.S. government has an opportunity to streamline processes, reduce costs, and create more appropriate incentives that will enable industry, academia, and others to contribute to the development of priority innovations for global health.

Recommendation 10: Accelerate the Development of Medical Products

U.S. government agencies should invest in a targeted effort to reduce the costs and risks of developing, licensing, and introducing vaccines, therapeutics, diagnostics, and devices needed to address global health priorities by enabling innovative approaches for trial design, streamlining regulation, ensuring production capacity, creating market incentives, and building international capacity for research and development. This effort should include the following:

- **Enabling innovative approaches for trial design:** The U.S. Food and Drug Administration (FDA), the Biomedical Advanced Research and Development Authority (BARDA), the U.S. Department of Defense (DoD), and the National Institutes of Health (NIH) should actively encourage public- and private-sector product development efforts using innovative product development approaches, including platform studies, adaptive trial designs, pragmatic trials, and improved biomarker development. BARDA should assess expanding its list of priority products for codevelopment with industry, taking into account global health priorities.
- **Streamlining regulation:** FDA should receive adequate resources to improve the tropical disease priority review voucher program and should assess the application of the provisions outlined in the Generating Antibiotic Incentives Now Act to neglected tropical diseases beyond those on the qualified pathogen list.
- **Ensuring production capacity:** BARDA should increase its efforts to promote adequate global manufacturing capacity for priority technologies (e.g., Centers for Innovation in Advanced Development and Manufacturing).
- **Creating market incentives:** The U.S. government should invest in generating and disseminating accurate and transparent market estimates and should use the purchasing power of U.S. government agencies and global partnerships such as Gavi, the Vaccine Alliance, and the Global Fund to Fight AIDS, Tuberculosis and Malaria, as well as such creative financing mechanisms as volume guarantees, to reduce market uncertainty for priority health products.
- **Building international capacity for research and development:** The U.S. Centers for Disease Control and Prevention, NIH, and DoD should increase the number of people and institutions in partner countries capable of conducting clini-

cal trials for global health priorities (e.g., through funding partnerships with academic institutions). This effort should encompass providing support for sustainable core capacities such as drug, vaccine, and diagnostic research capabilities and building the skills of principal investigators.

Development of Integrated Digital Health Infrastructure

Digital health efforts have shown promise in reducing costs and promoting health across the United States and the globe. However, many such investments have been siloed and shortsighted in their approach, often focusing on single diseases or sectors and missing opportunities to develop a sustainable, integrated platform. Growing mobile and internet connectivity worldwide, along with positive disruptive advances in the information and communications technology sector, provide a timely opportunity for the United States to reexamine its investment and development approaches to digital health efforts in other countries. A renewed focus should include goals of reducing fragmentation, improving integration of programs, and maximizing reusability to improve returns on investments. An emphasis on health systems innovation through technical assistance and public–private partnerships in digital health can lead to better care and more effective care delivery at lower cost.

Given the proliferation of digital health applications and platforms in countries across the world, created by public- and private-sector players alike, there is a need for a common digital health framework that can be applied to different country contexts, allowing for easier replication of best practices and information sharing. At the country level, cross-cutting digital health platforms should be interoperable and yet adaptable to local requirements and sovereignty. Such platforms should address each country's health care priorities during steady-state times, thereby incentivizing country coinvestment and ownership, while at the same time serving as a resilient system to facilitate controlled sharing of data across countries, thereby enhancing surveillance, coordinated responses, and delivery of services during an emergency. The U.S. government has the opportunity to leverage government content expertise and private-sector talent to build on recent and ongoing efforts, including legislation[8] aimed at improving and integrating efforts to incorporate internet access into education, development, and economic growth programs. Digital health efforts can be woven into each of those sectors with a holistic and cross-cutting perspective. New and existing U.S. investments should be buttressed by cross-cutting platforms and should assist in making these technological advances available to

[8] Digital Global Access Policy Act of 2017, H.R. 600, 115th Congress.

interested countries to improve their own health systems in a manner that is interoperable and scalable for future-minded solutions.

Recommendation 11: Improve Digital Health Infrastructure

Relevant agencies of the U.S. government should convene an international group of public and private stakeholders to create a common digital health framework that addresses country-level needs ranging from integrated care to research and development.

- **The U.S. Agency for International Development (USAID) and the U.S. Department of State should incentivize and support countries in building interoperable digital health platforms that can efficiently collect and use health data and analytic insights to enable the delivery of integrated services within a country.**
- **USAID's Global Development Laboratory should provide technical assistance to countries in the development and implementation of interoperable digital health platforms cofunded by the country and adaptable to local requirements.**
- **U.S. agencies should expand on the "build-once" principle of the Digital Global Access Policy Act and align U.S. funding in digital health by multiple agencies to reduce fragmentation and duplication, as well as maximize the effectiveness of investments. The provision of this funding should employ methods that reflect smart financing strategies to leverage private industry and country cofinancing (see Recommendation 13).**

Employ More Nimble and Flexible Financing Mechanisms

In the changing landscape of globalization and growth in middle-income countries, traditional aid models are also changing. As a global health leader, the United States should adapt its spending accordingly. Current U.S. global health financing is focused largely on immediate disease-specific priorities. This financial support is seen as development and humanitarian assistance for strategic partner countries. Instead, programs should focus on long-term goals of building global health systems and platforms that are disease-agnostic and can respond rapidly and flexibly to emerging threats that potentially impact the entire world, including the United States. There are innovative mechanisms for making present funds more effective, and opportunities exist for creative partnerships with new players and investors to develop better programs and goals. Existing platforms such as PEPFAR can be augmented through public–private partnerships to improve health outcomes in countries, such as efforts made in the last decade on generic drugs and strengthening of supply chains (Waning et al., 2010). There is also potential in incentivizing the private sector to invest in global health, both for social benefit and for positive long-term business outcomes. Governments can crowd-in additional funding sources by increasing the demand for goods through public funds, and sharing risk in various ways, which then catalyzes private investment that would not have otherwise taken place (Powers and Butterfield, 2014). Overall, by conducting more strategic and systematic assessments, the U.S. government can make long-term investments in global health that contribute to global public goods rather than short-term expenditures. These long-term investments should maintain a focus on global health security; disease prevention and control; cross-cutting health systems innovation; and R&D for essential vaccines, drugs, diagnostics, and devices.

In addition to pursuing more systematic spending, the United States needs to consider that many countries continue to grow economically, and their needs will change from direct support for the procurement of drugs, diagnostics, and other commodities to technical support and sustainable financing from multiple sources. Thinking more strategically about how to help growing middle-income countries transition out of bilateral aid programs and optimize their use of domestic resources in a sustainable way will be an important future role of the United States. Assisting interested countries in structuring debt ratios and tax initiatives, along with implementing other innovative mechanisms, can build stronger and more holistic health systems and provide multiple returns on investments. The U.S. government should review the wide variety of mechanisms that have been implemented by partners around the world as it explores options for expanding and diversifying U.S. global health funding to increase its effectiveness.

Recommendation 12: Transition Investments Toward Global Public Goods

> **The U.S. Agency for International Development, the U.S. Department of State, and the U.S. Department of Health and Human Services should, together, systematically assess their approach to global health funding with an eye toward making long-term investments in high-impact, country-level programs. The focus should be on programs that both build national health systems and provide the greatest value in terms of global health security (to prevent pandemics), as well as respond to humanitarian emergencies and provide opportunities for joint research and development for essential drugs, diagnostics, and vaccines that will benefit many countries, including the United States.**

Recommendation 13: Optimize Resources Through Smart Financing

Relevant agencies of the U.S. government should expand efforts to complement direct bilateral support for health with financing mechanisms that include results-based financing; risk sharing; and attracting funding from private investment, recipient governments, and other donors.

- **The U.S. Agency for International Development (USAID) and The U.S. President's Emergency Plan for AIDS Relief (PEPFAR) should structure their financing to promote greater country ownership and domestic financing. Assistance should be provided in developing innovative financing products/modalities and in working with the finance sector to push the envelope on innovative sources of financing, crowding in private-sector capital.**
- **USAID and PEPFAR should engage with ministries on system design and financing to assist in plan design, model refinement and expansion, return-on-investment analysis, and financial plan execution.**
- **USAID should expand the use and flexibility of such mechanisms as the Development Credit Authority, and the U.S. Department of the Treasury, the U.S. Department of State, and USAID should motivate the World Bank; the International Monetary Fund; the Global Fund to Fight AIDS, Tuberculosis and Malaria; and Gavi, the Vaccine Alliance, respectively, to promote transitioning to domestic financing, assist countries in creating fiscal space for health, leverage fiscal policies to improve health, and attract alternative financing sources.**

Maintain U.S. Global Health Leadership

Finally, given the extremely interconnected nature of the world today, it is critical for the United States to continue to be a leader in global health. Adequately protecting U.S. citizens at home and abroad requires not only investment in U.S. infrastructure, but also continued awareness of global issues and active engagement in the international global health arena. There have been continuing calls for management and operational reforms of WHO, and while the committee agrees on the need for reform, it also recognizes that WHO performs many essential functions—for example, setting such standards as International Health Regulations. In addition, many other UN agencies and international organizations and partnerships formed in the last few decades are crucial in providing support to countries around the world. The success of all of these multilateral entities, such as the Global Fund, will help the U.S. government accomplish its global health goals and maximize its returns on investments.

Many of the events and elements of the changing global health landscape described throughout this report have created an environment for a centralized and comprehensive strategy for U.S. global health diplomacy. The United States has an opportunity to solidify its leadership and take a more deliberate foreign policy approach, including the creation of a system to support a more sustainable global health workforce in the United States. The limited number of noncareer health appointments currently available abroad are ad hoc and do not facilitate institutional knowledge or a promising career track for health professionals. Also needed is better bidirectional communication between health and diplomacy professionals and increased cross-disciplinary training. Greater flexibility for U.S. health professionals to work abroad, with emphasis on country and cultural competence and understanding, can allow for better sharing of information and more coordinated response during an outbreak or other emergency. It also could enable long-term partnerships focused on developing cures for such diseases as HIV/AIDS and cancer. Strengthening relations with countries through a strong, centralized office of global health diplomacy can create a coordinating health role for U.S. embassies while also improving situational awareness and networking with other sectors connected to health, such as finance and energy.

Recommendation 14: Commit to Continued Global Health Leadership

To protect itself from global threats, benefit from successes achieved in global health programs, and maintain a strong research and development pipeline, the United States should commit to maintaining its leadership in global health and actively participating in global health governance, coordination, and collaboration. To this end, the U.S. Department of State and the U.S. Department of Health and Human Services (HHS) should do the following:

- **Use their influence to improve the performance of key United Nations agencies and other international organizations important to global health, particularly the World Health Organization (WHO). WHO is in need of greater resources to address the health challenges of the 21st century, and many of its priorities align with those of the U.S. government. However, U.S. government financial contributions to WHO should come with a requirement that**

the organization adopt and implement the much-needed management and operational reforms identified in recent reports.

- **Remain involved in and firmly committed to innovative global partnerships that further U.S. global health goals, such as the highly successful Gavi, the Vaccine Alliance, and the Global Fund to Fight AIDS, Tuberculosis and Malaria, as well as promising new entities such as the Global Health Security Agenda and the Global Financing Facility.**
- **Implement a more strategic approach to achieving global health goals. This new approach should include the commitment of the U.S. Department of State to creating a global health career track and congressional action to enable the establishment of a cadre of global health experts within HHS through an amendment to the Foreign Service Act. This would create the environment necessary to expand the health attaché program, particularly in middle-income countries.**

A BLUEPRINT FOR ACTION

The committee's 14 recommendations are directed toward a wide range of U.S. government entities. In Table 10-1, the recommendations pertinent to each entity are summarized to form a blueprint for action to achieve global health security and enhance productivity and economic growth worldwide.

TABLE 10-1 Report Recommendations Outlined by Entity

Entity	Recommendation Number	Action
Presidential Administration	1 (see Chapter 3)	Create a coordinating body for international public health emergency response that is accountable for international and domestic actions and oversee preparedness for and responses to global health security threats.
	6 (see Chapter 4)	Continue the commitment to the fight against malaria through the President's Malaria Initiative, working toward elimination.

TABLE 10-1 Continued

Entity	Recommendation Number	Action
	10 (see Chapter 8)	Invest in generating and disseminating accurate and transparent market estimates for priority health products, and use the purchasing power of U.S. government agencies and global partnerships, as well as such creative financing mechanisms as volume guarantees, to reduce market uncertainty for these products.
	14 (see Chapter 9)	Remain firmly committed to global partnerships that further U.S. global health goals, especially the Global Fund to Fight AIDS, Tuberculosis and Malaria.
Congress	4 (see Chapter 4)	Fund The U.S. President's Emergency Plan for AIDS Relief (PEPFAR) at current levels, and allow more flexibility within the program by continuing to relax specific funding targets.
	7 (see Chapter 5)	Increase funding to the U.S. Agency for International Development to augment investments in ending preventable maternal and child deaths.
	10 (see Chapter 7)	Ensure that the U.S. Food and Drug Administration receives adequate resources to improve the tropical disease priority review voucher program.
	14 (see Chapter 9)	Amend the Foreign Service Act to enable a cadre of global health experts within the U.S. Department of Health and Human Services.
Office of Management and Budget	1 (see Chapter 3)	Conduct an analysis to determine the appropriate levels for the three funding streams for preparedness, emergency response, and medical product development.
	11 (see Chapter 7)	Align U.S. funding in digital health by multiple agencies to reduce fragmentation and duplication while maximizing the effectiveness of investments.
U.S. Department of Defense	2 (see Chapter 3)	Continue investing in national capabilities and accelerate investment in international capabilities to detect, monitor, report, and combat antibiotic resistance.
	3 (see Chapter 3)	Expand training and information exchange efforts to increase the capacity of low- and middle-income countries to respond to both public health emergencies and acute mass casualty disasters.

continued

TABLE 10-1 Continued

Entity	Recommendation Number	Action
	10 (see Chapter 7)	Increase the number of people and institutions in partner countries capable of conducting clinical trials for global health priorities (e.g., through funding partnerships with academic institutions).
	10 (see Chapter 7)	Actively encourage public- and private-sector product development efforts using innovative product development approaches, including platform studies, adaptive trial designs, pragmatic trials, and improved biomarker development.
U.S. Department of Health and Human Services	2 (see Chapter 3)	Continue investing in national capabilities and accelerate the development of international capabilities to detect, monitor, report, and combat antibiotic resistance.
	12 (see Chapter 8)	Systematically assess its approach to global health funding with an eye toward making long-term investments that provide the greatest value in terms of global health security, humanitarian emergency assistance, and joint research and development for essential medical products.
	14 (see Chapter 9)	Use its influence to improve the performance of the World Health Organization.
	14 (see Chapter 9)	Establish a cadre of global health experts through amendment of the Foreign Service Act.
National Institutes of Health (NIH)	3 (see Chapter 3)	Expand training and information exchange efforts to increase the capacity of low- and middle-income countries to respond to both public health emergencies and acute mass casualty disasters.
	10 (see Chapter 7)	Actively encourage public- and private-sector product development efforts using innovative product development approaches, including platform studies, adaptive trial designs, pragmatic trials, and improved biomarker development.
	10 (see Chapter 7)	Increase the number of people and institutions in partner countries capable of conducting clinical trials for global health priorities (e.g., through funding partnerships with academic institutions).
National Institute of Allergy and Infectious Diseases (NIH)	5 (see Chapter 4)	Conduct a thorough global threat assessment of rising tuberculosis (TB) levels, including multidrug-resistant TB and extensively drug-resistant TB, and execute a plan of action.

TABLE 10-1 Continued

Entity	Recommendation Number	Action
U.S. Food and Drug Administration	10 (see Chapter 7)	Improve the tropical disease priority review voucher program, and assess applying Generating Antibiotic Incentives Now Act provisions to neglected tropical diseases.
	10 (see Chapter 7)	Actively encourage public- and private-sector product development efforts using innovative product development approaches, including platform studies, adaptive trial designs, pragmatic trials, and improved biomarker development.
U.S. Centers for Disease Control and Prevention	3 (see Chapter 3)	Expand training and information exchange efforts to increase the capacity of low- and middle-income countries to respond to both public health emergencies and acute mass casualty disasters.
	5 (see Chapter 4)	Conduct a thorough global threat assessment of rising tuberculosis (TB) levels, including multidrug-resistant TB and extremely drug-resistant TB, and execute a plan of action.
	9 (see Chapter 8)	Provide seed funding to facilitate the mobilization and involvement of the private sector in addressing cardiovascular disease and cancer at the country level.
	10 (see Chapter 7)	Increase the number of people and institutions in partner countries capable of conducting clinical trials for global health priorities (e.g., through funding partnerships with academic institutions).
Biomedical Advanced Research and Development Authority	10 (see Chapter 7)	Actively encourage public- and private-sector product development efforts using innovative product development approaches, including platform studies, adaptive trial designs, pragmatic trials, and improved biomarker development.
	10 (see Chapter 7)	Assess expanding its list of priority products for codevelopment with industry, taking into account global health priorities.
	10 (see Chapter 7)	Increase its efforts to promote adequate global manufacturing capacity for priority technologies.

continued

TABLE 10-1 Continued

Entity	Recommendation Number	Action
U.S. Department of State	9 (see Chapter 6)	Provide seed funding to facilitate the mobilization and involvement of the private sector in addressing cardiovascular disease and cancer at the country level.
	11 (see Chapter 7)	Incentivize and support countries in building digital health platforms.
	12 (see Chapter 8)	Systematically assess its approach to global health funding with an eye toward making long-term investments that provide the greatest value in terms of global health security, humanitarian emergency assistance, and joint research and development for essential medical products.
	13 (see Chapter 8)	Motivate the World Bank, the International Monetary Fund, the Global Fund, and Gavi to promote transitions to domestic financing, and assist countries in improving health through the use of fiscal policies.
	14 (see Chapter 9)	Use its influence to improve the performance of the World Health Organization.
	14 (see Chapter 9)	Commit to the creation of a global health career track.
The U.S. President's Emergency Plan for AIDS Relief (PEPFAR) (U.S. Department of State)	4 (see Chapter 4)	Ensure that national governments assume greater ownership of HIV/AIDS programs; adapt its delivery platform to become a chronic care system that is incorporated into each country's health system and priorities; rely on the Global Fund for functions where it has the comparative advantage; and enhance emphasis on primary prevention through multisector efforts.
	8 (see Chapter 5)	Support and incorporate proven, cost-effective interventions into its existing programs for ensuring that all children reach their developmental potential and become healthy, productive adults.
	13 (see Chapter 8)	Structure financing to promote country ownership and domestic financing, to include private-sector capital.
	13 (see Chapter 3)	Engage with country ministries on system design and financing to assist in planning, refinement, scaling, return-on-investment analysis, and financial plan execution.

TABLE 10-1 Continued

Entity	Recommendation Number	Action
U.S. Agency for International Development (USAID)	2 (see Chapter 3)	Leverage current supply chain partnerships with other countries to strengthen antibiotic supply chains, thus reducing the use of illegitimate pharmaceuticals and improving drug quality.
	2 (see Chapter 3)	Continue investing in national capabilities and accelerate the development of international capabilities to detect, monitor, report, and combat antibiotic resistance.
	3 (see Chapter 3)	Expand training and information exchange efforts to increase the capacity of low- and middle-income countries to respond to both public health emergencies and acute mass casualty disasters.
	5 (see Chapter 4)	Conduct a thorough global threat assessment of rising tuberculosis (TB) levels, including multidrug-resistant TB and extremely drug-resistant TB, and execute a plan of action.
	7 (see Chapter 5)	Augment investments in ending preventable maternal and child deaths.
	8 (see Chapter 5)	Support and incorporate proven, cost-effective interventions into its existing programs for ensuring that all children reach their developmental potential and become healthy, productive adults.
	9 (see Chapter 6)	Provide seed funding to facilitate the mobilization and involvement of the private sector in addressing cardiovascular disease and cancer at the country level.
	11 (see Chapter 7)	Convene an international group of stakeholders to create a common digital health framework; incentivize and support countries in building digital health platforms.
	12 (see Chapter 8)	Systematically assess its approach to global health funding with an eye toward making long-term investments that provide the greatest value in terms of global health security, humanitarian emergency assistance, and joint research and development for essential medical products.
	13 (see Chapter 8)	Structure financing to promote country ownership and domestic financing, to include private-sector capital.

continued

TABLE 10-1 Continued

Entity	Recommendation Number	Action
	13 (see Chapter 8)	Engage with country ministries on system design and financing to assist in planning, refinement, scaling, return-on-investment analysis, and financial plan execution.
	13 (see Chapter 8)	Expand the use and flexibility of the Development Credit Authority.
	13 (see Chapter 8)	Motivate the World Bank, the International Monetary Fund, the Global Fund, and Gavi, the Vaccine Alliance to promote transitions to domestic financing, and assist countries in improving health through the use of fiscal policies.
Global Development Lab (USAID)	11 (see Chapter 7)	Provide technical assistance to countries in developing and implementing interoperable digital platforms.
U.S. Department of Agriculture	2 (see Chapter 3)	Continue investing in national capabilities and accelerate the development of international capabilities to detect, monitor, report, and combat antibiotic resistance.
U.S. Department of the Treasury	13 (see Chapter 9)	Motivate the World Bank, the International Monetary Fund, the Global Fund, and Gavi, the Vaccine Alliance to promote transitions to domestic financing, and assist countries in improving health through the use of fiscal policies.

REFERENCES

Black, M. M., S. P. Walker, L. C. Fernald, C. T. Andersen, A. M. DiGirolamo, C. Lu, D. C. McCoy, G. Fink, Y. R. Shawar, J. Shiffman, A. E. Devercelli, Q. T. Wodon, E. Vargas-Baron, and S. Grantham-McGregor. 2017. Early childhood development coming of age: Science through the life course. *The Lancet* 389(10064):77-90.

Bloom, D. E., D. Canning, and D. T. Jamison. 2004. Health, wealth, and welfare. *Finance and Development* 41(1):10-15.

Burns, A., D. van der Mensbrugge, and H. Timmer. 2008. *Evaluating the economic consequences of avian influenza.* Washington, DC: World Bank.

CDC (U.S. Centers for Disease Control and Prevention). 2016. *CDC's response to the 2014–2016 Ebola epidemic—West Africa and United States.* Atlanta, GA: U.S. Centers for Disease Control and Prevention.

Daschle, T., and W. Frist. 2015. *The case for strategic health diplomacy: A study of PEPFAR* Washington, DC: Bipartisan Policy Center.

Ebola Vaccine Team B. 2016. *Plotting the course of Ebola vaccines: Challenges and unanswered questions.* Minneapolis: Center for Infectious Disease Research and Policy, University of Minnesota. http://www.cidrap.umn.edu/sites/default/files/public/downloads/ebola_team_b_report_2-033116-final.pdf (accessed January 10, 2017).

Epstein, S. B., and S. A. Lister. 2016. *Zika response funding: Request and congressional action.* Washington, DC: Congressional Research Service.

Epstein, S. B., S. A. Lister, A. Belasco, and D. J. Jansen. 2015. *FY2015 funding to counter Ebola and the Islamic State (IS).*Washington, DC: Congressional Research Service.

Fan, E. 2003. *SARS: Economic impacts and implications.* Manila, Philippines: Asian Development Bank.

Fan, V. Y., D. T. Jamison, and L. H. Summers. 2016. *The inclusive cost of pandemic influenza risk.* Cambridge, MA: National Bureau of Economic Research.

Frenk, J., and O. Gómez-Dantés. 2016. False dichotomies in global health: The need for integrative thinking. *The Lancet* 389(10069):667-670.

GAO (U.S. Government Accountability Office). 2017. *Defense civil support: DoD, HHS, and DHS should use existing coordination mechanisms to improve their pandemic preparedness.* Washington, DC: U.S. Government Accountability Office.

Gertler, P., J. Heckman, R. Pinto, A. Zanolini, C. Vermeersch, S. Walker, S. M. Chang, and S. Grantham-McGregor. 2014. Labor market returns to an early childhood stimulation intervention in Jamaica. *Science* 344(6187):998-1001.

Gold, J. 2014. "*Statement of Chancellor Jeff Gold, M.D. University of Nebraska Medical Center, Omaha, Nebraska before the Committee on Energy and Commerce Subcommittee on Oversight & Investigations*" (Date: 11/18/2014) Hearing on "*Update on the U.S. Public Health Response to the Ebola Outbreak.*" Available from: https://energycommerce.house.gov/hearings-and-votes/hearings/update-us-public-health-response-ebola-outbreak (accessed January 15, 2017).

Hotez, P. J., K. O. Murray, and P. Buekens. 2014. The Gulf Coast: A new American underbelly of tropical diseases and poverty. *PLOS Neglected Tropical Diseases* 8(5):e2760.

IOM (Institute of Medicine). 1997. *America's vital interest in global health: Protecting our people, enhancing our economy, and advancing our international interests.* Washington, DC: National Academy Press.

Iuliano, D. A., Y. Jang, J. Jones, T. C. Davis, D. E. Wentworth, T. M. Uyeki, K. Roguski, M. G. Thompson, L. Gubareva, A. M. Fry, E. Burns, S. Trock, S. Zhou, J. M. Katz, and D. B. Jernigan. 2017. Increase in human infections with avian influenza (H7N9) virus during the fifth epidemic—China, October 2016–February 2017. *Morbidity and Mortality Weekly Report (MMWR)* 66(9):254-255.

Jamison, D., L. Summers, G. Alleyne, K. Arrow, A. Binagwaho, F. Bustreo, D. Evans, R. Freachern, G. Ghosh, S. Goldie, Y. Guo, S. Gupta, R. Horton, M. Kruk, A. Mahmoud, L. Mohohlo, M. Ncube, A. Pablos-Mendéz, S. Reddy, H. Saxenian, A. Soucat, K. Ulltveit-Moe, and G. Yamey. 2013. Global health 2035: A world converging within a generation. *The Lancet.* 382(9908):1898-1955.

Kodjak, A. 2016. *Congress ends spat, agrees to fund $1.1 billion to combat Zika.* http://www.npr.org/sections/health-shots/2016/09/28/495806979/congress-ends-spat-over-zika-funding-approves-1-1-billion (accessed December 15, 2016).

Laurence, Y. V., U. K. Griffiths, and A. Vassall. 2015. Costs to health services and the patient of treating tuberculosis: A systematic literature review. *Pharmacoeconomics* 33(9):939-955.

Marmot, M. 2005. Social determinants of health inequalities. *The Lancet* 365(9464):1099-1104.

Marquez, P. V., and J. L. Farrington. 2013. *The challenge of non-communicable diseases and road traffic injuries in sub-Saharan Africa. An overview.* Washington, DC: World Bank.

Nieburg, P., T. Dubovi, and S. Angelo. 2015. *Tuberculosis: A complex health threat.* Washington, DC: Center for Strategic and International Studies.

OECD (Organisation for Economic Co-operation and Development). 2011. *Health reform: Meeting the challenge of ageing and multiple morbidities.*Washington, DC: Organisation for Economic Co-operation and Development.

Osterholm, M. T., and M. Olshaker. 2017. *Deadliest enemy: Our war against killer germs.* New York: Little Brown and Company.

PEPFAR (The U.S. President's Emergency Plan for AIDS Relief). 2017. *PEPFAR 2016 annual report to Congress.* Washington, DC: The Office of the U.S. Global AIDS Coordinator and Health Diplomacy, U.S. Department of State.

Pooran, A., E. Pieterson, M. Davids, G. Theron, and K. Dheda. 2013. What is the cost of diagnosis and management of drug resistant tuberculosis in South Africa? *PLOS ONE* 8(1):e54587.

Powers, C., and W. M. Butterfield. 2014. Crowding in private investment. In *Frontiers in development: Ending extreme poverty,* edited by R. Shah and N. Unger. Washington, DC: U.S. Agency for International Development.

Purdy, M., M. Robinson, K. Wei, and D. Rublin. 2013. The economic case for combating malaria. *The American Journal of Tropical Medicine and Hygiene* 89(5):819-823.

Reddy, S., F. Riahi, G. Dorling, R. Callahan, and H. Patel. 2016. *Innovative approaches to prevention: Tackling the global burden of cardiovascular disease.* Doha: World Innovation Summit for Health.

Stewart, B. W., and C. P. Wild. 2014. *World cancer report 2014.* Lyon, France: International Agency for Research on Cancer, World Health Organization.

Sudfeld, C. R., D. C. McCoy, G. Danaei, G. Fink, M. Ezzati, K. G. Andrews, and W. W. Fawzi. 2015. Linear growth and child development in low- and middle-income countries: A meta-analysis. *Pediatrics* 135(5):e1266-e1275.

UN (United Nations). 2016. *Draft political declaration of the high-level meeting of the General Assembly on Antimicrobial Resistance.* New York: United Nations.

UNAIDS (Joint United Nations Programme on HIV/AIDS). 2015a. *AIDS-related deaths (all ages).* Washington, DC: Joint United Nations Programme on HIV/AIDS.

UNAIDS. 2015b. *People living with HIV (all ages).* Washington, DC: Joint United Nations Programme on HIV/AIDS.

UNICEF (United Nations International Children's Emergency Fund). 2004. *Fact sheet: Malaria, a global crisis.* New York: United Nations International Children's Emergency Fund.

USAID (U.S. Agency for International Development). 2014. *Annual report to Congress: Global health programs FY2013.* Washington, DC: U.S. Agency for International Development.

USAID. 2017. *Maternal and child health.* https://www.usaid.gov/what-we-do/global-health/maternal-and-child-health (accessed March 28, 2017).

Wagner, Z., J. Barofsky, and N. Sood. 2015. PEPFAR funding associated with an increase in employment among males in ten sub-Saharan African countries. *Health Affairs (Project Hope)* 34(6):946-953.

Waning, B., M. Kyle, E. Diedrichsen, L. Soucy, J. Hochstadt, T. Bärnighausen, and S. Moon. 2010. Intervening in global markets to improve access to HIV/AIDS treatment: An analysis of international policies and the dynamics of global antiretroviral medicines markets. *Globalization and Health* 6(1):9-27

WEF (World Economic Forum). 2010. *Global risks 2010: A global risk network report.* Geneva, Switzerland: World Economic Forum.

WEF. 2017. *The global risks report 2017.* Geneva, Switzerland: World Economic Forum.

Wexler, A., S. Oum, and J. Kates. 2016. *The status of funding for Zika: The president's request, congressional proposals, & final funding.* Washington, DC: The Henry J. Kaiser Family Foundation.

WHO (World Health Organization). 2013. *World malaria report 2013*. Geneva, Switzerland: World Health Organization.

WHO. 2015a. *World malaria report 2015*. Geneva, Switzerland: World Health Organization.

WHO. 2015b. *Noncommunicable diseases fact sheet*. Geneva, Switzerland: World Health Organization. http://www.who.int/mediacentre/factsheets/fs355/en (accessed January 20, 2017).

WHO. 2016a. *Children: Reducing mortality fact sheet*. Geneva, Switzerland: World Health Organization. http://www.who.int/mediacentre/factsheets/fs178/en (accessed February 10, 2017).

WHO. 2016b. *Global tuberculosis report 2016*. Geneva, Switzerland: World Health Organization.

WHO. 2016c. *Maternal mortality fact sheet*. Geneva, Switzerland: World Health Organization. http://www.who.int/mediacentre/factsheets/fs348/en (accessed March 8, 2017).

WHO. 2016d. *World malaria report 2016*. Geneva, Switzerland: World Health Organization.

World Bank. 2012. *People, pathogens and our planet: The economics of One Health*. Washington, DC: World Bank.

World Bank. 2013. *Flu outbreaks reminder of pandemic threat*. http://www.worldbank.org/en/news/feature/2013/03/05/flu-outbreaks-reminder-of-pandemic-threat (accessed February 15, 2017).

APPENDIXES

Appendix A

Past Institute of Medicine Reports on Global Health

AMERICA'S VITAL INTEREST IN GLOBAL HEALTH: PROTECTING OUR PEOPLE, ENHANCING OUR ECONOMY, AND ADVANCING OUR INTERNATIONAL INTERESTS (1997)

The 1997 report presaged an international movement around the turn of the millennium toward promoting health, developing new interventions and strategies for treating diseases, ensuring global health security, and reducing inequities in health and in access to health care.[1] The report called for phasing out the distinction between domestic and international health issues and implementing cooperative efforts to deal with cross-border health threats, contending that "the direct interests of the American people are best served when the United States acts decisively to promote health around the world" (IOM, 1997). The recommendations made in the 1997 Institute of Medicine (IOM) report clustered around three broad ways that the United States would benefit from entering the global health arena—protecting the American people, enhancing the American economy, and advancing American international interests. These themes are presented in the report under the guiding principle that the United States should as-

[1] Programs and organizations launched include Médecins Sans Frontières' Campaign for Access to Essential Medicines (1999); World Health Organization's Global Outbreak Alert and Response Network (2000); the Bill & Melinda Gates Foundation (2000); Stop Tuberculosis Partnership (now housed by UNOPS) (2000); Gavi, the Vaccine Alliance (2000); the United Nations' Millennium Development Goals (2000); and the Global Fund to Fight AIDS, Tuberculosis and Malaria (2002).

sume a global health leadership role and lead from its strengths, particularly in the areas of medical science and technology.

Within the theme of "protecting our people" are recommendations in the areas of *health surveillance*, *information sharing*, *research*, and *collaboration*. The board advised the U.S. government, in partnership with the corporate sector, to facilitate the development of a global network to carry out biomedical surveillance for existing and emerging infectious diseases and to serve as an early warning system for global health threats, such as potential attacks with chemical or biological agents. This network was to be bolstered by efforts to more broadly share information among countries about efficient and equitable health care financing and delivery, to invest in further international collaborative health research and new product development, and to conduct research about the prevention of violence.

To enhance the U.S. economy, the committee recommended that the U.S. government incentivize biopharmaceutical industries to research and develop products aimed primarily at populations in low- and middle-income countries (LMICs),[2] with a view to strengthen the U.S. industry and improve the population health and economic prosperity of other countries. Furthermore, the committee advised the United States to broaden the scope of its investments in global health research and development toward preventing and controlling the greatest international health burdens and threats: infectious diseases, noncommunicable diseases (NCDs), substance abuse, injuries, and violence.

To advance the international interests of the United States, the committee advised the U.S. government to parlay partnerships and cost sharing with international governments and donors into increased investment in biomedical research and development linked to global health.

To build health workforce capacity, the report called for continued long-term federal investment to build on the U.S. strength in educating and training health providers, researchers, and policy makers toward establishing a sound global health infrastructure for preventing, detecting, and treating disease and other public health threats of international scope. In the areas of global leadership and the U.S. global health strategy, the committee recommended creating a governmental Interagency Task Force on Global Health to anticipate global health needs and coordinate responses, with the U.S. Department of Health and Human Services (HHS) taking a lead role in strategizing, setting priorities, and liaising among agencies and with other sectors (academia, nongovernmental organizations [NGOs], industries, and international agencies). The report also directed the government to expand

[2] Suggested incentives include allowing multi-tiered pricing of drugs and vaccines, protecting intellectual property rights, extending patents to encourage product development, and creating public–private partnerships to develop essential products for poor populations.

its sphere of international influence by paying its dues to the United Nations (UN) system and promoting the system's reform, as well as forming international, multisectoral, and multilateral health-focused partnerships to drive research, leverage expertise, and capitalize on limited resources.

THE U.S. COMMITMENT TO GLOBAL HEALTH (2009)

The Committee on U.S. Commitment to Global Health in 2009 noted that in the years since the 1997 IOM report discussed above, the United States vital self-interest in promoting global health and health security had been borne out and even heightened in the wake of burgeoning globalization and urbanization and cross-border health threats of infectious disease (such as the 2009 H1N1 influenza epidemic), as well as unhealthy consumer goods and the high prevalence of modifiable risk factors that are linked to chronic diseases and most premature deaths worldwide. The committee expanded on the definition of global health in the 1997 report by appending the "goal of improving health for all people by reducing avoidable disease, disabilities, and deaths" (IOM, 2009). The report's recommendations concentrate on ways the United States can lead by example in international collaborative efforts to develop, finance, and deliver essential, cost-effective health interventions to improve health on a worldwide scale, but with a particular focus on LMICs. The recommendations fall into four categories: increasing U.S. financial commitments to global health; scaling up existing health interventions; partnering to invest in people, institutions, and capacity building; and sharing knowledge to address health problems in LMICs.

The interim period between the two reports saw a marked increase in both the funding and priority afforded to global health, despite the relatively low level of overall overseas development assistance extended by the United States compared with other high-income countries. The committee urged the U.S. government to meet existing international aid commitments by investing $15 billion annually in global health by 2012,[3] with $13 billion of that directed to the health-related Millennium Development Goals and $2 billion toward NCDs and injuries. Related recommendations include designing a coordinated funding approach for global health research that leverages the HHS budget for research subsidies and the foreign affairs budget for innovative funding mechanisms to procure drugs and diagnostics; prioritizing donor aid; and providing support for developing sound country-led national health plans with appropriate monitoring, evaluation, and review.

[3] This would double U.S. annual commitments to global health between 2008 ($7.51 billion) and 2012.

To improve coordination across the U.S. government, the committee recommended creating a White House Interagency Committee on Global Health, chaired by a senior official designated by the president, to be tasked with leading, planning, prioritizing, and coordinating the budgeting for major U.S. government global health programs and activities. This was done through the launch of the Global Health Initiative (GHI) in 2009 by President Obama. However, with an initiative spanning so many agencies and health areas, its success depended on strong authority and budget given to the GHI organizers. Unfortunately, they received neither, and GHI had little more than a web presence coordinating priority area global health programs.

To achieve significant health gains by scaling up existing interventions, the committee recommended that the U.S. public and private sector lead through global partnerships to prepare for the emerging health challenges of the 21st century (e.g., infectious pandemic threats, NCDs, climate change, globalization, and urbanization), and to strengthen neglected health systems by leveraging disease-specific programs. The U.S. government's global health programs and other health organizations operating in low-income countries were advised to focus on strengthening and supporting national health systems by aligning sustained assistance with the priorities of each national health sector's human resource plans.

To generate and share knowledge about how to most effectively address the health problems that disproportionately affect LMICs, the committee recommended that the U.S. research sector collaborate with global partners to leverage its scientific and technical capabilities to study the basic mechanisms of those diseases, to examine new interventions for infectious diseases, to reduce health system bottlenecks, and to rigorously evaluate programmatic efforts. To empower researchers in LMICs to improve their populations' health, the report advised establishing global networks to disseminate and expedite sharing knowledge through improved access to scientific publications (e.g., in public digital libraries), research data, materials, and patented interventions.

To promote institutional capacity building, the U.S. government and private sector were advised to foster long-term reciprocally beneficial global partnerships with institutions (academia, research institutes, and health systems) in LMICs to further enable and financially support local problem solving and policy making.[4] At the time of the report the health workforce predicament in LMICs was of crisis proportions; thus, the committee rec-

[4] Specifically, by investing in training, creating an enabling institutional environment, funding a steady stream of diverse research grants, generating demand for scientific and analytical work that influences public policy, and contributing to the control of real and immediate health problems.

ommended exploring opportunities to support country-led health-sector workforce plans and explore potential opportunities to leverage the U.S. workforce (e.g., through a global health service corps).

The committee made several recommendations about how the United States could set the example of engaging in respectful partnerships and assume the role of international leader in global health. The committee advised that enabling countries to maintain ownership and accountability for their populations' health, as well as ensuring long-term sustainability, will require donors to support local capacity building and the development of outcome-oriented country-driven agreements to coalesce all partners (public and private sector) around a national health plan, a single monitoring and evaluation framework, and a unified review process. To that end, funding support should be proportionately greater for technically and financially sound country-led health plans coupled with transparent, agreed-upon implementation strategies.

The report advised the U.S. government to act as a global health leader by paying its fair share of the World Health Organization (WHO) budget and providing technical expertise to WHO as needed, but it also called for requesting a rigorous external review of WHO aimed at maximizing its effectiveness. The U.S. president was urged to highlight health as a pillar of U.S. foreign policy, given that acting in the global interest with priorities based on effectively attaining sustained health gains (rather than short-term strategic or tactical domestic benefits) will reap longer-term economic, diplomatic, and security rewards.[5]

KEY AREAS OF RECOMMENDATION AND ADVANCEMENTS TO DATE

Despite the change in the global health landscape between the two IOM reports, certain key areas of recommendation remained consistent: sharing information, health research collaboration, health workforce capacity, U.S. global health strategy, and the role of the United States as a global leader in this domain. The 1997 report made recommendations in the areas of surveillance, medical research and development, and violence research that were not prominent in the 2009 report, while the latter report provided explicit recommendations in the areas of institutional capacity building as well as financing and donor goals. Progress to date toward in each of those 10 areas is summarized in this section.

[5] The committee also suggested that the U.S. president convene world leaders for a summit meeting at the UN General Assembly General Debate and the 2009 G20 meeting to announce the commitment to the overall global health funding recommended in the report ($15 billion per annum) as well as highlighting the importance of improving food and water security.

In the area of information sharing, global knowledge networks have been supported across sectors through WHO, the World Bank, academic research centers, and NGOs. Other efforts to cooperatively and innovatively address complex global development challenges include the Global Knowledge Initiative (2009) and the U.S. Agency for International Development's (USAID's) Higher Education Solutions Network (2012),[6] although the latter is focused more generally on development.

Progress in health research collaboration includes the Partnerships for Enhanced Engagement in Research (2011), a competitive program that offers awards to scientists from LMICs (and partners them with U.S. government-funded researchers) to support research and capacity building; the program is administered by USAID but leverages funding across the U.S. government (USAID, 2016). Other USAID efforts include its Evaluation Policy (2011) (USAID, 2011) as well as the Global Development Lab (2014), which aims to strengthen the evidence base and leverage science and technology to improve development results, with a focus on ending extreme poverty by 2030 (USAID, 2017). The National Institute of Allergy and Infectious Diseases funded eight tropical research medicine centers in 2012 to support research on neglected tropical diseases in endemic areas.

Progress in health workforce capacity is evident on multiple fronts. The Medical Education Partnership Initiative was launched in 2010 by The U.S. President's Emergency Plan for AIDS Relief (PEPFAR), the Health Resources and Services Administration, and the National Institutes of Health (NIH) to address the severe shortage of skilled health workers, despite the resources mobilized by PEPFAR and others.[7] The Nursing Education Partnership Initiative (PEPFAR, n.d.) also supports PEPFAR by aiming to train at least 140,000 new health care professionals and paraprofessionals in the partner countries of the Democratic Republic of Congo, Ethiopia, Lesotho, Malawi, and Zambia. However, these programs concluded in 2015, and thus far have not been renewed. The U.S. Centers for Disease Control and Prevention (CDC)'s Division of Global Health Protection has delivered field epidemiology training programs since 1980 (currently in 70 countries) (CDC, 2016a), as well as a new initiative called Improving Public

[6] The Global Knowledge Initiative is an NGO that seeks to surmount global development challenges through collaborative innovation and knowledge sharing by connecting innovative stakeholders with resources, expertise, and financing. See more at http://globalknowledgeinitiative.org (accessed April 17, 2017). The USAID Higher Education Solutions Network is a partnership between USAID and seven universities designed to foster cooperative scientific innovation. See more at https://www.usaid.gov/hesn (accessed April 17, 2017).

[7] MEPI addressed these shortages by improving the quality of graduates, promoting retention of graduates where they are most needed, improving capacity for regionally relevant research, building communities of practice within Africa and globally, and ensuring sustainability (NIH, 2017).

Health Management for Action (CDC, 2016c), which trains public health managers. The Global Health Service Partnership, established in 2012, is a public–private partnership between Seed Global Health, the Peace Corps, PEPFAR, and the Global Health Service Corps to send doctors and nurses to LMICs facing health care provider shortages as medical educators (Peace Corps, n.d.; Seed Global Health, 2017).

Efforts related to the U.S. global health strategy include the GHI (2008), a presidential initiative that was launched with great fanfare, but did not receive anticipated funding, attributable at least in part to a lack of clear leadership or hierarchy. The Global Health Security Agenda (2014) (GHSA, n.d.) is a partnership that seeks to build country-level capacity to address the threat of infectious disease and maintain global health security through implementation of the International Health Regulations (2005). Currently, the President's National Security Council serves the coordinating role in calling for interagency policy committees as needed for specific topics or initiatives.

Progress toward the United States assuming a global leadership role as requested through multilateral engagement in health is less apparent. As of 2015, the United States was assessed at 28 percent of the UN peacekeeping budget and 22 percent of the regular budget (UN, 2016, 2017), and 22 percent of the overall WHO budget (WHO, 2015). However, a significant proportion of this funding still is unpaid (WHO, 2017). The 2009 G20 meeting included food security but not water; however, at the 2009 G8 summit President Obama announced plans for increased investment in global food security.[8]

In surveillance, a focus of the 1997 report's recommendations, progress at the global level includes the International Health Regulations (established in 2005) and the CDC Country Partnerships for Integrated Disease Surveillance and Response Implementation, which seeks to make surveillance and laboratory data more usable by public health managers and other decision makers in improving detection and response to health problems in African countries (CDC, 2017). The Global Outbreak Alert and Response Network (WHO, n.d.) (2000) is a collaboration to guide technical expertise on the ground during disease outbreaks that pose an international threat.[9]

---

[8] For example, Feed the Future (2012), is a whole-of-government approach led by USAID to address extreme poverty, undernutrition, and hunger. See more at https://www.feedthefuture.gov/about (accessed April 17, 2017).

[9] In addition to these sources of surveillance data, there are informal sources, including the International Society for Infectious Diseases–Program for Monitoring Emerging Diseases (ISID, 2014), the Global Public Health Intelligence Network via Health Canada (Government of Canada, 2016), the CDC Global Disease Detection Operations Center (CDC, 2016b), and HealthMap (HealthMap, n.d.).

The 2016 publication *The Neglected Dimension of Global Security* recommended that WHO should generate a high-priority "watch list" of outbreaks to be released to national focal points on a daily basis and on a weekly basis to the public. However, the commission noted that reporting by countries will need to be incentivized by International Health Regulations toward a broader aim of fostering transparency in information sharing (GHRF Commission, 2016). At the national level, Homeland Security Presidential Directive 10 (2004) addresses biodefense for the 21st century (Bush, 2004). However, according to a 2016 Blue Ribbon Study Panel on Biodefense, the U.S. Department of Homeland Security (DHS) National Biosurveillance Integration Center (DHS, 2016) has been unable to meet its mandate of "integrating and analyzing data relating to human health, animal, plant, food, and environmental monitoring systems" (Blue Ribbon Study Panel on Biodefense, 2015). Thus, while much progress has been made since 1997 in surveillance at national and global levels, the 2009 H1N1 outbreak and the 2014–2015 Ebola outbreak illustrate that there is still a long way to go before countries are able to rapidly detect and report disease outbreak.

In the area of medical research and development, another focus of the 1997 report, the Office of the Assistant Secretary for Preparedness and Response established the Biomedical Advanced Research and Development Authority in 2006 through the Pandemic and All-Hazards Preparedness Act,[10] which incentivizes cost sharing through Centers of Innovation for Advanced Development and Manufacturing partnerships between the U.S. government and the private sector for collaboration, development, cost sharing, and ensuring surge capacity for vaccine manufacturing (ASPR, 2007). The U.S. Food and Drug Administration's (FDA's) Priority Review Voucher program (2007) spurs development by allowing for expedited FDA review of certain types of new drugs (i.e. neglected diseases, medical countermeasures, and rare pediatric diseases), which can translate into millions in dollars of profits (Gaffney et al., 2016). The U.S. Patent and Trademark Office's Patents for Humanity program awards patents to innovators striving to address global humanitarian challenges (USPTO, 2016). In addition to these programs, the U.S. supports key public–private partnerships—product development partnerships—that are instrumental in incentivizing the innovation of diagnostics drugs that target poverty-related diseases.

To advance violence research as recommended in the 1997 report, the U.S. Department of State and USAID have funded sexual- and gender-based violence prevention and response projects (2012).[11] CDC, the United

[10] H.R. 307, 113th Congress.

[11] Pursuant to Section 7061 of the Conference Report accompanying the U.S. Department of State, Foreign Operations, and Related Programs Appropriations Act, 2012 (Div. I, Public Law 112-74).

Nations Population Fund, and the Office of the United Nations High Commissioner for Refugees have conducted population-based studies in Liberia, East Timor, and Uganda to examine violence against women, and NIH has funded research grants addressing partner violence in the context of human immunodeficiency virus (HIV) programming.

Institutional capacity building, as well as donor goals and financing, were areas of recommendation for the 2009 IOM report. To the former, the CDC Global Disease Detection Program works in 50 countries through 10 centers to develop six core capacities[12] formulated to achieve compliance with International Health Regulations (CDC, 2016b). The Health Systems 20/20 Project (2008–2012) was USAID's global health flagship project designed to strengthen health systems though integrative approaches to addressing financing, governance, operational, and capacity-system constraints (USAID, 2013). The USAID Collaborative Support for Health program in Liberia seeks to strengthen the health system's resilience in emergency contexts (MSH, 2017).

With respect to donor goals and financing, funding did increase slightly after 2008 but not to the extent recommended in the IOM report; it hovered around $9 billion annually from 2009 to 2016 (Salaam-Blyther, 2013).[13] There has been an ideological shift toward country ownership reflected in the change in terminology from *aid* to *partnership* and a new emphasis on government-to-government funding, which will become clear in the 2017 committee report recommendations as well.

REFERENCES

ASPR (Assistant Secretary for Preparedness and Response). 2007. *Pandemic and All-Hazards Preparedness Act: Progress report.* Washington, DC: Assistant Secretary for Preparedness and Response (ASPR), U.S. Department of Health and Human Services.

Blue Ribbon Study Panel on Biodefense. 2015. *A national blueprint for biodefense: Leadership and major reform needed to optimize efforts.* Washington, DC.

Bush, G. 2004. *Biodefense for the 21st century.* Washington, DC.

CDC (U.S. Centers for Disease Control and Prevention). 2016a. *Field epidemiology and training program (FETP).* https://www.cdc.gov/globalhealth/healthprotection/fetp (accessed March 20, 2017).

CDC. 2016b. *Global disease detection program: About us.* https://www.cdc.gov/globalhealth/healthprotection/gdd/about.html (accessed March 21, 2017).

[12] Core capacities: emerging infectious disease detection and response; training in field epidemiology and laboratory methods; pandemic influenza preparedness and response; zoonotic disease investigation and control; health communication and information technology; laboratory systems and biosafety.

[13] Appropriated U.S. funding for global health between 2009 and 2016 fluctuated: $8.46 billion in 2009, $9.016 billion in 2010, $8.86 billion in 2011 (Salaam-Blyther, 2013), $9.8 billion in 2012, $9.6 billion in 2013, $10.2 billion in 2014, $10.2 billion in 2015, and 10.2 billion in 2016 (Valentine et al., 2016).

CDC. 2016c. *Improving Public Health Management for Action (IMPACT)*. https://www.cdc.gov/globalhealth/healthprotection/impact/index.html (accessed March 20, 2017).

CDC. 2017. *Integrated disease surveillance response (ISDR)*. http://www.cdc.gov/globalhealth/healthprotection/idsr/index.html (accessed March 20, 2017).

DHS (U.S. Department of Homeland Security). 2016. *National Biosurveillance Integration Center*. https://www.dhs.gov/national-biosurveillance-integration-center (accessed March 20, 2017).

Gaffney, A., M. Mezher, and Z. Brennan. 2016. *Regulatory explainer: Everything you need to know about FDA's Priority Review Vouchers*. http://www.raps.org/Regulatory-Focus/News/2015/07/02/21722/Regulatory-Explainer-Everything-You-Need-to-Know-About-FDA%E2%80%99s-Priority-Review-Vouchers (accessed February 13, 2017).

GHRF Commission (Commission on a Global Health Risk Framework for the Future). 2016. *The neglected dimension of global security: A framework to counter infectious disease crises*. doi: https://doi.org/10.17226/21891.

GHSA (Global Health Security Agenda). n.d. *What is GHSA?* https://www.ghsagenda.org/. (accessed March 20, 2017).

Government of Canada. 2016. *About GHPIN*. https://gphin.canada.ca/cepr/aboutgphin-rmispenbref.jsp?language=en_CA (accessed December 10, 2016).

HealthMap. n.d. *About*. http://www.healthmap.org/site/about (accessed December 10, 2016).

IOM (Institute of Medicine). 1997. *America's vital interest in global health: Protecting our people, enhancing our economy, and advancing our international interests*. Washington, DC: National Academy Press.

IOM. 2009. *The U.S. commitment to global health: Recommendations for the public and private sectors*. Washington, DC: The National Academies Press.

ISID (International Society for Infectious Diseases). 2014. *About promed-mail*. https://www.promedmail.org/aboutus (accessed December 15, 2016).

MSH (Management Sciences for Health). 2017. *USAID Collaborative Support for Health program*. https://www.msh.org/our-work/projects/usaid-collaborative-support-for-health-program (accessed December 19, 2016).

NIH (National Institutes of Health). 2017. *Medical Education Partnership Initiative (MEPI)*. https://www.fic.nih.gov/programs/pages/medical-education-africa.aspx (accessed December 10, 2016).

Peace Corps. n.d. *Global Health Service Partnership*. https://www.peacecorps.gov/volunteer/is-peace-corps-right-for-me/global-health-service-partnership (accessed March 20, 2017).

PEPFAR (The U.S. President's Emergency Plan for AIDS Relief). n.d. *Nursing Education Partnership Initiative (NEPI)*. http://www.pepfar.gov/partnerships/initiatives/nepi (accessed March 20, 2017).

Salaam-Blyther, T. 2013. *U.S. global health assistance: Background issues for the 113th Congress*. Washington, DC: Congressional Research Service.

Seed Global Health. 2017. *History*. http://seedglobalhealth.org/about/history/#.WP5B6PnyvRZ (accessed April 24, 2017).

UN (United Nations). 2016. *Assessment of member states' contributions to the United Nations regular budget for the year 2017*. New York: United Nations General Assembly.

UN. 2017. *Peacekeeping fact sheet*. http://www.un.org/en/peacekeeping/resources/statistics/factsheet.shtml (accessed April 17, 2017).

USAID (U.S. Agency for International Development). 2011. *Evaluation: Learning from experience*. Washington, DC: U.S. Agency for International Development.

USAID. 2013. *Health systems 20/20*. https://www.usaid.gov/node/50731 (accessed December 18, 2016).

USAID. 2016. *Higher Education Solutions Network (HESN)*. https://www.usaid.gov/hesn (accessed March 20, 2017).

USAID. 2017. *The U.S. Global Development Lab*. https://www.usaid.gov/globaldevlab (accessed March 20, 2017).

USPTO (U.S. Patent and Trade Office). 2016. *Patents for humanity*. https://www.uspto.gov/patent/initiatives/patents-humanity (accessed December 15, 2016).

Valentine, A., A. Wexler, and J. Kates. 2016. *The U.S. Global Health Budget: Analysis of the fiscal year 2017 budget request*. http://kff.org/global-health-policy/issue-brief/the-u-s-global-health-budget-analysis-of-the-fiscal-year-2017-budget-request (accessed January 26, 2017).

WHO (World Health Organization). 2015. *Scale of assessments for 2016-2017*. Geneva, Switzerland: World Health Organization.

WHO. 2017. *Assessed contribution status report as at 31 March 2017*. Geneva, Switzerland: World Health Organization.

WHO. n.d. *Global Outbreak Alert and Response Network (GOARN)*. http://www.who.int/ihr/alert_and_response/outbreak-network/en (accessed March 20, 2017).

B

Global Health Organizations Referenced in This Report[1]

A

Acting on the Call: Ending Preventable Child and Maternal Deaths
Parent organization: U.S. Agency for International Development (USAID)
Website: https://www.usaid.gov/ActingOnTheCall
Category: U.S. government program
Area of focus: women's and children's health

ASPR: Assistant Secretary for Preparedness and Response
Parent organization: U.S. Department of Health and Human Services (HHS)
Website: https://www.phe.gov/about/aspr/pages/default.aspx
Category: U.S. government program
Area of focus: preparedness

B

BARDA: Biomedical Advanced Research and Development Authority
Parent organization: U.S. Department of Health and Human Services (HHS)
Website: https://www.phe.gov/about/BARDA/Pages/default.aspx
Category: U.S. government program
Area of focus: drug development and discovery

[1] This glossary is meant to provide additional information on the organizations and agencies working in global health mentioned in this report. Please note this is just a representative sample of the many successful programs in global health and is not meant to be an exhaustive list.

C

CARB-X: Combating Antibiotic-Resistant Bacteria Biopharmaceutical Accelerator
Website: http://www.carb-x.org/home
Category: public–private partnership
Area of focus: antibiotic resistance

CDC: U.S. Centers for Disease Control and Prevention
Website: https://www.cdc.gov
Category: U.S. government department
Area of focus: public health

CEPI: Coalition for Epidemic Preparedness Innovation
Website: http://cepi.net
Category: public–private partnership
Area of focus: research and development for pandemics

D

DREAMS: Determined, Resilient, Empowered, AIDS-free, Mentored, and Safe women
Parent organization: The U.S. President's Emergency Plan for AIDS Relief (PEPFAR)
Website: https://www.pepfar.gov/partnerships/ppp/dreams
Category: public–private partnership
Area of focus: AIDS prevention in young women

E

The End TB Strategy
Parent organization: World Health Organization (WHO)
Website: http://www.who.int/tb/post2015_strategy/en
Category: nongovernmental organization program
Area of focus: tuberculosis

Every Woman Every Child
Parent organization: United Nations
Website: https://www.everywomaneverychild.org
Category: nongovernmental organization program
Area of focus: women's and children's health

F

FETP: Field Epidemiology Training Program
Parent organization: U.S. Centers for Disease Control and Prevention (CDC)
Website: https://www.cdc.gov/globalhealth/healthprotection/fetp
Category: U.S. government–sponsored program
Area of focus: epidemiology, outbreak response

FHI 360: Family Health International
Website: https://www.fhi360.org
Category: nongovernmental organization
Area of focus: global health development

FP2020: Family Planning 2020
Website: http://www.familyplanning2020.org
Category: nongovernmental organization
Area of focus: family planning, women's health

G

Gavi, the Vaccine Alliance
Website: http://www.gavi.org
Category: public–private partnership
Area of focus: immunization coverage

GFF: Global Financing Facility
Parent organization: World Bank
Website: https://www.globalfinancingfacility.org
Category: public–private partnership
Area of focus: women's and children's health financing

GHSA: Global Health Security Agenda
Website: https://www.ghsagenda.org
Category: public–private partnership/multilateral organization
Area of focus: global health security

Global Development Lab
Parent organization: U.S. Agency for International Development (USAID)
Website: https://www.usaid.gov/GlobalDevLab/about
Category: U.S. government organization program
Area of focus: global health innovation

Global Fund to Fight AIDS, Tuberculosis and Malaria
Website: http://www.theglobalfund.org/en
Category: nongovernmental organization
Area of focus: AIDS, tuberculosis, and malaria

H

Health Attaché Program
Parent organization: U.S. Department of Health and Human Services (HHS)
Website: https://www.hhs.gov/about/agencies/oga/global-health-diplomacy/health-attaches/index.html
Category: U.S. government organization program
Area of focus: global health diplomacy

HHS: U.S. Department of Health and Human Services
Website: https://www.hhs.gov
Category: U.S. government organization
Area of focus: many areas of global health

L

The *Lancet* Commission on Investing in Health
Parent organization: *The Lancet*
Website: http://www.thelancet.com/global-health/commissions/global-health-2035
Category: journal commission
Area of focus: economics of health

M

MDGs: Millennium Development Goals
Website: http://www.un.org/millenniumgoals
Category: nongovernmental organization program
Area of focus: global development

MEPI: Medical Education Partnership Initiative
Parent organization: The U.S. President's Emergency Plan for AIDS Relief (PEPFAR)
Website: https://www.pepfar.gov/partnerships/initiatives/index.htm#
Category: U.S. government program
Area of Focus: workforce strengthening

MSF: Médecins Sans Frontières
Website: http://www.msf.org
Category: nongovernmental organization
Area of focus: health aid and emergency health response

N

NEPI: Nursing Education Partnership Initiative
Parent organization: The U.S. President's Emergency Plan for AIDS Relief (PEPFAR)
Website: https://www.pepfar.gov/partnerships/initiatives/index.htm#
Category: U.S. government program
Area of Focus: workforce strengthening

NIH: National Institutes of Health
Parent organization: U.S. Department of Health and Human Services (HHS)
Website: https://www.nih.gov
Category: U.S. government organization
Area of focus: medical research and development

O

OECD: Organisation for Economic Co-operation and Development
Website: http://www.oecd.org/about
Category: nongovernmental organization
Area of focus: economic development

P

PACCARB: Presidential Advisory Council on Combating Antibiotic-Resistant Bacteria
Parent organization: U.S. Department of Health and Human Services (HHS)
Website: https://www.hhs.gov/ash/advisory-committees/paccarb
Category: U.S. government program
Area of Focus: antimicrobial resistance

PATH
Website: http://www.path.org
Category: nongovernmental organization
Area of focus: global health innovation

PCAST: President's Council of Advisors on Science and Technology
Website: https://obamawhitehouse.archives.gov/administration/eop/ostp/pcast/about
Category: U.S. government council
Area of focus: science and technology

PEPFAR: The U.S. President's Emergency Plan for AIDS Relief
Parent organization: U.S. Department of State
Website: https://www.pepfar.gov
Category: U.S. government program
Area of focus: HIV/AIDS

PHEMCE: Public Health Emergency Medical Countermeasures Enterprise
Parent organization: U.S. Department of Health and Human Services (HHS)
Website: https://www.phe.gov/Preparedness/mcm/phemce/Pages/default.aspx
Category: U.S. government program
Area of focus: research and development for medical countermeasures

PMI: President's Malaria Initiative
Website: https://www.pmi.gov
Category: U.S. government program
Area of focus: malaria

PRRR: Pink Ribbon Red Ribbon
Website: http://pinkribbonredribbon.org
Category: nongovernmental organization
Area of focus: women's cancers

S

Saving Mothers, Giving Life Partnership
Parent organization: U.S. Agency for International Development (USAID)
Website: https://www.usaid.gov/what-we-do/global-health/maternal-and-child-health/projects/saving-mothers-giving-life
Category: U.S. government program
Area of focus: maternal mortality and child mortality

SDGs: Sustainable Development Goals
Website: https://sustainabledevelopment.un.org/sdgs
Category: nongovernmental organization program
Area of focus: global development

U

UKAID: United Kingdom Department for International Development
Website: https://ukaiddirect.org
Category: U.K. government organization
Area of focus: foreign aid and development

UN: United Nations
Website: http://www.un.org/en/index.html
Category: nongovernmental organization
Area of focus: global governance

UNAIDS: Joint United Nations Programme on HIV/AIDS
Parent organization: United Nations
Website: http://www.unaids.org
Category: nongovernmental organization
Area of focus: HIV/AIDS

UNICEF: United Nations International Children's Emergency Fund
Parent organization: United Nations
Website: https://www.unicef.org
Category: nongovernmental organization
Area of focus: children's health

USAID: U.S. Agency for International Development
Website: https://www.usaid.gov
Category: U.S. government organization
Area of focus: foreign aid and development

W

WHO: World Health Organization
Website: http://www.who.int/en
Category: nongovernmental organization
Area of focus: global health governance

World Bank
Website: http://www.worldbank.org
Category: nongovernmental organization
Area of focus: global health financing

World Economic Forum
Website: https://www.weforum.org
Category: nongovernmental organization
Area of focus: global economic issues

Appendix C

Public Meeting Agendas

COMMITTEE MEETING ONE
September 29, 2016
Washington, DC

1:00–1:10 pm **Welcoming Remarks**
Jendayi Frazer, Co-Chair
Valentin Fuster, Co-Chair

1:10–2:45 pm **Sponsor Briefing: Discussion of the Committee's Charge**
Ariel Pablos-Méndez
Assistant Administrator for Global Health, U.S. Agency for International Development

Vikas Kapil
Associate Director for Science and Chief Medical Officer, Center for Global Health, U.S. Centers for Disease Control and Prevention

Leslie Ball
Assistant Commissioner for International Programs, Office of International Programs, U.S. Food and Drug Administration

	Roger Glass Director, Fogarty International Center, National Institutes of Health
	David Smith Deputy Assistant Secretary of Defense for Health Readiness Policy and Oversight, U.S. Department of Defense
	Summer Galloway Senior Policy Advisor, U.S. Department of Defense
	Christian Hassell Deputy Assistant Secretary of Defense for Chemical and Biological Defense Programs, U.S. Department of Defense
	Paurvi Bhatt (via teleconference) Senior Director for Global Access, Medtronic Philanthropy
2:45–3:15 pm	**Discussion with Committee**
3:15–3:30 pm	**Break**
3:30–4:15 pm	**Global Health and the United States—Past and Future Directions** Thomas Bollyky Senior Fellow for Global Health, Economics, and Development, Council on Foreign Relations
	Rebecca Katz Director, Center for Global Health Science and Security, Georgetown University
	Helene Gayle Cochair, CSIS Task Force on Women's and Family Health; CEO, McKinsey Social Initiative
4:15–4:30 pm	**Discussion with Committee**

4:30–5:30 pm	**Public Comment Period** Any additional input/feedback from participants
5:30 pm	**Adjourn**

COMMITTEE MEETING TWO
December 6, 2016
Washington, DC

10:00–10:10 am	**Welcome and Introduction** Jendayi Frazer, Co-Chair Valentin Fuster, Co-Chair
10:10–11:00 am	**Overview and Programs: A Changing Landscape** Jimmy Kolker Assistant Secretary for Global Affairs, U.S. Department of Health and Human Services Chris Elias (via videoconference) President, Global Development Program, Bill & Melinda Gates Foundation Mark Dybul (via videoconference) Executive Director, Global Fund Loyce Pace Executive Director, Global Health Council
11:00 am–12:00 pm	**Discussion with Committee**
12:00–1:00 pm	**Lunch**
1:00–1:45 pm	**Future Financing Strategies for Global Health** Mariam Claeson Director, Global Financing Facility Natasha Bilimoria Director, U.S. Strategy, Gavi, the Vaccine Alliance

	Claire Qureshi Office of the United Nations Special Envoy for Health in Agenda 2030 and for Malaria; Interim Project Director, Financing Alliance for Health
1:45–2:45 pm	**Discussion with Committee**
2:45–3:00 pm	**Break**
3:00 pm	**Innovation to Build Capacity and Improve Health** Peter Singer (via videoconference) CEO, Grand Challenges Canada Kirsten Gagnaire Managing Director, Global Health and Digital Development, FSG Ed Seguine CEO, Clinical Ink Sarah Glass Director for Special Projects, U.S. Global Development Lab, U.S. Agency for International Development
4:00 pm	**Discussion with Committee**
5:00 pm	**Adjourn**

Appendix D

Committee Member Biosketches

Jendayi E. Frazer, Ph.D. (*Co-Chair*), is adjunct senior fellow for Africa studies at the Council on Foreign Relations (CFR). Dr. Frazer was a distinguished public service professor at Carnegie Mellon University from 2009 to 2014, where she was on the faculty of Heinz College's School of Public Policy and Management. Her research focused on strengthening regional security cooperation and economic and political integration in Africa. She was the director of Carnegie Mellon's Center for International Policy and Innovation (CIPI), which focuses on using technology and applying innovative solutions to core issues of development and governance in Africa. The author of and contributor to a number of articles, journals, and books, she is the co-editor of *Preventing Electoral Violence in Africa* (2011), which grows out of her work with CIPI. Dr. Frazer served as the U.S. assistant secretary of state for African affairs from 2005 to 2009. She was special assistant to the president and senior director for African affairs at the National Security Council from 2001 until her swearing-in as the first woman U.S. ambassador to South Africa in 2004.

She previously served in government from 1998 to 1999 as a CFR International Affairs Fellow, first at the Pentagon as a political-military planner with the Joint Chiefs of Staff, working on West Africa during Nigeria's transition to civilian rule, and then as director for African affairs at the National Security Council, working on Central and East Africa. Dr. Frazer was also an assistant professor of public policy at the Harvard Kennedy School of Government and assistant professor at the University of Denver's Graduate School of International Studies. She has been awarded the Distinguished Service Medal, the highest award bestowed by the Secretary of State in recognition of her public service. In 2010, she was given the distinction of Dame Grand Commander in the Humane Order of African Redemption by Liberian President Ellen Johnson Sirleaf. She was also honored with the 2008 Distinguished Leadership Award from Boston University's African Presidential Archives and Research Center. Frazer received her B.A. in political science and African and Afro-American studies, M.A. in international policy studies and international development education, and Ph.D. in political science, all from Stanford University.

Valentin Fuster, M.D. (*Co-Chair*) serves the Mount Sinai Medical Hospital as physician-in-chief, as well as director of Mount Sinai Heart, the Zena and Michael A. Wiener Cardiovascular Institute, and the Marie-Josée and Henry R. Kravis Center for Cardiovascular Health. He is also the Richard Gorlin, MD/Heart Research Foundation Professor, Icahn School of Medicine at Mount Sinai. Dr. Fuster was the President of Science and is now the General Director of the Centro Nacional de Investigaciones Cardiovasculares Carlos III (CNIC) in Madrid, Spain, and is also chairman of the Science, Health and Education Foundation (SHE). The innumerable positions he has held include those of president of the American Heart Association, president of the World Heart Federation, member of the National Academy of Medicine, member of the U.S. National Heart, Lung, and Blood Institute, and president of the training program of the American College of Cardiology. Dr. Fuster received his medical degree from the University of Barcelona. He has served as professor in medicine and cardiovascular diseases at the Mayo Medical School and the Medical School of Mount Sinai Hospital, and professor of medicine at Harvard Medical School and chief of cardiology at the Massachusetts General Hospital, Boston.

In 1994, he was named director of the Cardiovascular Institute at Mount Sinai, a post he has combined since 2012 with that of physician-in-chief of the hospital. Dr. Fuster has been named Doctor Honoris Causa by 33 universities around the world, and has earned three of the most important awards from the National Institutes of Health (NIH). He is an author of more than 900 scientific articles in international medical journals, and has published as lead editor of two leading books on clinical cardiology and research. He was also named editor-in-chief of the journal *Nature Reviews in Cardiology*. Dr. Fuster, in addition to his dedication to research, is strongly committed to his responsibility to communicate to the public. This commitment has in the last 4 years produced six books. His vocation and the clear need to promote healthy lifestyle habits recently led to Dr. Fuster launching the Science, Health and Education Foundation (SHE), which is directed at improving public health, especially in the young.

Gisela Abbam, M.B.A., is global executive director for government affairs and policy for General Electric (GE) Healthcare. Ms. Abbam is responsible for the strategic direction of government affairs and policy for GE Healthcare, the $18 billion business unit of General Electric that provides transformational medical technologies and solutions to health customers in more than 100 countries. She works in collaboration with the World Health Organization (WHO) and other international organizations to improve health outcomes. Furthermore, Ms. Abbam leads and drives a broad range of legislative and policy issues to shape global health policies. She is focused on addressing health needs of various countries. Ms. Abbam has written more than 40 briefings on various policy issues including health reform. Ms. Abbam is also currently the chair of the Global Diagnostic Imaging, Healthcare IT & Radiation Therapy Trade Association (DITTA) WHO Working Group. Ms. Abbam was previously head of government affairs for GE Healthcare for the United Kingdom and Ireland and successfully initiated an Early Diagnosis Campaign in collaboration with several charities (NGOs) to improve early diagnosis in the United Kingdom across all diseases, which gained attention by the prime minister and key members of Parliament. Due to her leadership, GE Healthcare won its first ever award for its contribution to improving stroke management. Ms. Abbam joined GE Healthcare in 2007 after 13 years working in the National Health Service and Local Government in the United Kingdom. Ms. Abbam was on the leadership team that set up the Centre for Public Health Excellence at the internationally acclaimed National Institute for Health and Clinical Excellence (NICE). She developed the Operating Model and Structure for the Centre. Until April 2010, Ms. Abbam served on the board of Dimensions UK (formerly Adepta), a health charity. She is currently a nonexecutive Director for Strong Tower Missionaries. Ms. Abbam holds an M.B.A. and an honors degree in education.

Amie Batson, M.B.A., is the chief strategy officer and vice president of strategy and learning at PATH. Ms. Batson is responsible for guiding PATH's strategy, strengthening their partnerships and business relationships in the global health community, and contributing to their advocacy and policy priorities. Ms. Batson's 20-year career in global health includes positions with WHO, the United Nations International Children's Emergency Fund (UNICEF), the World Bank, and most recently, the U.S. Agency for International Development (USAID), where she served as senior deputy assistant administrator for global health. During her 3-year appointment with USAID, Ms. Batson led the agency's engagement in the president's Global Health Initiative, represented the U.S. government on the board of the Gavi Alliance, and led the U.S. government team in co-convening the Child Survival Call to Action, which launched the global vision to end preventable child deaths. Throughout her career in global health, Ms. Batson has been a leader in innovation. Her contributions to immunization and vaccine financing at the World Bank resulted in billions of dollars in new funding for global health and the vaccination of millions of children against polio, pneumonia, and other vaccine-preventable causes of death. Ms. Batson earned a B.A. in economics from the University of Virginia and an M.B.A. from the Yale University School of Management.

Frederick M. Burkle, Jr., M.D., M.P.H., DTM, is senior fellow and scientist, the Harvard Humanitarian Initiative, Harvard University, and Harvard School of Public Health, and senior associate faculty and research scientist, the Center for Refugee & Disaster Response, Johns Hopkins University Medical Institutes. Since 2008 he has served as a senior international public policy scholar, Woodrow Wilson Center for International Scholars, Washington, DC. He served as deputy assistant administrator for the Bureau of Global Health at USAID, U.S. Department of State. He is currently an adjunct professor at Monash University Medical School, Melbourne, and James Cook University, Queensland, in Australia and Uniformed Services University of Health Sciences, and retired professor of surgery, pediatrics, and tropical medicine at the University of Hawaii. Dr. Burkle is a graduate of Saint Michael's College (1961) and the University of Vermont College of Medicine (1965), and holds a master's degree in public health.

He is board qualified in Emergency Medicine, Pediatric Emergency Medicine, Pediatrics, Psychiatry, Public Health, and Tropical Medicine. He is a Fellow of the American College of Emergency Physicians and the American Academy of Pediatrics. Dr. Burkle has worked in and consulted on numerous humanitarian emergencies and large-scale international disasters in Asia, Africa, the Middle East, and Eastern Europe, and is currently a consultant for WHO-Health Action in Crises. Dr. Burkle was elected to the National Academy of Medicine in 2007. He is a member of the Board of Directors of the International Rescue Committee and the Scientific Advisory Board of the American Red Cross. A retired captain in the U.S. Naval Reserve he completed combat tours in the Vietnam (1968) and the Persian Gulf Wars with the 1st, 2nd, and 3rd Marine Divisions, and with the U.S. Central Command in Somalia.

Lynda Chin, M.D., is currently chief innovation officer and associate vice chancellor for health affairs, director of the Institute for Health Transformation at the University of Texas System. Dr. Chin is focusing on addressing the rising chronic disease burden that is threatening the health and productivity of Americans and the solvency of its health care system through innovative technology and business solutions and public–private partnerships. Throughout her career, Dr. Chin has championed a model of integration, collaboration, and cooperation between the research and clinical care enterprises, as well as between public and private sectors. She was the scientific director of the Belfer Institute for Applied Cancer Science at Dana-Farber Cancer Institute and subsequently the Institute for Applied Cancer Science at the MD Anderson Cancer Center, an organization designed to bring together the best attributes of academia and industry in a new organizational construct to rapidly translate cancer genomics knowledge into effective therapeutic endpoints. In her current endeavor, Dr. Chin has been the architect behind a digital health infrastructure built on interconnected technology and service platforms developed by AT&T, IBM, and PwC, designed to support secure and private sharing of contextualized patient health profiles synthesized from not only electronic health record (EHR) data, but also real-world clinical data, patient-generated health data, and other data sources. Through such connectivity, Dr. Chin is convening an ecosystem of technology, service, retail, and health care stakeholders in both public and private sectors to collaborate in tackling the challenges of diabetes in an underserved community in South Texas.

Dr. Chin graduated with an M.D. degree from Albert Einstein College of Medicine and is a board-certified dermatologist. She conducted her clinical and scientific training at Columbia Presbyterian Medical Center and the Albert Einstein College of Medicine, where she completed in parallel her residency training in the hospital and postdoctoral fellowship in the laboratory. For 13 years, Dr. Chin was a professor of dermatology at Dana-Farber Cancer Institute and Harvard Medical School and a senior associate member of the Broad Institute of the Massachusetts Institute of Technology and Harvard. Her research program spans the fields of transcription, telomere biology, cancer genomics, and personalized cancer medicine. Dr. Chin held multiple leadership roles in *The Cancer Genome Atlas*. She is a member of the Scientific Steering Committee of the International Cancer Genome Consortium. Dr. Chin joined the MD Anderson Cancer Center in 2011 as the founding chair for the Department of Genomic Medicine, with a mission to bring to bear on the cancer crisis not only the transformative potential of genomics, but also of data, technologies, and innovative strategies. She led the development of MD Anderson Oncology Expert Advisor, an example of a cognitive expert system for democratization of clinical expertise for evidence-based care. Dr. Chin was elected a member of the National Academy of Medicine in 2012.

Stephanie L. Ferguson, Ph.D., R.N., FAAN, is a consulting associate professor in the Stanford in Washington Program at Stanford University, professor of nursing in the School of Health Science and Human Performance at Lynchburg College, and frequent consultant and facilitator for WHO and the Pan American Health Organization (PAHO). Since 2000, Dr. Ferguson has contributed to various WHO resolutions and initiatives on "Strengthening Nursing and Midwifery," progress reports, and recently the development of the Global Strategic Directions for Nursing and Midwifery (SDNM) 2016–2020. Dr. Ferguson is currently working with WHO to develop the Monitoring and Evaluation Framework for the SDNM 2016–2020 and the PAHO Strategic Direction for Nursing in the Americas. She is also Honorary Council Board Member for the G4 Alliance for Safe Surgical Care. Dr. Ferguson is a board member of the Bon Secours Health System, Inc.; member of the National Academy of Medicine; distinguished practitioner in the National Academies of Practice; and fellow of the American Academy of Nursing; where she serves as the chair of its Institute for Nursing Leadership's National Advisory Council. Dr. Ferguson is a member of the *Nursing Economic$* journal's editorial board and the director of its Global Health Department, which includes the regularly featured column, "Global Health."

She was the former director of the International Council of Nurses' (ICN) Leadership for Change Program and the ICN-Burdett Global Nursing Leadership Institute. In 1996 and 1997, Dr. Ferguson was appointed a White House Fellow and worked with the Honorable Secretary Donna E. Shalala at the U.S. Department of Health and Human Services (HHS). HHS Secretary Tommy Thompson appointed her in 2001 to serve on the Advisory Council of the National Institute of Nursing Research (NINR) at NIH. Dr. Ferguson also served on the HHS's Health Resources and Services Administration Task Force for examining nursing's workforce issues related to racial, ethnic, and gender diversity. She was selected by the U.S. Department of Defense in 2001 to attend its Airforce Air War College's National Security Forum. In 2010–2011, HHS, the U.S. Department of State, and NINR/NIH appointed her to serve on the Global Advances in Practice and Research in Nursing (GAPRIN) program. GAPRIN was designed to build nurse capacity globally through evidence-based practice for President Obama's Global Health Initiative (GHI). She was elected as a member of the Board of Trustees for the U.S. Catholic Health Association (CHA) and she served as a member of the Catholic Medical Mission Board (CMMB). Dr. Ferguson is a widely sought after consultant and keynote speaker worldwide addressing various nursing, health professional, and global and domestic health issues. She has worked in the U.S. addressing global health issues with many federal agencies and organizations such as the Veterans Health Administration, the U.S. Navy, the U.S. Army Nurse Corps, the U.S. Public Health Nurse Corps, and the American Red Cross.

Lia Haskin Fernald, Ph.D., M.B.A., is a professor in the School of Public Health at the University of California, Berkeley. She holds a Ph.D. in international nutrition and child development from the University of London and an M.B.A. from the University of California, Berkeley, with a focus on health management. Dr. Fernald was a Fulbright Scholar in Jamaica and has been working in the field of public health nutrition for more than 20 years focusing specifically on children in developing countries. Her work has focused primarily on how inequalities in socioeconomic position contribute to growth and developmental outcomes in mothers, infants, and children, and on how interventions can address socioeconomic and health disparities. Much of her work for the past two decades has centered on looking at the effects of interventions (e.g., conditional cash transfer programs, parenting programs, microcredit interventions, and community-based nutrition interventions) on child development and maternal mental health, particularly focused on low- and middle-income countries. She recently worked with a team of authors to write two review papers for *The Lancet* about strategies to address poor development among infants and children in low- and middle-income countries.

Peter Lamptey, M.D., Dr.P.H., is based in Accra, Ghana, and is a distinguished scientist/president emeritus at Family Health International 360 (FHI 360). He serves on the FHI 360 executive team that provides managerial, financial, and strategic leadership to FHI 360's development programs in more than 55 low- and middle-income countries. Dr. Lamptey is also a part-time professor of Global NCD (noncommunicable disease) at the London School of Hygiene & Tropical Medicine (LSHTM). He serves on the LSHTM Global NCD Advisory Board as the lead for the West Africa Hub on NCD for the LSHTM. He has served as a consultant to the WHO Global Coordinating Mechanism/NCD on the integration of NCD with HIV; sexual and reproductive health; maternal, neonatal, and child health; and primary health care. Dr. Lamptey is an internationally recognized public health physician and expert in communicable diseases and NCDs in low- and middle-income countries. With a career at FHI 360 spanning more than 30 years, Dr. Lamptey has been instrumental in establishing FHI 360 as one of the world's leading international nongovernmental organizations in implementing communicable and noncommunicable programs in LMICs. He has a medical degree from the University of Ghana, an M.P.H. from the University of California, Los Angeles, and a Dr.P.H. from the Harvard School of Public Health. Dr. Lamptey serves on the *Lancet* Commission on the Future Health of Africa and served on the 2010 U.S. Institute of Medicine Committee on Preventing the Global Epidemic of Cardiovascular Disease: Meeting the Challenges in Developing Countries.

Ramanan Laxminarayan, Ph.D., M.P.H., is director and senior fellow at the Center for Disease Dynamics, Economics & Policy (CDDEP) in Washington, DC, and a senior research scholar and lecturer at the Princeton Environmental Institute at Princeton University. He is also a distinguished professor of public health at the Public Health Foundation of India, and affiliate professor at the University of Washington. Since 2005, Dr. Laxminarayan has worked to improve the understanding of antibiotic resistance as a problem of managing a shared global resource. His work encompasses extensive peer-reviewed research, public outreach, and direct engagement in 11 countries in Asia and Africa through the Global Antibiotic Resistance Partnership. In 2003 and 2004, he served on the Institute of Medicine Committee on the Economics of Antimalarial Drugs and subsequently helped create the Affordable Medicines Facility for malaria, a novel financing mechanism for antimalarials. In 2014, Dr. Laxminarayan served on the U.S. President's Council of Advisors on Science and Technology's antimicrobial resistance working group. Currently, he is a voting member of the U.S. Presidential Advisory Council on Combating Antimicrobial Resistance. He is a series editor of the *Disease Control Priorities for Developing Countries*, 3rd edition. An economist and epidemiologist by training, his research integrates the use of epidemiological models of infectious disease and drug resistance into the economic analysis of public health problems.

Michael H. Merson, M.D., is the founding director of the Duke Global Health Institute and the Wolfgang Joklik Professor of Global Health at Duke University. In addition, Dr. Merson is the university's vice president and vice provost for global affairs and from 2010 to 2016 served as its vice chancellor for Duke-National University of Singapore affairs. Dr. Merson graduated from Amherst College (B.A.) and the State University of New York, Downstate Medical Center. After serving as a resident at Johns Hopkins Hospital, he worked in the Enteric Diseases Branch at the Centers for Disease Control in Atlanta and then served as the chief epidemiologist at the Cholera Research Laboratory in Dhaka, Bangladesh. His research focused on the etiology and epidemiology of acute diarrheal diseases, including cholera, in developing countries and on the cause of travelers' diarrhea in persons visiting these countries. In 1978, he joined WHO as a medical officer in the Diarrheal Diseases Control Program. He served as director of that program from January 1980 until May 1990, from 1987 to 1990 as director of the WHO Acute Respiratory Infections Control Program, and from 1990 to 1995 as director of the WHO Global Program on AIDS.

In April 1995, he was appointed the first dean of the Yale School of Public Health, a position he held until December 2004. From 1999 to 2006, he was director of the Center for Interdisciplinary Research on AIDS at Yale University. Dr. Merson has authored more than 175 articles, primarily in areas of disease prevention and global health policy. He is the lead editor of *Global Health: Disease, Programs, Systems, and Policies*, a leading global health textbook in the United States. He has served in advisory capacities for various United Nations agencies, international organizations, and foundations and on several NIH review panels and academic advisory committees. He is a recipient of two honorary degrees and the Surgeon General's Exemplary Service Medal and is a member of the National Academy of Medicine.

Vasant (Vas) Narasimhan, M.D., is the global head of drug development and chief medical officer for Novartis. He is a member of the Executive Committee of Novartis. Dr. Narasimhan joined Novartis in 2005 and has held numerous leadership positions in development and commercial functions. Since 2014 he has been global head of development, Novartis Pharmaceuticals, a role he continues to hold alongside his other responsibilities. Dr. Narasimhan also served as global development head at Novartis Vaccines and earlier he led the Sandoz biosimilars and oncology injectables business unit where he oversaw the Sandoz biosimilars pipeline. Dr. Narasimhan also held commercial and strategic roles at Novartis. He was region head, Novartis Vaccines North America, and United States country president for Novartis vaccines and diagnostics. Before joining Novartis, Dr. Narasimhan worked at McKinsey & Company. Dr. Narasimhan received his medical degree from Harvard Medical School and obtained a master's degree in public policy from Harvard University's John F. Kennedy School of Government. He received his bachelor's degree in biological sciences from the University of Chicago. Dr. Narasimhan is an elected member of the National Academy of Medicine.

Michael T. Osterholm, Ph.D., M.P.H., is an internationally recognized expert in infectious disease epidemiology. At the University of Minnesota, he serves as a professor in the Schools of Public Health, College of Science and Engineering, and Medicine, and also serves as the director of the Center for Infectious Disease Research and Policy. From 2001 through 2005, Dr. Osterholm served as a special advisor to then-HHS Secretary Tommy G. Thompson on issues related to bioterrorism and public health preparedness. He was also appointed to the Secretary's Advisory Council on Public Health Preparedness. During his 15 years as state epidemiologist at the Minnesota Department of Health, he led investigations into infectious disease outbreaks. Dr. Osterholm has been an international leader on the critical concern regarding preparedness for an influenza pandemic. Dr. Osterholm has also been an international leader on the growing concern regarding the use of biological agents as catastrophic weapons. He serves on the editorial boards of several scholarly journals and is a frequent consultant to WHO, NIH, the U.S. Food and Drug Administration (FDA), the U.S. Department of Defense, and the U.S. Centers for Disease Control and Prevention. He is a fellow of the American College of Epidemiology and the Infectious Diseases Society of America. He is a member of the National Academy of Medicine.

Juan Carlos Puyana, M.D., is a professor of surgery, critical care medicine and clinical translational science; and a trauma/acute care surgeon at the University of Pittsburgh. He is a clinical investigator and has been the principal investigator of several programs on capacity building and eHealth from the Fogarty International Center of NIH. He has worked extensively in Latin America over the past 20 years. He was the secretary of the Pan-American Trauma Society from 2003 to 2010 and president of that society from 2011 to 2012. He is an international leader in trauma, injury and emergency surgery and has a wide understanding of barriers and possible solutions to conduct research in emergency, trauma, and acute care settings in low- and middle-income countries. He has actively participated in surveillance and registry designs for trauma in acute care surgery in Central and South America. He has had active projects and collaborative academic interactions with trauma and emergency experts in countries such as Colombia, Paraguay, Mexico, Ecuador, Honduras, and Guatemala, and most recently in Kenya and Mozambique. Dr. Puyana was a co-director of the surgical intensive care unit at the Brigham and Women's Hospital Boston. Dr. Puyana was born in Colombia where he finished medical school at Javeriana University before completing his residency training at McGill University in Montreal, Canada, and his trauma fellowship at Yale University. Dr. Puyana is an active trauma and critical care surgeon working at the largest level 1 trauma center and acute care center in Pennsylvania. He participates in fellowship, resident, and student mentoring. He serves as vice chairman for Pennsylvania on the Committee on Trauma of the American College of Surgeons. Dr. Puyana is involved in promoting research, educational opportunities, and clinical collaboration in Latin America.